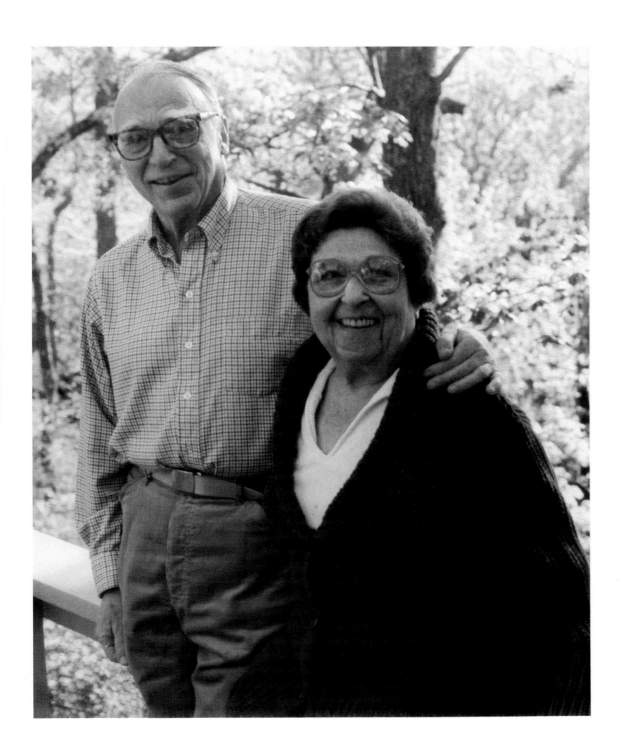

Current Practice of Surgical Stapling

Current Practice of Surgical Stapling

Edited by

Mark M. Ravitch, M.D.
Honorary President

Felicien M. Steichen, M.D.
Co-President

Roger Welter, M.D.
President

Second International Symposium and First European
Congress on Stapling in Surgery

 LEA & FEBIGER   *Philadelphia • London • 1991*

Lea & Febiger
200 Chester Field Parkway
Malvern, Pennsylvania 19355-9725
U.S.A.
(215) 251-2230
1-800-444-1785

Lea & Febiger (UK) Ltd.
145a Croydon Road
Beckenham, Kent BR3 3RB
U.K.

Library of Congress Cataloging-in-Publication Data

International Symposium on Stapling in Surgery (2nd: 1988: Luxembourg, Luxembourg)
    Current practice of surgical stapling/edited by Mark M. Ravitch, Felicien M. Steichen,
      Roger Welter.
       p.   cm.
    "Second International Symposium and First European Congress on Stapling in Surgery."
    ISBN 0-8121-1328-4
    1. Staplers (Surgery)—Congresses. 2. Suturing—Congresses. I. Ravitch, Mark M.,
      1910–1989. II. Steichen, Felicien M., 1926–   . III. Welter, Roger. IV. European
      Congress on Stapling in Surgery (1st: 1988: Luxembourg, Luxembourg) V. Title.
    [DNLM: 1. Surgical Staplers—congresses. 2. Suture Technics—instrumentation—
      congresses. WO 162 I61c 1988]
    RD73.S75I58   1988
    617'.9178—dc20
    DNLM/DLC
    for Library of Congress   90-5932
                                                                CIP

PRINTED IN THE UNITED STATES OF AMERICA

Print No. 5   4   3   2   1

Acknowledgments

We are very grateful to H.R.H. Grand Duchess Joséphine-Charlotte and H.I.R.H. Princess Marie-Astrid, who graciously honored the proceedings of this First European Congress and Second International Symposium on Stapling with their presence and active interest in all the events of the convention.

Mr. Gaston Thorn, former President of the General Assembly of the United Nations and of the European Community Commission, affirmed his long-standing friendship by participating in the opening session and making possible the concert given by the Symphony Orchestra of Radio-Television Luxembourg under the direction of Leopold Hager, with Leon Fleisher playing the piano concerto in D for left hand by Maurice Ravel. We thank all of them for having elevated the routine activities of a scientific meeting by their artistic inspiration.

The Prime Minister of Luxembourg and the members of the government were represented by his Excellency Benny Berg, Minister of Health. He presided over the inaugural session and delivered a special message from him and his colleagues for success of the Symposium and happy days in Luxembourg.

The Honorable Lydie Polfer, charming and energetic Mayor of the city of Luxembourg, distinguished by her presence many of the scientific sessions and presided with grace over the banquet held for all the participants in the Atrium of the Municipal Theatre of Luxembourg. The atmosphere of open hospitality was heightened by the musical contribution of the Chamber Orchestra "Soloists of Luxembourg" under the direction of Mr. Battistella and with the participation of Mr. Philippe Koch, violinist.

A special tribute should be paid to the impeccably planned organization guided by Roger Welter, expertly supervised by Ms. Julie Dettori, and enthusiastically executed by the members of the organizing team. Charm combined with competence and selfless service were the hallmarks of this team, which included specialists in five languages and the personnel of the auditorium of the European Parliament in Luxembourg. The resources and cooperation of so many friends of this team, only possible within the inner circle of a small country, provided the organizational aspects of this meeting with the talent of many unsung volunteers, among them a surgeon who substituted as the Italian interpreter.

Our very sincere thanks go to Turi Josefsen and U.S. Surgical Corporation, who gave generous support to this Congress and without whose help the entire undertaking would have been impossible. The assistance by members of their European and international staffs in solving many unexpected surprises that seem to arise during any meeting was especially appreciated.

Our thanks also go to Mr. Carroll Cann, Executive Editor of Lea & Febiger, who deserves our gratitude for accepting this work for publication and extending the deadline for submission of manuscripts. Special thanks go also to Jack Daniel, who did an outstanding job of copy editing, and Thomas J. Colaiezzi, Production Manager, who showed great imagination in counseling us for the overall design.

We would also like to thank our Secretary, Ruthlyn Haynes, for her patience in typing and retyping the corrections of these 51 manuscripts, and keeping the editors on target for the publication date.

Thoughts on Mark M. Ravitch

By a Friend

Mark Ravitch the private person is best understood through his partnership with Irene, his wife and loyal companion of 57 years. Together they created a home for family, friends, and visitors that was full of unrestricted hospitality and great generosity of mind and matter favoring intellectually stimulating encounters. Material goods were appreciated for the comfort and enjoyment of life they provided and for the pleasure they gave in sharing them with family and friends; they never were a prime motivating force in the Ravitchs' household. From this home base, Mark felt an unwavering support in the quest for excellence in his professional life. It was Mark Ravitch's strongly held opinion that just as physical exercises can strengthen the body, mental exercises can maintain and enrich the brain.

While politically and socially his views were those of an unabashed liberal, his personal code of conduct was guided by the highest ethics, dignity, and respect for tradition in education, and by the belief that each individual has a responsibility to realize his or her given endowment of talent. These values may seem conservative, even reactionary to some contemporary free spirits.

He was impatient with those who did not live up to their promise or responsibilities and yet he could show genuine understanding and compassion for people with intellectual and physical limitations. Nowhere was this more apparent than on hospital rounds, where a duty dereliction by a resident or nurse could bring him to a quick boil. Only moments later, this would be followed by the most considerate approach to a sick patient, especially if this patient was a child.

For those of us who found the road to the Ravitchs' home through the more formal professional route, the obvious joy of life there and reciprocal respect and admiration between family members became an adventure that was difficult to resist.

Mark Ravitch would show the same rapt attention to a brilliant exposé by a famous visitor as he would to the latest exploits and opinions of his own children and, later, grandchildren (including the children of this writer, for whom he has always been a stand-in grandfather). Mark Ravitch, the leader and the human being, represented to all of us the best traditions of the Sage of a yeshiva, the Scholar of a medieval library, and the Philosopher of a Greek city-state: He was a man for all seasons. On March 1, 1989, we all suddenly felt very lonely.

Felicien M. Steichen, M.D.

La chirurgie, cette discipline ou matière grise et dextérité
s'allient au plus haut niveau pour aboutir
a une performance humaine sans rivale.

("Surgery is the endeavour where intellect and dexterity meet at the highest level in the creation of a peerless human accomplishment.")

R. Schaus, M.D.

Practicing Internist and Author, in book review on "Stapling in Surgery"

"While instruments may be mechanized, the surgeon is in no danger of becoming a mechanic, nor will more or less automatic instruments make a safe craftsman of the tyro."

M.M. Ravitch, M.D.

in: "Second Thoughts of a Surgical Curmudgeon"

Preface

Following the first International Symposium on Stapling in Surgery held at the University of Pittsburgh in April 1986, Mark Ravitch and Felicien Steichen contemplated with measured enthusiasm the organization of a second International Symposium at a "later date in a different place." The satisfaction born from the success of this first symposium was understandably tempered by the memory of the time and energy spent to organize it, as well as by the need for creative funding that all international conventions appear to require.

During the trip to the meeting of the American Surgical Association at the Homestead Hotel, following the first symposium, Mark Ravitch and Felicien Steichen were joined in their discussions by Roger Welter, M.D., of Luxembourg. With an almost euphoric amnesia for all the hurdles that were only days behind them and stimulated by the exchange of ideas and a selective memory for the accomplishments of these international contacts, these three men rapidly advanced the outline of a second symposium from a possible to an authentic planning stage.

The city of Luxembourg was chosen as the Congress site because of its central location in Europe, its international vocation, and perhaps also the recognition that Luxembourg surgeons had very early and enthusiastically accepted stapling techniques. Above all, the readiness of Roger Welter to undertake all the details of an intricate organization was decisive in this choice.

What had been envisioned as a meeting for 180 to 250 participants bloomed into a congress of some 800 participants from 27 different countries on five continents. The international character of the symposium was underlined by the cooperation of the *Association Européenne de Chirurgie Viscérale* (founded by R. Welter) and the University of Pittsburgh School of Medicine as the organizing institutions, given support and help by the European Community Commission, the government of the Grand Duchy of Luxembourg, and the administration of the City of Luxembourg. In addition, the *Association Française de Chirurgie*, the *Deutsche Gesellschaft für Chirurgie*,

the *Association Française de Viscéro-Synthèse*, and the *Société des Sciences Médicales du Grand-Duché de Luxembourg* participated actively in organizing and moderating the proceedings. The *Association Française de Viscéro-Synthèse* held their third annual meeting in conjunction with the Luxembourg symposium, under the presidency of Prof. P. Cubertafond.

The international class of the meeting was assured by the willingness of leading surgeons from all over the world to participate as teachers or students, most often in both capacities—international gatherings of this type so happily reveal all that is good, noble, and valued in human beings of different backgrounds.

The presentations made by the authors from all corners of the earth gave a clear picture of their present-day practices in stapling techniques as well as honest assessments of the results obtained by them in operations on the lungs, esophagus, and gastrointestinal tract. The contributions made by our colleagues represent the state of the art world-wide, and are especially pertinent since they show potential intra-operative and postoperative complications and ways to avoid them. Because of Mark Ravitch's untimely death, the date of publication has been somewhat delayed. However, the authors and editors have made every effort to upgrade descriptions of techniques in which newer instruments are now used, as well as of clinical studies and results that have been extended since the meeting.

Our colleagues have taken great care to explain individual approaches to a given technical challenge, to analyze results, and to make suggestions for improvements, if necessary. Because of the expanding field of stapling techniques in surgery, minimal if any duplication of subjects is presented in these chapters. It is gratifying to see that great thought continues to be given to the creation of new instruments and methods to join the bowel, and that no effort is spared to study tissue healing with mechanical means of closing and joining viscera. Complications with stapling are better understood as time passes; methods to avoid them emerge quite clearly from the recommendations of our colleagues. They have once again approached the overall subject as surgeons and scientists, and have presented their analyses from both a technical and a scientific vantage point, with great emphasis on general surgical principles, selection and preparation of patients, appropriate operative management, and critical evaluation of postoperative results. As presented at the Congress and documented by the contents of this book, this approach to the subject of stapling makes possible the writing of a textbook of operative surgery with mechanical suturing techniques by recognized masters the world over. We are very grateful for their generous contributions.

New York
Luxembourg

Felicien M. Steichen
Roger Welter

Contributors

M. Adloff, M.D.
Centre Médico-Chirurgical
University of Strasbourg
19 Rue Pasteur,
Strasbourg, France 67300

Hiroshi Akiyama, M.D.
Toranomon Hospital
222 Toranomon
Minatoku, Japan 105

G. Antypas, M.D.
Department of Thoracic Surgery and Anesthesia
Metaxa Memorial Hospital
Athens, Greece

R.V. Bardini, M.D.
Clinica Chirurgica I
Ospedale Policlinico
Via Gustiniani 2
Padova, Italy 35128

R. Bares, M.D.
Surgical Clinic of the Technical University
Aachen, West Germany

J.A. Barra, M.D.
Departments of Surgery and Anatomy
Faculty of Medicine
Brest, France

S. Bathrellou
Department of Thoracic Surgery and Anesthesia
Metaxa Memorial Hospital
Athens, Greece

R.W. Beart, M.D.
Mayo Clinic W. 6B
Rochester, Minnesota, USA 55905

H.D. Becker, M.D.
Eberhard-Karls-Universität Tübingen
Chirurgische Klinik
Calwer Strasse 7
Tübingen, West Germany 7400

G. Bell
Western Infirmary
Dunbarton Road
Glasgow, Great Britain, G11 6NT

E. Benizri, M.D.
Department of Surgery
Hopital St. Roch
5 Rue Pierre Devoluy
Nice, France 06006

Ph. Bérard, M.D.
Hotel Dieu
1 Place De L'Hôpital
Lyon, France 69288

Peter A. Beyer, M.D.
Department of General Surgery
The Johann Wolfgang Goethe
University of Frankfurt/Main
Germany

J. Block, M.D.
Department of Surgery
Hopital St. Roch
5 Rue Pierre Devoluy
Nice, France 06006

U. Bull, M.D.
Surgical Clinic of the Technical University
Aachen, West Germany

L. Boemi, M.D.
Direttore Istituto III Clinica Chirurgica
Universita Degli Studi (La Sapienza)
Rome, Italy 00161

Ph. Breil, M.D.
4, Bis, Passage Legrand
Boulogne, France 92100

S. Broun, M.D.
Surgical Department of "Diakonissen" Hospital
D-7000 Stuttgart -1, West Germany

J. Cady, M.D.
Service de Chirurgie Digestive
Clinique Geoffroy Saint Hilaire
Rue Geoffroy Saint Hilaire
Paris, France 75005

A. Cancrini, M.D.
Direttore Istituto III Clinica Chirurgica
Universita Degli Studi (La Sapienza)
Rome, Italy 00161

Valdemar M.B. Cardoso, M.D.
Department of Surgery, Fourth Service
Hospital De S. Joao
University of Oporto School of Medicine
Oporto, Portugal

S. Castle-Dupont
Departments of Surgery and Anatomy
Faculty of Medicine
Brest, France

M. Celerier
Hopital St. Louis
Service de Chirurgie Viscerale
1 Avenue Claude Vellefaux
Paris, France 75010

Eduardo O.P. Cernadas, M.D.
Department of Surgery
Fourth Service
Hospital De S. Joao
University of Oporto School of Medicine,
Oporto, Portugal

Maryalice Cheney, M.D.
Division of Colorectal Surgery
Thomas Jefferson University
1100 Walnut Street, Suite 700
Philadelphia, Pennsylvania 19107

M. Chir
Colorectal Research Unit
Basingstoke District Hospital
Basingstoke, Hampshire
Great Britain, RG24 9NA

J.M. Collard, M.D.
Département de Chirurgie
Université Catholique de Louvain
Avenue Hippocrate 10
Bruxelles, Belgique 1200

J. Dartois, M.D.
Department of Surgery
Hopital St. Roch
5 Rue Pierre Devoluy
Nice, France 06006

E. De Antoni, M.D.
Direttore Istituto III Clinica Chirurgica
Universita Degli Studi (La Sapienza)
Rome, Italy 00161

Panagiotis Delikaris, M.D.
Second Surgical Department
"G. Papanikolaou" General Hospital
Thessaloniki, Greece

Theodoros Diamantis, M.D.
Second Surgical Department
"G. Papanikolaou" General Hospital
Thessaloniki, Greece

G. Di Matteo, M.D.
Direttore Istituto III Clinica Chirurgica
Universita Degli Studi La Sapienza
Rome, Italy 00161

Mr. Raymund J. Donnelly
Regional Adult Cardiothoracic Unit
Broadgreen Hospital
Thomas Drive, Liverpool, L 14 3LB
England

F.W. Eigler, M.D.
Department of Surgery
University of Essen
Germany 4300

P. Fabiani
Department of Surgery
Hôpital St. Roche
Nice, France 06031

J. Fass, M.D.
Surgical Clinic of the Technical University
Aachen, West Germany

V.W. Fazio, M.D.
Cleveland Clinic Foundation
9500 Euclid Avenue
Cleveland, Ohio, USA 44106

K.H. Fuchs, M.D.
Department of Surgery
Christian-Albrechts University
Marschionini Strasse 40
Kiel, West Germany 2300

F. Gaillard, M.D.
Department of Pathology
Faculty of Medicine
University of Nantes, France

D.J. Galloway
Western Infirmary
Dunbarton Road
Glasgow
Great Britain G11 6NT

F.M.D. Gaujoux, M.D.
Department of Surgery
Hotel Dieu Hospital
Lyon, France 69288

M. Gavioli-Ferrari, M.D.
Centre Médico-Chirurgical
University of Strasbourg
19 Rue Pasteur,
Strasbourg, France 67300

Bryce Gayet, M.D.
Hopital Beaujon
100, Boulevard General Leclerc
Paris, France 92118

W.D. George
Western Infirmary
Dunbarton Road
Glasgow
Great Britain G11 6NT

D. Le Goff, M.D.
Highland Clinic
1035 Creswell Street
Shreveport, LA, USA 71101

Scott Goldstein, M.D.
Division of Colorectal Surgery
Thomas Jefferson University
1100 Walnut Street, Suite 700
Philadelphia, Pennsylvania, USA 19107

B. Gouboux
Department of Surgery
Hôpital St. Roche
Nice, France 06031

F.D. Griffen, M.D.
Highland Clinic
1035 Creswell Street
Shreveport, Louisiana, USA 71101

Greg Groglio, M.D.
Washington Hospital Center
Washington D.C., USA

E. Gross, M.D.
Department of Surgery
Hamburg City Hospital
Hamburg, Germany 2000

J. Gugenheim, M.D.
Department of Surgery
Hopital St. Roch
5 Rue Pierre Devoluy
Nice, France 06006

Joaquim Guimares, M.D.
Department of Surgery
Fourth Service
Hospital de S. Joao
University of Oporto School of Medicine
Oporto, Portugal

C. Guoillat, M.D.
Department of Surgery
Hotel Dieu Hospital
Lyon, France 69288

Jin Guoxiang, M.D.
Department of Surgery
Changhai Hospital
Shanghai, China

H. Hamelmann, M.D.
Department of Surgery
Christian-Albrechts University
Marschionini Strasse 40
Kiel, West Germany 2300

A. Hatzinis, M.D.
Department of Thoracic Surgery and Anesthesia
Metaxa Memorial Hospital
Athens, Greece

R.J. Heald
Colorectal Research Unit
Basingstoke District Hospital
Basingstoke, Hampshire
Great Britain RG24 9NA

E. Hoffman, M.D.
Chirurgische Universssitatsklinik Dusseldorf
Deutschland 4000

Christer Stael Von Holstein, M.D.
Department of Surgery
Lund University
Lund, Sweden 22185

Xiao-Mai Huang, M.D.
Department of Thoracic Surgery
Chinese Pla General Hospital
301 Hospital, Military
Post Graduate School
Beijing, People's Republic of China

Nguyen Huu, M.D.
Departments of Surgery and Anatomy
Faculty of Medicine
Brest, France

Olof Jansson, M.D.
Department of Surgery
Lund University
S-2215, Lund, Sweden

Bo Joelsson, M.D.
Department of Surgery
Lund University
Lund, Sweden, 22185

Folke Johnsson, M.D.
Department of Surgery
Lund University
Lund, Sweden, 22185

Th. Junginger, M.D.
Department of General and Abdominal Surgery
Johannes-Gutenberg University
Mainz, Germany 6500

Li-Yuan Kang, M.D.
Department of Thoracic Surgery
Chinese Pla General Hospital
301 Hospital, Military
Post Graduate School
Beijing, People's Republic of China

M. Kantarzis, M.D.
St. Josef Hospital
Department of Surgery
University of Dusseldorf
D-5600 Wuppertal 1, Germany

David Kaplan
Regional Adult Cardiothoracic Unit
Broadgreen Hospital
Thomas Drive, Liverpool, L 14 3LB
England

N. Katkhouda, M.D.
Hopital Saint Roch
5 Rue Pierre Devoluy
Nice, France 06006

John M. Keshishian, M.D.
3 Washington Circle, N.W.
Washington D.C., USA 20037

P.J. Kestens, M.D.
Département de Chirurgie
Université de Louvain
Avenue Hipprocate 10
Bruxelles, Belgium 1200

P. Keszler, M.D.
Bacjy Zsilinszky Hospital
1475 Budapest, Hungary

C.D. Knight, Sr. M.D.
Highland Clinic
1035 Creswell Street
Shreveport, Louisiana, USA 71101

C.D. Knight, Jr.
Highland Clinic
1035 Creswell Street
Shreveport, Louisiana, USA 71101

N. Kockel
Chirurgische Klinik Gerresheim
Gerresheim, Graulingerstrasse 120
Dusseldorf, Deutchland 4000

Konstantinos Karamoscos
Second Surgical Department
"G. Papanikolaou" General Hospital
Thessaloniki, Greece

Gustavo G. Kuster, M.D.
10666 N. Torrey Pines Rd.
La Jolla, California, USA 92037

P.A. Lehur, M.D.
Centre Hospitalier Régional
Universitaire de Nantes
Hôpital Guillaume et René Laënnec
B.P. 1005 Nantes, France, 44035

G. Leoni, M.D.
Clinica Chirurgica I
Ospedale Policlinico
Via Gustiniani 2
Padova, Italy 35128

J. Lersmacher, M.D.
Chirurgische Universsitatsklinik Dusseldorf
Deutschland 4000

Chen Libing
Department of Surgery
Changhai Hospital
Shanghai, China

J. Logie
Western Infirmary
Dunbarton Road
Glasgow, Great Britain, G11 6NT

J. McGregor
Western Infirmary
Dunbarton Road
Glasgow, Great Britain G11 6NT

O. Meinicke, M.D.
Department of Surgery
University Hospital
Kiel 23, West Germany

Ph. Mondine, M.D.
Departments of Surgery and Anatomy
Faculty of Medicine
Brest, France

J. Monod, M.D.
Departments of Surgery and Anatomy
Faculty of Medicine
Brest, France

I. Morrice
Western Infirmary
Dunbarton Road
Glasgow, Great Britain G11 6NT

J. Mouiel, M.D.
Department of Surgery
Hopital St. Roch
5 Rue Pierre Devoluy
Nice, France 06006

Derek D. Muehrcke
Regional Adult Cardiothoracic Unit
Broadgreen Hospital
Thomas Drive, Liverpool, L 14 3LB
England

A. Munro
Western Infirmary
Dunbarton Road
Glasgow, Great Britain G11 6NT

J. Cl. Ollier, M.D.
Centre Medico-Chirurgical
University of Strasbourg
Schiltigheim, Strasbourg
France 67300

J.B. Otte, M.D.
Département de Chirurgie
Université de Louvain
Avenue Hipprocate 10
Bruxelles, Belgium 1200

G. Palazzini, M.D.
Direttore Istituto III Clinica Chirurgica
Universita Degli Studi (La Sapienza)
Rome, Italy 00161

Luca Pecchioli
Division of Colorectal Surgery
Thomas Jefferson University
1100 Walnut Street, Suite 700
Philadelphia, Pennsylvania, USA 19107

A. Peracchia, M.D.
Clinica Chirurgica I
Ospedale Policlinico
Via Gustiniani 2
Padova, Italy 35128

Giuseppe Pezzuoli, M.D.
First Surgical Clinic
Ospedale Maggioro
University of Milan
Via Francesco Sforza 35
Milan, Italy 20122

Amadeu P.A. Pimenta, M.D.
Department of Surgery
Fourth Service
University of Oporto School of Medicine
Hospital de S. Joao
Oporto, Portugal

Chen Qinglan, M.D.
Department of Surgery
Changhai Hospital
Shanghai, China

Y. Raut, M.D.
Departments of Surgery and Anatomy
Faculty of Medicine
Brest, France

Mark M. Ravitch
Department of Surgery
Montefiore Hospital and
University of Pittsburgh
Pittsburgh, Pennsylvania, USA

Carlo Rebuffat, M.D.
First Surgical Clinic
Ospedale Maggioro
University of Milan
Via Francesco Sforza 35
Milan, Italy 20122

G. Reginato, M.D.
Clinica Chirurgica I
Ospedale Policlinico
Via Gustiniani 2
Padova, Italy 35128

M. Reynaert, M.D.
Département de Chirurgie
Université de Louvain
Avenue Hipprocate 10
Bruxelles, Belgium 1200

H. Rinecker, M.D.
Chirurgische Klinik Rinecker
Isartal Strasse 82
D-800 Munich 70
West Germany

Jacqueline Ritchie
Western Infirmary
Dunbarton Road
Glasgow
Great Britain G11 6NT

Meng Ronggui, M.D.
Department of Surgery
Changhai Hospital
Shanghai, China

Ricardo Rosati, M.D.
First Surgical Clinic
Ospedale Maggioro
University of Milan
Via Francesco Sforza 35
Milan, Italy 20122

F. Sandei, M.D.
Clinica Chirurgica I
Ospedale Policlinico
Via Gustiniani 2
Padova, Italy 35128

Andreas Schmidt-Matthiesen, M.D.
Department of General Surgery
The Johann Wolfgang Goethe
University of Frankfurt/Main
Germany

S. Schroeder, M.D.
Department of Surgery
Christian-Albrechts University
Kiel 23, West Germany

V. Schumpelick, M.D.
Surgical Clinic of the Technical University
Aachen, West Germany

Rainer M. Seufert, M.D.
Department of General Surgery
The Johann Wolfgang Goethe
University of Frankfurt/Main
Germany

K.W. Steegmuller, M.D.
Surgical Department of "Diakonissen" Hospital
Stuttgart -1, West Germany

F.M. Steichen, M.D.
130 East 77 Street
New York, NY, USA 10021

O. Stremme, M.D.
Department of Surgery
Friedrich Ebert Krankenhaus
Neumunster, Germany 2350

B. Sugden
Western Infirmary
Dunbarton Road
Glasgow, Great Britain G11 6NT

Yu-E Sun
Department of Thoracic Surgery
Chinese Pla General Hospital
301 Hospital, Military
Post Graduate School
Beijing, People's Republic of China

A. Thiede, M.D.
Department of Surgery
Friedrich Ebert Krankenhaus
Neumunster, Germany 2350

Masahiko Tsurumaru, M.D.
Toranomon Hospital
222 Toranomon
Minatoku, Japan 105

B. Ulrich, M.D.
Chirurgische Klinik Gerresheim
Gerresheim, Graulingerstrasse 120
Düsseldorf, Deutchland 4000

Stefano Valabrega, M.D.
Division of Colorectal Surgery
Thomas Jefferson University
1100 Walnut Street, Suite 700
Philadelphia, Pennsylvania, USA 19107

Nguyen Hoan Vu, M.D.
Departments of Surgery and Anatomy
Faculty of Medicine
Brest, France

A. Van Der Tol
Roman Catholic Hospital
Groningen
The Netherlands

Bruno S. Walther, M.D.
Department of Surgery
Lund University
Lund, Sweden, 22185

Roger Welter, M.D.
Hopital Princess Marie-Astrid
187 Avenue de la Liberté, Differdange
G.D. de Luxembourg 4602

J.M. Whitaker, M.D.
Highland Clinic
1035 Creswell Street
Shreveport, Louisiana, USA 71101

Richard I. Whyte
Regional Adult Cardiothoracic Unit
Broadgreen Hospital
Thomas Drive, Liverpool, L 14 3LB
England

J. Winter
Chirurgische Universssitatsklinik
Dusseldorf,
Deutschland 4000

Tu Yue, M.D.
Department of Surgery
Changhai Hospital
Shanghai, China

Yu Dehong, M.D.
Department of Surgery
Changhai Hospital
Shanghai, China

Thomas Zilling, M.D.
Department of Surgery
Lund University
Lund, Sweden, 22185

Contents

Part V
Morbidity and Mortality Associated with Stapling Procedures

Part VI
Stapling in Pulmonary Surgery

Part VII
Stapling in Esophageal Surgery

Part VIII
Stapling in Operations at the Esophago-gastric or Esophago-jejunal Junction

Part IX
Stapling in Gastric Surgery

Part X
Stapling in Colo-rectal Surgery

Part I

History and Principles
of
Stapling in Surgery

CHAPTER 1

HISTORICAL PERSPECTIVE AND PERSONAL VIEWPOINT

Mark M. Ravitch

When we visited Kiev (Fig. 1-1) in 1958, almost by chance we became the guests of Dr. N.M. Amosov (Fig. 1-2) at the Thoracic Surgical Institute. We were startled to see a series of patients who had had segmental resections, lobectomies, and pneumonectomies with staples (Fig. 1-3) instead of sutures and saw the extraordinary simplicity and efficiency of the instruments in Dr. Amosov's hands during operations. We visited the Institute in Moscow (Figs. 1-4, 1-5), where the staplers had been developed, and were very well received. We were shown the rather large range of instruments they had developed for all purposes, from the suture of blood vessels to the stapling of bone or even suturing of corneal grafts. We were unsuccessful in finding any government office, organization, or bureau through which these staplers could be purchased.

During a café conversation in Leningrad, a young university student, on being told that the stapling instruments were one of the things that had impressed us thus far in our trip, commented that they were made in the Red Guard factory just outside of Leningrad. That struck a responsive chord in my memory. I immediately recalled that, earlier that very day as we had been driving down the Nevskii Prospect, I had tucked away for future consideration a

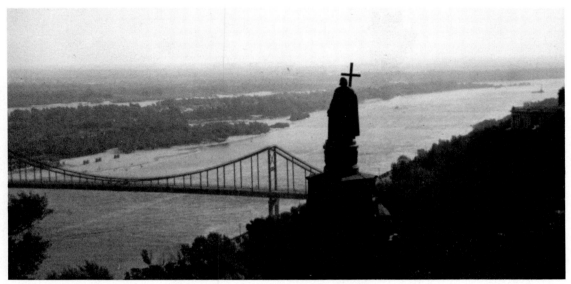

Fig. 1-1. Dnieper River and statue of St. Valadimir, photographed from Valadimir Hills in Kiev by M.M. Ravitch in 1958.

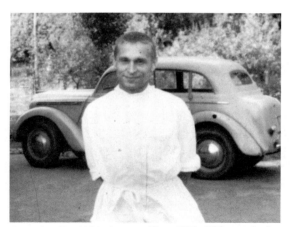

Fig. 1-2. Dr. N.M. Amosov, Kiev, 1958. (Photography by M.M. Ravitch.)

sign above an ordinary store window that said "Surgical Instruments and Apparatus." All hospitals in the Soviet Union are government hospitals, and all surgeons are government surgeons, and though there was a certain amount of licit and illicit private practice, this did not extend to the performance of surgical procedures outside of government hospitals. What, therefore, could be the purpose of the sale of surgical instruments from a store in a business district? In any event, we went to that store the next morning and found that in fact they were selling all sorts of instruments and apparatus, and that they did have stapling instruments. Somewhat to our surprise,

they were perfectly willing to sell an instrument to me for cash even though, quite unnecessarily I am sure, I identified myself plainly as an American. The only instrument they had in stock that day was the bronchial stapler with which the row of staples was placed across the bronchus with the bar of each staple in the axis of the bronchus. This was designed to preserve the circulation at the end of the bronchus and, as a matter of fact, employed the same reasoning many of us had long used in placing manual sutures for bronchial closure in exactly the same way (Fig. 1-6).

The personnel at the Institute in Moscow were delighted that we had been able to secure an instrument. They calibrated it for us and checked us out on the details of its operation and maintenance. Returning to Baltimore, we at once set about using the instruments for bronchial closure in a series of dogs. There was no question but that the closure was perfectly secure and that the healing was beautiful. We then began a series of pulmonary resections, mostly for tuberculosis. Several years later, we were able to secure the more universally applicable UKL, which placed two staggered lines of staples with the bar in the direction of the staple line. We switched over to this instrument exclusively for the bronchus, the pulmonary vessels, and the pulmonary parenchyma.

We then began exploring the applications of the UKL to closure of portions of the gastro-intestinal tract. We were absolutely delighted with it, and found, as we should have expected, that the stapled mucosa-to-mucosa closure of stomach, duodenum or

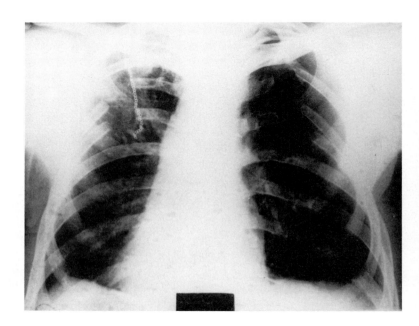

Fig. 1-3. Postoperative radiographic examination showing a line of staples in the apex of the right chest. Original x-ray film was given to Mark Ravitch by Dr. N.M. Amosov in 1958.

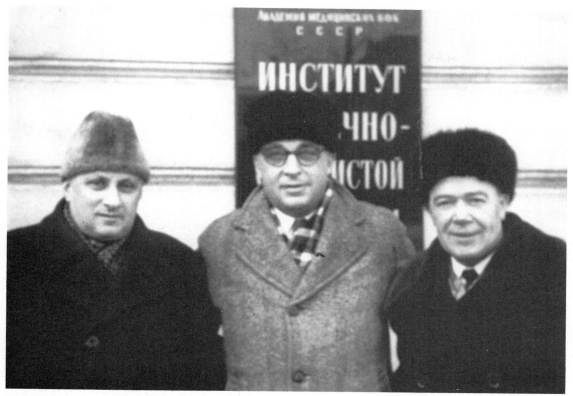

Fig. 1-4. Photo taken in front of the Institute of Cardiac and Vascular Surgery of the Academy of Medical Sciences of the USSR. From right to left: Prof. Androsov, Prof. Mark M. Ravitch, and a person identified as Tsintsiper, probably a member of the staff doubling as a guide (1958).

intestine without inversion or suture reinforcement was as uniformly safe and secure as the similar closure of the bronchus.

About this time we were visited in our laboratory by a group of Soviet surgeons who demonstrated the UKZh, which was the instrument for gastro-intestinal anastomosis. The demonstration was not flawless, and I came to the swift and totally erroneous conclusion that this was an ingenious instrument to perform awkwardly what could be done more skillfully by hand. Nevertheless, when I obtained an instrument of this kind (the progenitor of the GIA), I became convinced of its extraordinary utility and adaptability after a few trials. Interestingly enough, a number of American manufacturers, knowing of our interest, visited our laboratories and operating rooms to see how the staplers performed, but for one reason or another decided there was no future in stapling—to their later expressed regret!

The American manufacturers who secured from the Russians the right to reproduce or modify Russian instruments had already made faithful replicas of the Russian UKL (Fig. 1-7). These American manufactur-

ers were told that although these instruments functioned well, they were a little heavy, had an awkward balance, required hand loading of the fine staples and partial disassembling of the instrument to reload them and, finally, had too many parts and were difficult to clean and maintain. It was suggested that we needed disposable, preloaded, presterilized, and color-coded staple cartridges. The makers responded not only by providing those staple cartridges and modifying the balance of the instruments, but by making the moving parts within the instrument, particularly the fins that served as staple drivers, a part of the disposable cartridge—a great advance. The result was that the instrument itself was reduced to the simple driving mechanism that pushed forward the bar in the cartridge to which the staple driving fins were attached; this essentially removed all the complexity from the instrument and made it easy to maintain and clean.

The delay in working on, modifying, and perfecting the cylindric end-to-end anastomosing instrument, the EEA, was due to my own gross miscalculation of the extent to which such an instrument might be

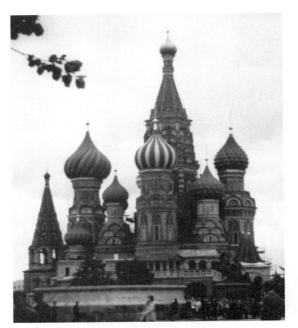

Fig. 1-5. Photograph of St. Basil's Cathedral in Moscow, taken by M.M. Ravitch in 1958.

used. I had tried for a number of years to persuade the American manufacturers that the Russian instrument for end-to-end anastomosing had some extremely attractive features: if it were supplied with a double row of staples instead of a single row, and if it incorporated all the concepts of the previously made American instruments—now including the GIA, which had two rows of staples instead of the Russian equivalent's one and in which, again, the staples, activating mechanism, and knife were disposable—it would be extremely attractive and useful to surgeons performing lower rectal (and perhaps other) anastomoses (Fig. 1-8). When I was asked how many times a year I or others might use such an instrument, I underestimated the potential to an extraordinary degree. The result was that the manufacturers said a very special instrument of this kind could never recover the enormous costs involved in its development. Nevertheless, after some years and many representations, they were persuaded to undertake the manufacture of the instrument, and you know of its success.

In Russia, we had found that the instruments were anything but universally employed: in some major institutions they were not used at all, whereas in other institutions, with surgeons of equal repute, they were regularly used. In the United States the reception was slow. Resistance to adoption of the staplers arose from several factors. Surgeons are craftsmen; they are proud of their art and reluctant to believe that an automatic instrument can do things as well as they can, let alone better. Like all good craftsmen, surgeons enjoy the exercise of their skills and decry anything that diminishes that pleasure, or that levels the difference between the results of the master craftsman and those of, let us say, the average one. There was also concern that if these instruments really were useful and effective, surgeons would forget how to sew and be unable to do so in critical situations in which the instruments were perhaps not

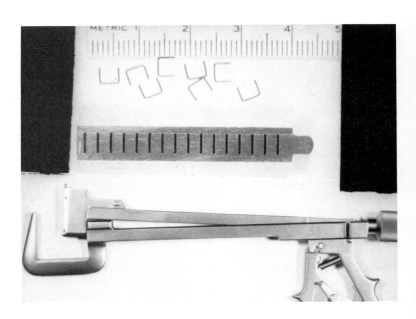

Fig. 1-6. Instrument (brought to Baltimore by Mark M. Ravitch in 1958) and slide marked "My own UKB."

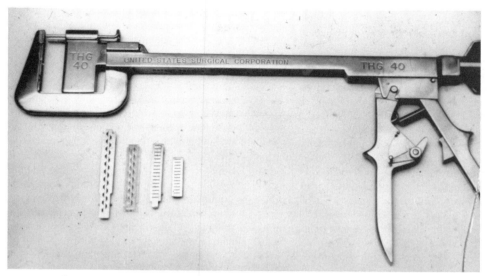

Fig. 1-7. The UKL instrument in its first American version.

applicable. This particularly concerned the teachers of surgery with respect to the training of young surgeons. Finally, there was concern about the expense.

I think it is fair to say that the first surgeons in the United States to adopt stapling enthusiastically were the thoracic surgeons, who immediately saw the increase in facility and safety and the improvement in results with closures of the bronchus and parenchyma. Very shortly, there was universal acceptance of the fact that the old-fashioned anatomic segmental dissection—technically demanding and therefore heartwarming to the skilled surgeon despite such factors as bleeding and air leaks—had been superseded entirely by the stapled resection technique termed

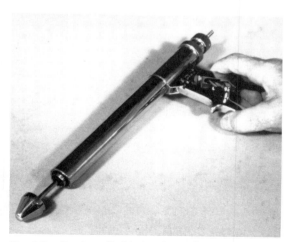

Fig. 1-8. Russian cylindrical end-to-end anastomosing instrument, held by Mark M. Ravitch.

by Amosov "the economical resection." This technique involved resecting the diseased tissue, whether only a part of a segment, all of a segment, or all or part of one segment with parts of adjacent segments, ignoring segmental boundaries. Interestingly enough, there are still a good many thoracic surgeons in the United States who are very happy with the bronchial and parenchymal closures but distrustful of the closures of the pulmonary artery and pulmonary veins, a distrust based on a priori fears and not on experience. More and more general surgeons are using the stapling instruments routinely for nearly all procedures on the gastro-intestinal tract.

It is an interesting sociologic phenomenon (and one that was predicted) that the surgeons first adopting the use of staplers were surgeons in private hospitals, usually smaller private hospitals. The major clinics and universities were much slower to adopt them, probably because a private practitioner could buy the instruments for himself if he thought they would be better for his patients or would provide him an opportunity to do more operations in a day, or even to simply prove that he was more of an innovator than his competitors. Also, if the chairman of a department of surgery in a university hospital or in a major clinic was uncertain about stapling or prejudiced against it, he could simply decree that staples would not be used. It is my impression that in the universities and in the major clinics it was upward pressure from below—from the house staff, from the younger staff surgeons—that gradually brought stapling into general use in the major centers. The result, of course, is that now the new generation of surgeons everywhere is trained in stapling. It is an interesting sidelight that the EEA. was readily accepted because it produced an *in*verting anastomosis. Many surgeons who had been unwilling to use the mucosa-to-mucosa closures with the linear staplers were seduced by the EEA, and then led into adopting the linear stapler.

Although the results in pulmonary surgery clearly have been superior with stapling, it has generally been possible to state only that in abdominal surgery, stapling is at least as safe as manual sutures. One of the problems, of course, has been that those with the most stapling experience are so convinced of the superiority of stapling that they have been unwilling to mount elaborate prospective clinical trials of gastrectomy or colonic anastomosis or whatever. In any case, complications are not numerous, and very large numbers would be required. By and large, surgeons who are proficient with staplers and also proficient with sutures are unequivocally convinced that a substantial amount of time is saved with stapling. Although time is not extraordinarily important, it relates to the duration of anesthesia and to the duration of possible

contamination, whether from within or without. Here and there are isolated reports of comparative series in which little or no time is alleged to have been saved by stapling. Since I can do a stapled functional end-to-end anastomosis of the bowel in something under 60 seconds, it is hard for me to credit those who say either that they can sew faster than they can staple or that they staple more slowly than they sew. It turns out, of course, that precisely in the two areas in the gastro-intestinal tract in which suturing is most difficult—the lower and upper ends, the rectum and the esophagus—there appears to be considerable uniformity of judgement, even among the great experts, that stapling is somewhat superior to manual suture in freedom from leakage. I suppose that few will doubt this; therefore, the results of those who are not among the "great experts" will necessarily be better with stapling than with manual suture.

We would be the first to say, and we have always insisted, that stapling is not a technique that will make a surgeon out of a mechanic; that the basic rules of surgery—gentle handling of tissue, careful atten-

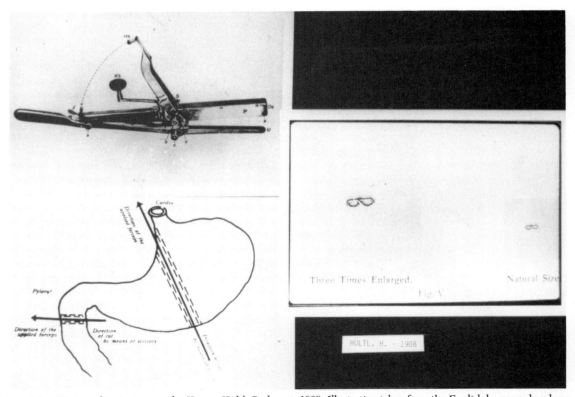

Fig. 1-9. First stapling instrument by Humer Hültl, Budapest, 1908. Illustration taken from the English language brochure of the instrument used by Dr. Grausman from Mount Sinai Hospital in New York. He had worked with Hültl in 1923 and 1924 and visited him in 1928 and 1932. This instrument was donated by Dr. Grausman to the Library of the New York Academy of Medicine.

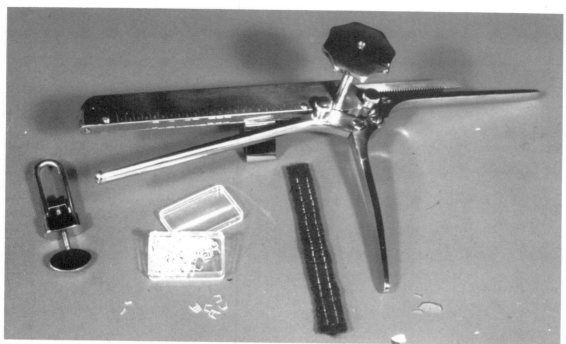

Fig. 1-10. Stapling instrument developed by Aladar Von Petz, Budapest, 1921 and 1924.

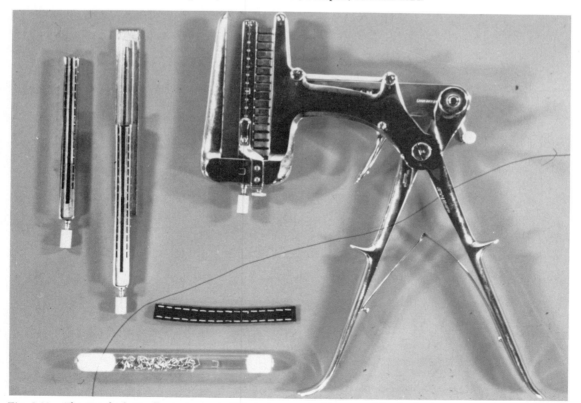

Fig. 1-11. The Friedrich-Neuffer instrument. This instrument had been used by Prof. Phemister at the University of Chicago. In 1969 it found a temporary home at Montefiore Hospital of the University of Pittsburgh.

tion to blood supply, assurance that suture lines are not placed through diseased tissue, avoidance of excessive tension—are as important with staplers as with manual suture. Furthermore, it is important to remember that because the instruments are large and long, undue leverage can easily be exerted. A good deal of judgement and skill must still be employed to avoid injury to the tissue.

The matter of cost has yet to be settled and is in many ways difficult to measure. For instance, if you can save 15 to 30 minutes in each of several successive operations, you will save enough time in one 8-hour shift for an additional operation with the same nursing and operating room personnel: that saves money for the hospital. If, as in the United States, patients are charged for use of the operating room by increments of time and the anesthetist similarly charges by increments of time, then the patient or the third-party payer is saved a significant amount of money. By and large, I think the discussion of cost is moot. It is almost irrelevant. The reason is that surgeons the world over have come to the conclusion that stapling instruments are better for them and bet-

ter for patients. Over the centuries, surgeons have insisted that they be provided with the instruments they believe will do the best job for their patients.

This is not to say that I do not have some nostalgic regrets. I loved to sew. I loved to place my fine curved needles correctly and turn my wrists in exactly the right way so that no strain was placed on either the tissues or the needles. I loved to be able to pick up just the right thickness of tissue. I loved to have the responsibility of tying my knots so that they would be tight enough but not too tight and so that they would be secure. Happily, one still has to do that once in a while, and of course we insist that all of our residents have ample experience with suture closures and suture anastomoses. If there is not sufficient operative material for a resident to learn both techniques, then there is probably not sufficient operative material to justify a residency program.

One of the remarkable things is that, by and large, the stapling instruments we use today differ only in details and not in principles from the one devised by Hültl in Hungary over 80 years ago (Fig. 1-9). I believe it is reasonable to presume that mechanical su-

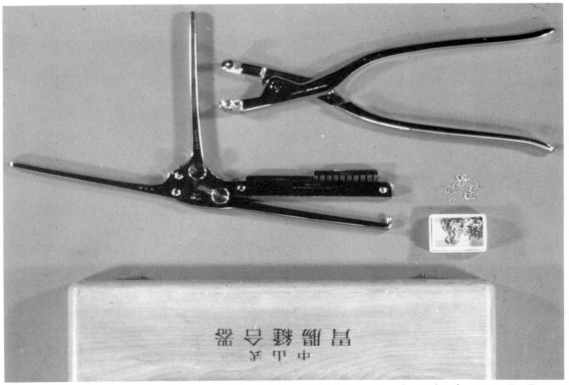

Fig. 1-12. The Nakayama stapling instrument. This particular model had been given by Prof. Nakayama to Dr. Denton Cooley, who was easily convinced by Dr. Ravitch that it should join the developing museum of such instruments in Pittsburgh (late 1970s, early 1980s).

turing devices will be produced that are quite different from those we have at hand, but I think we can accept the fact that mechanical suturing is here to stay.

Note: A "mini museum" of the early stapling instruments, representative examples of the vast range of Russian instruments (including all staplers shown in Figures 1-6 through 1-8 and in Figures 1-10 through 1-12, as well as a replica of Hültl's stapler, shown in Figure 1-9, and all models of the first generation of American instruments was shown by Mark M. Ravitch and F.M. Steichen at the Clinical Congress of the American College of Surgeons in San Francisco in 1972. This scientific exhibit has since been donated by the U.S. Surgical Corporation and its authors to the Smithsonian Institutions in Washington.

CHAPTER 2

INSPIRATION AND RATIONALE FOR THE DEVELOPMENT OF MECHANICAL SUTURES

Felicien M. Steichen

Until the beginning of the nineteenth century, surgeons had not clearly recognized the fact that all wound healing is based on the same principles, regardless of the anatomic location, tissue composition, and etiologic agent of the wounding. The need for hemostasis by ligature rather than by deep cautery, as well as the need for wound debridement and preservation and gentle handling of viable tissue during the reconstructive phase, had been studied and progressively accepted for wounds of the soft tissues and bones since Ambroise Paré (1510–1590).[1] This came about because flesh wounds and traumatic amputations were the mainstay of surgical practice and the basis for understanding the relation between treatment and results through clinical observation. However, healing of visceral wounds within the body cavities was poorly understood, in no small part because of the fact that if the patient survived the initial insult, infection—invariably the result of deep injuries and of surgical manipulations limited in scope and understanding—was much more threatening than superficial soft tissue and extremity wounds. Success in the treatment of intestinal wounds, for instance, was anecdotal; the variety of approaches was dictated by circumstances rather than by a surgeon's plan, and was always based on the possible occurrence of a fistula channeled to the outside by a variety of creative techniques, with the name of each surgeon attached to a successful outcome.

An additional factor was the fear that hollow viscera might heal by collapse of the scar—by analogy with solid tissue scars. This led to many ingenious suture modalities to satisfy the formation of a directed fistula, as well as to maintain the caliber of the lumen, often by invaginating the bowel ends at the anastomosis. As late as 1889 the concern for bowel patency found expression in the decalcified bone plates of Senn,[2,3] Abbe's catgut rings (1889),[4,5] Sachs' decalcified bone buttons (1890),[6] and a host of modifications of these anastomotic devices.

With the passage of time, as surgeons learned that healthy hollow viscera would heal primarily if the bowel walls were joined by a reliable technique, it seems that little attention was paid to the modality of either manual suture or a mechanical device, as long as the final result was reliable healing. Therefore, in a short period of time—as so often happens in research and development when an idea is ripe—the two basic modalities of hollow visceral closure and bowel anastomosis were described: the everting manual suture by Benjamin Travers in 1812[7] and the inverting manual suture by Antoine Lembert in 1826[8] (Fig. 2-1). Parallel to these two surgeons, Denans,[9,10] in 1826, presented ferrules, or rings, joining inverted bowel ends compressed by an expanding intraluminal cylinder (Fig. 2-2). Also in 1826, Henroz[11] experimentally used articulated metal rings to join everted bowel ends (Fig. 2-3). Both of these devices were mechanical means to achieve anastomosis. Henroz's external rings illustrate the concern to maintain a patent lumen. However, Henroz and Travers did demonstrate that healthy everted bowel ends, joined mu-

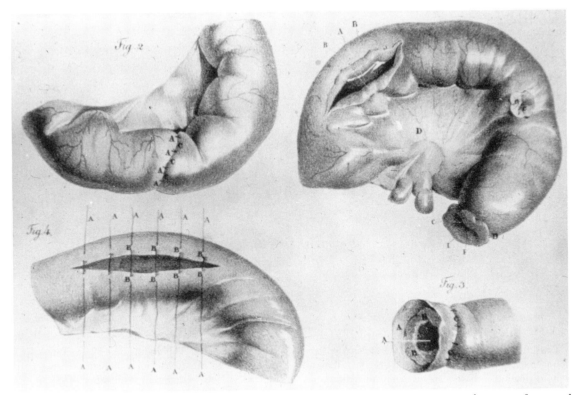

Fig. 2-1. Original illustrations of Antoine Lembert's inverting sutures, apposing serosa-to-serosa, in the repair of intestinal wounds and in circular anastomosis of bowel. In Figure 2-3, Lembert shows a definite circular ridge of inverted bowel ends, and he warned that excessive tissue inversion could lead to prolonged obstruction.[8] Lembert's technique found universal acceptance as the fundamental basis for successful intestinal closure and anastomosis, in spite of the earlier work by Benjamin Travers on everting sutures (1812).[7]

Fig. 2-2. Illustration of the second model of the Denans instrument for sutureless compression anastomosis.[10] The bowel ends, inverted around two rings, are slipped over a cylindric metal spring that holds the bowel ends in apposition and achieves a compression anastomosis. A few widely spaced sutures hold the bowel ends. After anastomosis the rings and cylindric stent are eliminated with bowel movements.

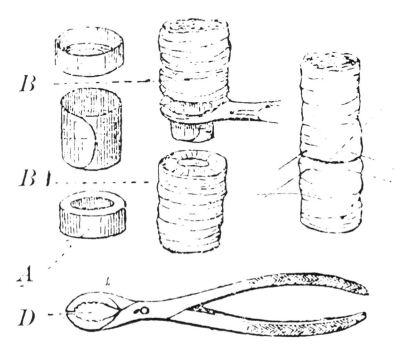

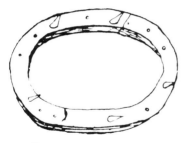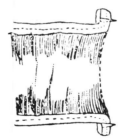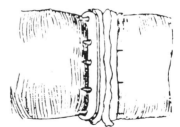

Fig. 2-3. Illustration of the Henroz articulated metal rings of alternating pins and holes, used experimentally and successfully for everting compression anastomosis.[11] These illustrations are from Nicholas Senn, who ignored Henroz's success and came to the pre-conceived conclusion that "It must have proved a failure."[3]

cosa-to-mucosa with a continent anastomotic line, would heal—a lesson soon lost and only rediscovered with surprise and some reluctance in recent times. Denans, in spite of a coarse instrument based on the available materials of his time, clearly described the principle of sutureless, compression anastomosis, later perfected by John B. Murphy (1892),[12,13] Adalbert Ramaugé (1893)[14] (Figs. 2-4, 2-5), and the many modifications inspired by their very original contri-

butions. At present, sutureless compression anastomosis, facilitated by newer materials and state-of-the-art instruments, is enjoying a well deserved renaissance[15–18] (Figs. 2-6, 2-7, 2-8).

However, because it was technically simpler than the other methods then available to individual surgeons, and because of the clean, solid appearance, which inspired confidence, bowel closure and anastomosis with inversion as described by Lembert be-

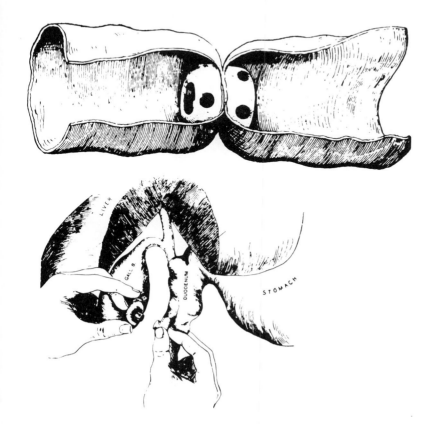

Fig. 2-4. End-to-end inverting compression bowel anastomosis and side-to-side cholecystoduodenostomy for obstructive jaundice with the Murphy button.[12,13]

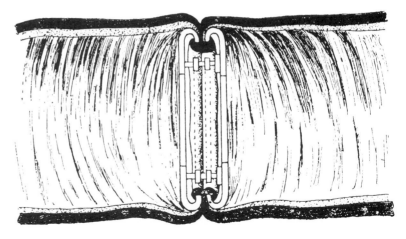

Fig. 2-5. End-to-end inverting compression bowel anastomosis with the elegant, slender Ramaugé rings, requiring no purse-string sutures of the bowel ends.[14] However, even a later sophisticated model of Ramaugé's instrument never gained the popularity of Murphy's button.

came the method of choice. This development was enhanced by W.S. Halsted's demonstration in 1887 that the tough submucosa was the all-important layer, to be included for maximum strength in all bowel sutures[19] (Table 2-1).

Control of pain—as brought about by Wells and nitrous oxide in 1844,[20] Morton and ether in 1846,[21,22,23] and Simpson and chloroform in 1847[24]—as well as the recognition of the importance of antisepsis (Joseph Lister, 1867)[25,26,27] and later asepsis, allowed surgeons to expand beyond the passive role of mending penetrating injuries of the bowel, and of removing gangrene from strangulating herniations, to enter the field of elective, planned surgical procedures in the treatment of cancer and benign conditions resisting non-operative treatment. These procedures were perhaps most brilliantly demonstrated by Theodore Billroth and the Vienna School of Gastro-Intestinal Surgery before and around the turn of the century. Although manual inverting sutures were the standard for many surgeons, the various anastomotic compression devices clearly constituted not just another method of achieving an anastomosis, but a competing one, with its predictable, reproducible quali-

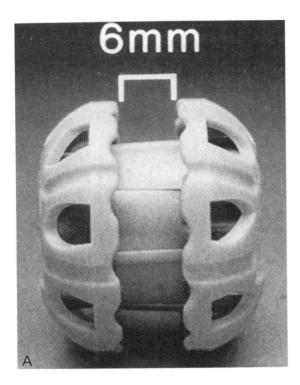

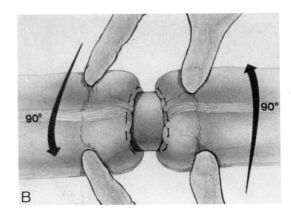

Fig. 2-6. *A, B.* Modern version of a modified compression anastomotic ring, or button, made of absorbable polyglycolic acid and 12% barium sulphate. Following anastomosis the ring breaks up into small fragments and is evacuated with bowel movements.[15]

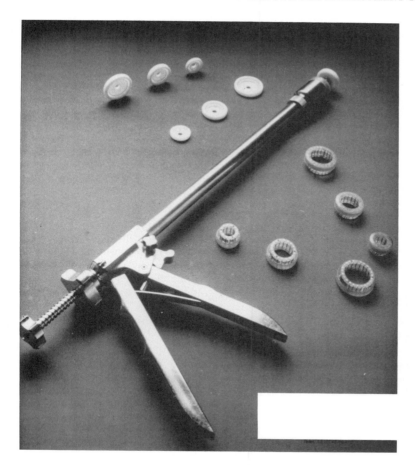

Fig. 2-7. The Russian AKA-2 apparatus uses the mechanism of the SPTU stapler to place two interdigitating plastic rings, which are held together by a circle of fine hooks. Between these rings the pursestringed bowel ends are held circumferentially and excised centrally by an advancing annular blade, just as for the circular stapling instruments and are compressed by a third, intermediate ring.[16,17]

ties in the hands of surgeons at various levels of technical competence. Prof. Jeannel[14] of Paris was inspired to say the following in 1893:

I believe I know how to sew, yet I side with the "boutonnistes." The ranks of the "suturistes" include only the prestidigitators of our profession. But I beg these skilled men to consider that they are the exception, that they cannot have a monopoly of intestinal surgery. Is it to be denied

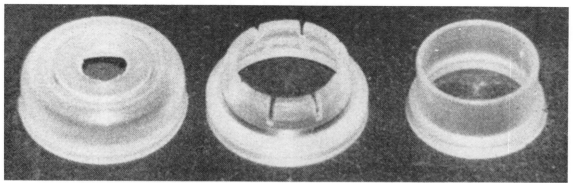

Fig. 2-8. Modern version of the Denans principle, for circular compression anastomosis, placed with circular anastomosing instruments. The pursestringed bowel ends are invaginated into each other and held in that position by two cylinders of plastic material. The inner, compressible cylinder is advanced and held by a third cylinder, which is activated by the circular instrument's mechanism.[18]

Table 2-1. Mechanical Devices: Goals

Achieve anastomosis
and
Maintain patent lumen
through
Sutureless compression instruments
of technical simplicity

that for the average surgeon it is easier to apply an anastomotic button, than to suture an anastomosis? And friends, when the suturists point to the failures of the buttons, have they forgotten their own failures? Who would dare say that suturing has not had and will not have more victims than the buttons?

Anastomotic buttons had the disadvantage of necessitating evacuation through the intestinal tract, but the stage was set for a controversy that continues to enliven surgical meetings today.

The next step, the creation of a true mechanical suture, was inspired by Humer Hültl[28] of Budapest in his concern for reducing to a minimum intraoperative contamination from an open gastric or intestinal lumen, or eliminating it altogether (1908). Speed was a consideration only if it resulted in diminished exposure of the open abdominal wound and was not a goal in itself. Hültl was known for his com-

pulsive isolation of the operative field with pads and towels (called abdominal wall papering by him), his use of sterile gloves and face masks, and his insistence on touching the same needle and holder only once, requiring a large number of needles and holders during a given anastomosis (Fig. 2-9).

Although all subsequent instruments did use the tissue- and vessel-sparing B-shaped staple, and although Friedrich (1934)[29] (Fig. 2-10) and Tomoda (1937)[30] developed instruments with varying tissue compression, no thought seems to have been given to relying on staple closures only; the lines were always reinforced with manual sutures. Motivation for the instruments of von Petz[31] (Fig. 2-11), Friedrich,[29] Sandor,[32] Tomoda,[30] and Nakayama,[33] which all delivered single, mostly linear staple lines, was still reduction or elimination of contamination from an open gastro-intestinal lumen, a challenge of engineering and manufacturing improvements (not always clearly achieved) and greater efficiency in overall execution of operative steps (Table 2-2).

With the interest and accomplishments of Russian surgeons and scientists in mechanical sutures during and after World War II, this emphasis changed somewhat. During a period when surgeons with various levels of training and experience had to cover the vast territory of the Soviet Union, mechanical sutures were felt to provide standardization of techniques and results, with greater safety for technical operative

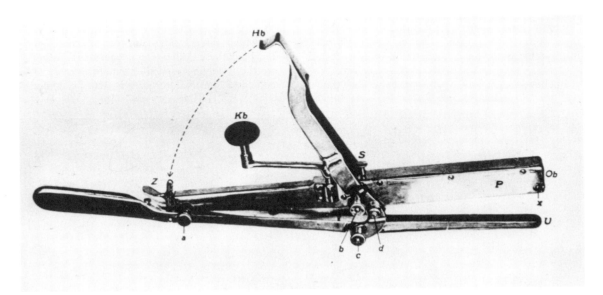

Fig. 2-9. The first stapling instrument by Humer Hültl, 1908, incorporated all the principles of modern surgical stapling: closure of the instrument produced tissue compression and immobilization in the first step; the fine wire staples were then driven through the tissues in four staggered rows with each staple assuming the classic B-shape. The viscus was divided, leaving two rows of staples on each side.[28]

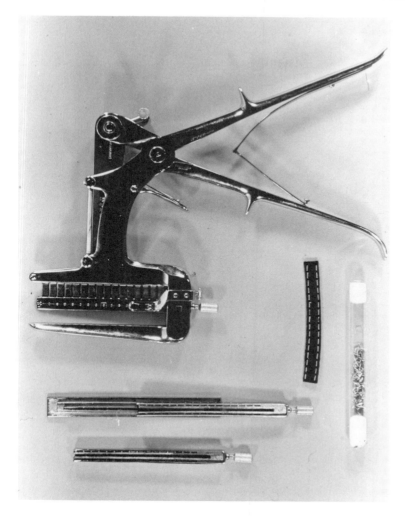

Fig. 2-10. The stapling instrument by H. Friedrich (1934) provided surgeons with real advances in mechanical suturing such as interchangeable cartridges, variable tissue compression, and a single mechanism for tissue compression and staple placement. A disadvantage was the heavy staples first used by Von Petz and placed in two single, indian-file rows.[29]

steps in treating the acutely sick patient who needed the expertise, and yet could not be transported over great distances to a center with optimal human and material resources.[34] In fact, this public health speculation led to the innovative development of linear and circular suturing and anastomosing instruments, and was fully vindicated by the collective results obtained. In addition, the Russians also applied linear staplers to pulmonary surgery with significant improvements in the safety and reliability of bronchial and pulmonary vascular closures; they also saw technical simplification and functional improvements in pulmonary parenchymal resections, to the point where even surgeons in large centers became convinced of the worth of mechanical sutures in operations on the lungs (Table 2-3).

The original American contribution, by now 30 years old, was guided by Mark M. Ravitch, who returned from a trip to the Soviet Union with a bronchial stapler.[35] This particular instrument allowed the placement of staples in the long axis of the bronchial stump, held together for healing in a mucosa-to-mucosa (everting) fashion. The 1942 publication of Rienhoff, Gannon, and Sherman[36] had demonstrated that the bronchus healed from the cut end. The sutures, in fact, only maintained occlusion until the transected bronchus healed at the end.

In retrospect, several factors—the improved bronchial healing in a series of operations for tuberculosis with this original Russian stapler,[37] the knowledge of Travers' earlier work with mucosa-to-mucosa closures and extensive experimental studies in visceral closures with double staple lines, and placement of the bar of the staple at a right angle to the long axis of bronchus or bowel—facilitated our acceptance of the concept of mucosa-to-mucosa staple closure without need for reinforcement of any kind.

The American effort developed in two directions:

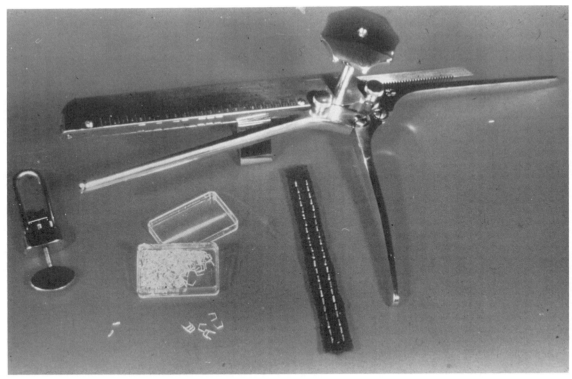

Fig. 2-11. The Von Petz instrument, based on the Hültl principles, was mechanically much simpler and technically easier to handle during a surgical procedure. While it inaugurated the use of the coarse, flat, "New Silver" staples—perhaps a step backward from the fine wire staples—this Von Petz instrument did become synonymous with surgical stapling until the advent of the Russian instruments.

advanced engineering and state of the art manufacturing with new materials have stimulated changes in some basic concepts of surgical technique. The engineering and manufacturing changes consisted of new designs and mechanical improvements for existing instruments, as well as the continued creation of totally new instruments. In the first family of instruments, complicated transfer mechanisms, from the compression of the instruments' handles or pusher bars to the actual formation of staples, were all moved from the instruments into disposable, pre-loaded, sterilized cartridges, providing great versatility and ease of use.[38] Since then, completely disposable instruments have become available with hardly a generation gap between models, it seems. Evolving engineering concepts and designs facilitate continued refinements in surgical applications.[41]

Conversely, progressive changes in surgical techniques—often inspired by the basic principles of mechanical suturing—and entire areas of operative surgery new to stapling methods, have stimulated continued improvements in the instrumentation, or entirely new creations. This interchange between surgeon and engineer-manufacturer was the base for success of the very first stapler through the Hültl-Fischer collaboration, and has continued through the various Hungarian, German, Japanese, Russian, and American developments; it will bear fruit as long as such mutual relationships persist.[39,40]

With the demonstration that staples were the equivalent of manual sutures and required no rein-

Table 2-2. Historical Stapling Instruments: Goals

1. Reduce duration of open bowel and exposure to contamination
2. Improve efficiency of operative techniques
3. Accept bioengineering challenge

Table 2-3. Soviet Stapling Instruments: Goals

1. Create reproducible standards for safe techniques with optimal end results at all levels of surgical talent
2. Improve existing and develop new instruments and concepts
3. Extend field of application to broncho-pulmonary surgery

forcement in most comparable instances, came also the recognition that the fine wires and B-formation used by Hültl and again in the Russian and American instruments reduced tissue trauma and maintained vessel patency and viability to the cut end of the respective viscus, while the duration of exposure to the open bowel was even more limited. In addition to fine wire staples and their B-formation, the variable tissue compression is of paramount importance in using staples as independent sutures. Before 1950, compression by the instruments was severe and invited tissue necrosis; thus the protective inversion (Table 2-4). Tomoda's and Friedrich's instruments did provide variable tissue compression, but they used heavy, broad staples in single Indian-file rows that could not be relied on for permanent closure. The Russian reports continued to emphasize tissue inversion of the staple lines, except for the bronchus, which was covered with pleura.

A discussion of the philosophy of stapling or mechanical suturing in general cannot be concluded without returning to the time when the goal of safe closure or anastomosis of viscera was so desperately sought.

History repeats itself, if only because improved ways and means allow a better realization of a time-honored principle. The concept of the sutureless anastomosis by compression—first used by Denans serendipitously to solve a practical problem—has taken on new importance with the realization that the mechanical device maintains coaptation while the natural tissue resources assure firm union of bowel ends. The materials and the techniques of application have changed, but the basic principle of compression anastomosis remains the same.[15–18] Denans, were he to return to this international meeting, could rightfully exclaim: "Plus ça change, plus c'est la même chose."[42] The only real change from his presentation at the Royal Society of Medicine in Marseilles (1826)[9] and at the Royal Academy of Paris (1836)[10] would be the simultaneous translation of his communication into five languages, which in itself represents a real advance in international goodwill and reflects the accomplishments in surgical techniques the world over. Denans and Hültl would most of all understand and applaud the motivation underlying the effort to find

the "ideal" suture method, which is the desire—highly developed in surgeons—to accept challenges and to create new and better ways to attain them.

REFERENCES

1. Paré A: The Apology and Treatise of Ambroise Paré. London: Falcon Educational Books, 1951; Birmingham: Classics in Surgery, 1984.
2. Senn N: Intestinal Surgery. Chicago: WT Keener, 1889.
3. Senn N: Enterorrhaphy: its history, technique and present status. JAMA 21:217, 1893.
4. Abbe R: Complete obstruction of the colon successfully relieved by using Senn's plates. A proposed substitute of catgut rings. NY Med J 49:314, 1889.
5. Abbe R: Intestinal anastomosis. The Medical News (Philadelphia) 54:589, 1889.
6. Sachs W: Drei Kleine Beiträge zur Darmchirurgie. Zentralbl Chir 17:753, 1890.
7. Travers B: An Inquiry Into the Process of Nature in Repairing Injuries of the Intestines. London: Longman, 1812:128–135, 180–189.
8. Lembert A: Mémoire sur l'entéroraphie. Rep Gen d'Anat et de Physiol Pathol II:101, 1826.
9. Denans F-N: Nouveau procédé pour la guérison des plaies des intestins. Recueil de la Société Royale de Médecine de Marseille [Séance du 24 fev. 1826, rédigé par M.P. Roux], Imprimerie d' Archard, Marseille, Tome I:127–131, 1827.
10. Denans F-N: Lettre avec envoi d'un système de viroles qu'il propose en remplacement de la ligature pour la réunion des plaies transversales de l'intestin. Bulletin de l'Académie Royale de Médecine [Séance du 15 mai 1836, Rapporteur Emery] Paris, 1837–38, p. 719.
11. Henroz JHF: Dissertatio inauguralis critica Medico-Chirurgica de Methodis ad Sananda Intestina Divisa Adhibitis. In: Qua Nova Sanationis Methodus Proponitur. Universitate Leodiensi, June 1826: PJ Collardin, Typographi Academici, 1826.
12. Murphy JB: Cholecysto-intestinal, gastro-intestinal, entero-intestinal anastomosis, and approximation without sutures (original research). Medical Record, New York 42:665, 1892; Chicago Medical Record XIII:803, 1892.
13. Murphy JB: Intestinal approximation: its pathological histology of reunion, and statistical analysis. Medical Record, New York 65:650–663; 684–692; 721–722, 1894: Chicago Clinical Review III:479–558, 1893–1894.
14. Ramaugé A: Entéroplexie. Considérations préliminaires. Mémoire presenté et couronné au Concours de Medicine International Sud-Américain, pp. 5–32, 20 January, 1893.
15. Hardy TG Jr, Pace WG, Maney JW, Katz AR, Kaganov AL: A Biofragmentable ring for sutureless bowel anastomosis. Dis Colon Rectum 28:484, 1985.
16. Gross E, Eigler FW: Die nahtlose Kompressionsanastomose am distalen Kolon und Rektum. Methode und Ergebnisse. Chirurgische Gastroenterologie Mit Interdisziplinären Gesprächen. Hameln, West Germany: TM-Verlag, 1986:125–130.
17. Tanos G, Gewalt R: Kolon-Kompressionsanastomosen ohne Nadel-und Fremdmaterial, Chirurgische Gastroenterologie Mit Interdisziplinären Gesprächen. Hameln, West Germany: TM-Verlag, 1986:133–135.
18. Rosati R, Rebuffat C, Pezzuoli G: A new mechanical

Table 2-4. American Stapling Instruments: Goals

1. Improve mechanical features and create new instruments for easier handling and greater operative versatility
2. Recognize staples and manual-suture equivalent with reduced tissue trauma, limited contamination, and preservation of vascular supply

device for circular compression anastomosis. Ann Surg 207:245, 1988.

19. Halsted WS: Circular suture of the intestine—an experimental study. Am J Med Sci XCIV:436, 1887.
20. Garrison FH: An Introduction to the History of Medicine. 4th Ed. WB Saunders, 1929:505, 723.
21. Bigelow HJ: Boston Medical and Surgical Journal 35:309, 379, 1846–1847.
22. Morton TW: Morton's Letheon (circular). Boston, 1846.
23. Morton TW: Remarks on the proper mode of administering sulfuric ether. Boston, 1847.
24. Simpson JY: Account of a new anesthetic agent. Edinburgh, 1847.
25. Lister J: On a new method of treating compound fracture, abscess, etc. with observations on the conditions of suppuration. Lancet I:326, 357, 387, 507; II:95, 1867.
26. Lister J: On the antiseptic principle in the practice of surgery. British Medical Journal II:246, 1867.
27. Lister J: Illustrations of the antiseptic system of treatment in surgery. Lancet II:668, 1867.
28. Hültl H: II Kongress der Ungarischen Gesellschaft für Chirurgie, Budapest, May 1908. Pester Med Chir Presse 45:108–110, 121–122, 1909.
29. Friedrich H: Ein neuer Magen-Darm—Nähapparat. Zentralbl Chir 61:504, 1934.
30. Tomoda M: Ein neuer Magen-Darmnähapparat. Zentrabl Chir 64:1455, 1937.
31. Von Petz A: Zur Technik der Magenresektion. Ein neuer Magen-Darmnähapparat. Zentrabl Chir 51:179, 1924.
32. Sándor S: Magen-Darmnaht mit Metalklammern nach

Hültl und ein neues Nähinstrument. Zentrabl Chir 63:1334, 1936.
33. Nakayama K: Simplification of the Billroth I gastric resection. Surgery 35:387, 1954.
34. Gritsman JJ: Mechanical suture by Soviet apparatus in gastric resection: use in 4000 operations. Surgery 59:663, 1966.
35. Ravitch MM, Brown IW, Daviglus GF: Experimental and clinical use of the Soviet bronchus stapling instrument. Surgery 46:97, 1959.
36. Rienhoff WF Jr, Gannon J Jr, Sherman I: Closure of the bronchus following total pneumonectomy. Experimental and clinical observations. Trans Am Surg Assoc 60:481, 1942.
37. Ravitch MM, Steichen FM, Fishbein RH, Knowles PW, Weil P: Clinical experiences with the Soviet mechanical bronchus stapler (UKB-25). J Thorac Cardiovasc Surg 47:446, 1964.
38. Steichen FM, Ravitch MM: Stapling in Surgery. Chicago: Year Book, 1984.
39. Welter R, Patel J-Cl: Chirurgie Mécanique Digestive. Paris: Masson, 1985.
40. Ravitch MM, Steichen FM: Principles and Practice of Surgical Stapling. Chicago: Year Book, 1987.
41. Knight CD, Griffen FD: An improved technique for low anterior resection of the rectum using the EEA stapler. Surgery 88:710, 1980.
42. Karr Alphonse, 1808–1890: Journaliste, Écrivain Directeur du Figaro (1839), dans revue satirique "Les Guêpes" en 1849.

CHAPTER 3

CHANGING CONCEPTS IN SURGICAL TECHNIQUES

Felicien M. Steichen

As increasing experience with mechanical sutures demonstrated to surgeons that the fine B-shaped wire staples were the equivalent of individual, interrupted manual sutures, it became progressively apparent that staples would change some of the time-honored traditional concepts in operative surgery (Table 3-1).[1–3] First among these was the renewed recognition that everting, mucosa-to-mucosa staple closures of the transected or incised organ, at all levels of the gastro-intestinal tract, would heal without reinforcing manual sutures. This firmly established the technique of the functional end-to-end anastomosis by eliminating the need for a row of sutures over the everting terminal closure of the GIA placement site or exit gap (Fig. 3-1).

Following acceptance of this change, a second, almost parallel development occurred with the crossing of staple lines, preferably in the same plane, avoiding the creation of blind corners with diminished blood supply, tissue necrosis, and subsequent leaks. This technique is not acceptable with manual sutures where transecting suture lines tend to leak. The safe overlapping of staple lines make the closure of the GIA introduction sites for functional end-to-end, end-to-side, and side-to-side anastomoses feasible (Fig. 3-1).

The next step, the logical consequence of staple line crossing and overlapping, was the intersection of a linear staple line by a circular, end-to-end, anastomosing ring of staples. At first this technique was considered potentially hazardous, but it has been proven safe and reliable by its experimental study and clinical application. The use in one stage of this technique, intersecting a fresh linear TA line in the rectum with a circular EEA line and blade in low anterior resections, was pioneered by Charles Knight of Shreveport, Louisiana[4] and was then extended to esophago-gastrostomy and gastro-duodenostomy; it has also become standard technique for the second-stage Hartmann operation. In fact, circular staple lines may also be transected by linear GIA lines in the creation of various gastric tubes (see Fig. 3-15) and in the fully mechanically sutured Duhamel procedure. Parallel to these clinical developments, Julian and Ravitch studied the behavior of staples encountered by the EEA blade and experimentally established the safety of this approach.[3] Finally, by using the entire potential of the new premium CEEA stapler, the separated anvil and central rod are placed into the proximal colon, which is then closed with a sagittal linear staple line. The cartridge containing the retracted trocar is advanced transanally into the previously transversely closed rectal stump; the trocar is then advanced through the center of the linear rectal staple closure. Similarly, the central rod is advanced through the center of the proximal colon closure. After removal of the trocar, the central rod is joined into

Table 3-1. New Concepts in Operative Surgery with Modern Stapling Techniques

Everting, mucosa-to-mucosa visceral suture
Crossing, overlapping staple lines
Intersecting staple lines
Variable anastomotic cross-section
Sequential anastomosis-resection
Creation of substitute organs and preservation of function

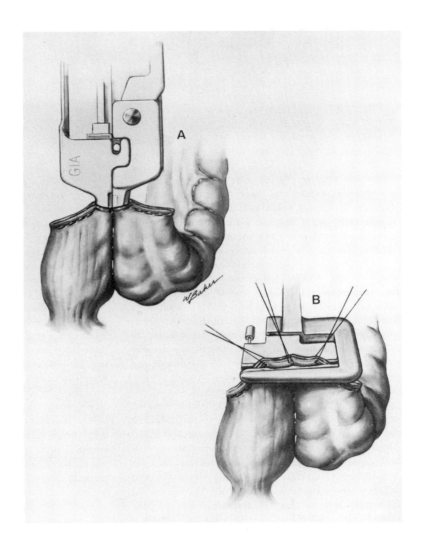

Fig. 3-1. *A*. Example of mucosa-to-mucosa bowel closure. Also shown is crossing and overlapping of staple lines at various angles but in the same plane (*A, B*). No reinforcing manual sutures are needed. We place reinforcing sutures only if the GIA staples have been used on both (thicker) gastric walls in the construction of various gastric tubes.

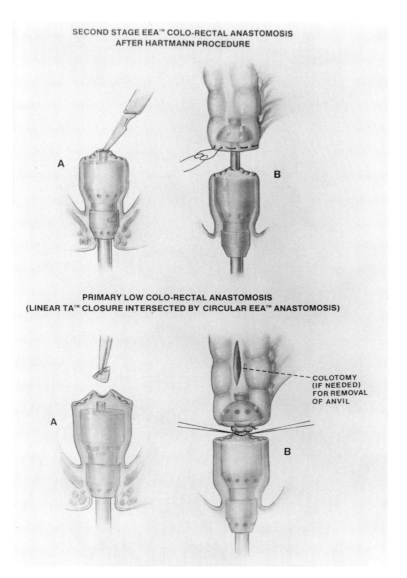

SECOND STAGE EEA™ COLO-RECTAL ANASTOMOSIS AFTER HARTMANN PROCEDURE

PRIMARY LOW COLO-RECTAL ANASTOMOSIS (LINEAR TA™ CLOSURE INTERSECTED BY CIRCULAR EEA™ ANASTOMOSIS)

COLOTOMY (IF NEEDED) FOR REMOVAL OF ANVIL

Fig. 3-2. *Top.* Example of linear staple line intersected by a circular, anastomosing ring of staples first used in the second-stage colorectal reconstruction through a healed rectal stump after the Hartmann procedure. *Bottom.* Knight extended the use of this approach to primary, one-stage intersection of the linear rectal closure by a circular anastomosis in anterior resections.

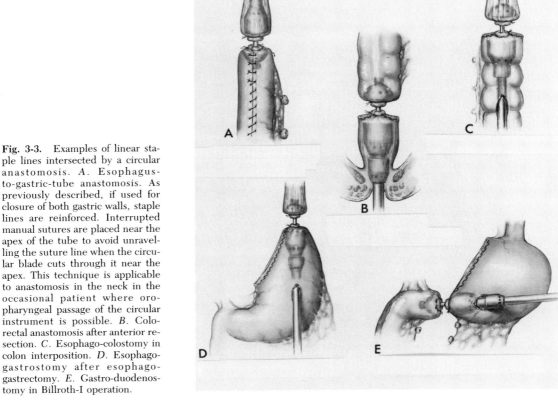

Fig. 3-3. Examples of linear staple lines intersected by a circular anastomosis. *A*. Esophagus-to-gastric-tube anastomosis. As previously described, if used for closure of both gastric walls, staple lines are reinforced. Interrupted manual sutures are placed near the apex of the tube to avoid unravelling the suture line when the circular blade cuts through it near the apex. This technique is applicable to anastomosis in the neck in the occasional patient where oropharyngeal passage of the circular instrument is possible. *B*. Colorectal anastomosis after anterior resection. *C*. Esophago-colostomy in colon interposition. *D*. Esophagogastrostomy after esophagogastrectomy. *E*. Gastro-duodenostomy in Billroth-I operation.

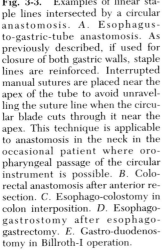

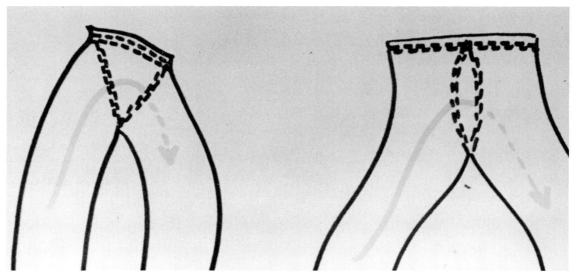

Fig. 3-4. Modification of the anastomotic cross section with the GIA-TA functional anastomosis, depending on the closure of the GIA exit gap in a V-shape (*A*) or oval form (*B*). The V-shape can increase the cross-sectional anastomotic surface almost 3-fold, and prevents the raw GIA linear lines from healing across and creating a stricture.

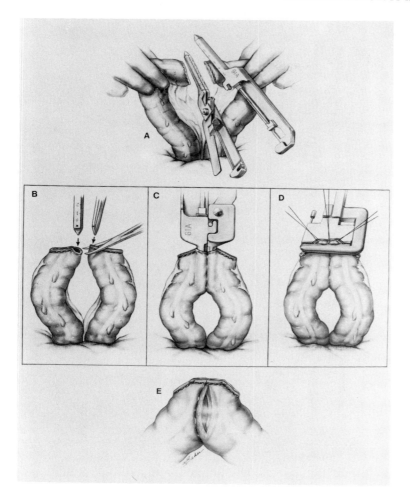

Fig. 3-5. Illustration of a functional end-to-end colo-colostomy demonstrating many of the stapling concepts, such as everting (*A*, *B*) and overlapping (*D*, *E*) lines, as well as the O-shaped anastomotic configuration in a colon resection (*C*, *E*). With time, the anastomotic site will return to the tubular configuration of the colon (*E*).

the central shaft, and circular anastomosis is performed through two linear staple lines arranged in a cross-like fashion. This technique has been extended by us to esophago-gastrostomy, esophago-jejunostomy and Billroth I gastro-duodenostomy (Figs. 3-2, 3-3).

A fourth concept, made possible mostly by the use of the GIA-TA functional end-to-end anastomosis, is the calculation of the cross-sectional surface of this anastomosis and its comparison with circular manual or mechanical end-to-end anastomoses. In a standard, double-row, inverting, end-to-end manual anastomosis, properly performed in healthy and viable tissue, a temporary or possibly prolonged obstruction can occur if excessive amounts of intestine have been inverted—a potential danger described by Lembert in 1826.[5] With the use of stapling instruments, the amount of tissue inversion or eversion is limited and rigorously reproducible, and the ratio of inversion or eversion to the functioning diameter of the intestinal lumen can be calculated based on the type and size of instrument used. Of the two main anastomotic techniques with stapling instruments, we prefer the GIA-TA functional end-to-end anastomosis for intraperitoneal procedures, and the circular EEA end-to-end anastomosis where the instrument can be placed through a natural body orifice or through the open end of the bowel preserved for the purpose of anastomosis and then resected close to it: that is to say, for reconstruction of the esophagus or rectum (see Fig. 3-16A).

The functional end-to-end anastomosis is technically simple and can be accomplished expeditiously with minimal contamination, optimal preservation of blood supply, and ultimate return of the anastomotic passage to the shape of the tubular "host organ."

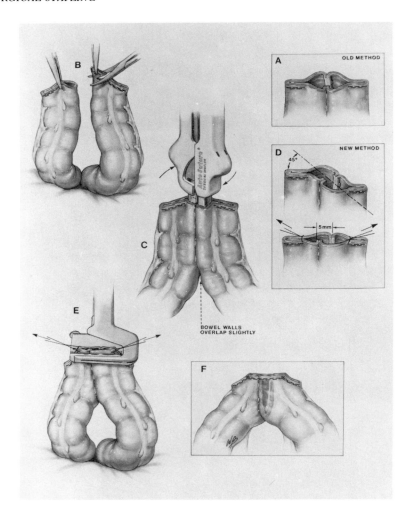

Fig. 3-6. Illustration of the offset closure of the GIA exit gap (*A–D*) resulting in a narrow V-shape (*F*), midway between the wide V and the oval shapes. This technique results in a moderate increase of anastomotic cross-section and prevents healing of the GIA lines to each other. Eversion and overlapping are additional steps shown with this technique (*E, F*).

With this technique it is possible to increase the size of the anastomotic cross-section 2 to 3 times, depending on the shape given to the anastomotic design by the terminal linear closure of the GIA introduction site, by fashioning either an oval or V-shaped passage through the anastomosis; the wide open V-shape accounts for the threefold increase.[3,6] (Figs. 3-4 through 3-7).

If the EEA instrument is used for end-to-end anastomosis and an ideal fit within the intestinal lumen is obtained, the anastomotic cross-section will be slightly smaller than that of the bowel; it will be the size of the circular knife, with a diameter varying from 11.4 mm for the 20.9-mm cartridge to a diameter of 21.2 mm for the 31.6-mm cartridge. The GIA-TA functional end-to-end anastomosis represents the only technique in which the anastomotic lumen can vary in size according to requirements that may become obvious to the surgeon intra-operatively.

Stapling techniques also contribute to the technical ease and safety needed to accomplish difficult operative steps. In areas of narrow or deep anatomic access, manual anastomoses are facilitated by maintaining gentle traction on the specimen while placing the posterior row of the anastomosis before resecting the specimen and completing the anastomosis anteriorly. With the GIA-TA functional end-to-end or end-to-side techniques, it is possible to achieve the entire anastomosis first; traction on the specimen facilitates placement of the GIA linear instrument in a challenging area, such as above or below the clavicle and the diaphragm, or deep in the pelvis.[1–3] After completion of the anastomosis, the now common GIA introduction site and exit gap, and the lumen of the specimen,

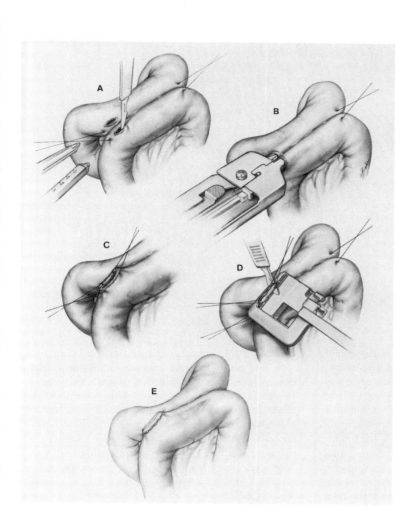

Fig. 3-7. Illustration of a side-to-side entero-enterosostomy demonstrating the separation of both GIA lines at the exit gap, resulting in a wide V-shape (*A–E*). This technique avoids the creation of a critically narrow passage at this point of the anastomosis (*E*).

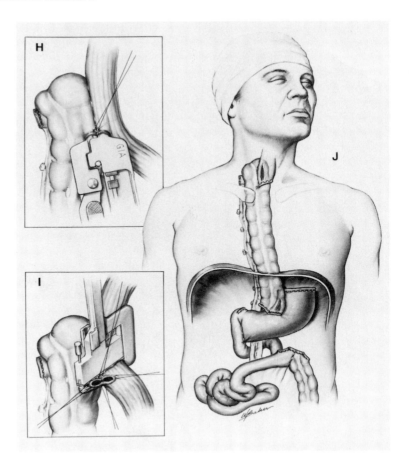

Fig. 3-8. Example of sequential anastomosis first, resection second ("anastomose-résection intégrée") in cervical esophago-colostomy (*top insert*) followed by TA closure and esophagectomy (*bottom insert*) in esophago-coloplasty. (Technique of F.N. Steichen)

are closed by one application of the TA linear stapler. The specimen is excised using the TA stapler as a guide for resection on the specimen side. The concept of sequential anastomosis first and resection second, with the specimen temporarily left in continuity at the anastomotic site for better exposure and greater safety, popularized by R. Welter, has found a special application in the Barcelona technique of Ravitch, in which continuity is temporarily maintained at both ends of the looped specimen while anastomosis is performed. These techniques reduce the duration of open bowel exposure and, by their design or operative planning, will conform to the V-mode of the functional end-to-end or end-to-side anastomosis (Figs. 3-8 through 3-12).

In radical extirpative procedures, surgical stapling techniques facilitate reconstruction during the same operation, which adds both great versatility in the creation of substitute organs and flexibility in the adaptation of organs to various anatomic locations and unexpected technical challenges. Structurally reli-

able autologous organ replacements can be created with low morbidity and mortality rates in all age groups to replace the function of resected organs. Replacement of the esophagus with various gastric tubes or colon segments, of the stomach with jejunal reservoirs, of the bladder with ileal or colon loops, and of the colon with ileal pouches are examples of this approach[1,3] (Figs. 3-13 through 3-16).

At other times, stapling instruments facilitate preservation of function without the need for a substitute organ; this is most vividly demonstrated by the primary colo-rectal anastomosis in the very low anterior rectal resection. Although the movement away from abdomino-perineal amputation, in favor of anterior resection and sphincter preservation, was well on its way by the time the circular anastomosing instrument arrived, there is no doubt that this instrument and the various techniques it has inspired make the low anastomosis easier and safer.

At times a two-stage approach is required, as in sigmoid resection for diverticulitis with localized per-

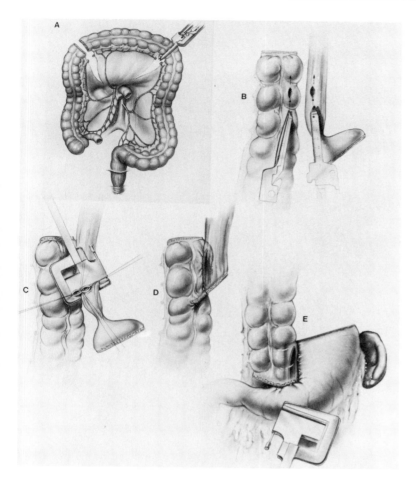

Fig. 3-9. Example of sequential anastomosis first, resection second in mid-thoracic esophago-colostomy (*A, B*) followed by esophago-gastrectomy (*C, D*) in colon interposition (*E*). (Technique of F.N. Steichen)

foration and abscess formation, with no generalized peritonitis. Following excision of the diseased sigmoid colon, the two colon ends can be joined—local and general conditions permitting—with the long GIA-90 linear anastomosing stapler (9 cm) in a functional side-to-side fashion, rather than performing a Hartmann procedure. For protection of this anastomosis, the common open bowel ends, having served for the intraluminal placement and exit of the GIA-90 (normally closed transversely with the linear TA instrument in a classic functional end-to-end anastomosis), are exteriorized on the abdominal wall in Mikulicz colostomy fashion. After a few bowel movements through this double colostomy, the patient will pass feces and flatus per rectum, and the colostomy opening will shrink to the size of a mucous fistula. Some 2 to 3 months later it can be closed extraperitoneally under local anesthesia with a linear stapler or by hand, on an ambulatory basis.

CONCLUSIONS

It can be stated that in one area—the sutureless compression anastomosis—we have now come full circle with the rejuvenation of instruments and operative techniques that had until recently been considered of historical interest only, reserved for scholarly considerations and concerns.

As to the apparent antagonism between manual and mechanical sutures, such a position is highly arguable and does not correspond to the realities of clinical practice. Neither system satisfies all modern technical operative requirements completely and optimally enough to allow exclusion of one by the other. Present-day operative surgery requires teaching and learning both methods. Beyond that, ease and improved results with stapling techniques recommend their use in difficult reconstructions, creation of autologous organs, all broncho-pulmonary surgery, and

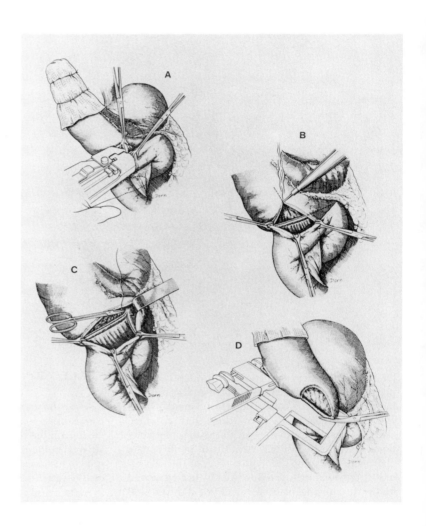

Fig. 3-10. Example of sequential anastomosis first, resection second in gastro-jejunostomy (*A–C*) followed by distal gastrectomy (*D*) in Billroth-II procedure (technique of R. Welter, M.D.).

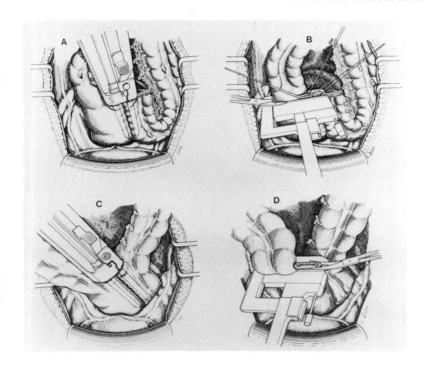

Fig. 3-11. Example of sequential anastomosis first, resection second in functional end-to-end (*A*, *B*) and Bajonet side-to-side (*C*, *D*) colo-rectal anastomoses followed by left-sided colon resection (*B*, *D*) (technique of R. Welter, M.D.).

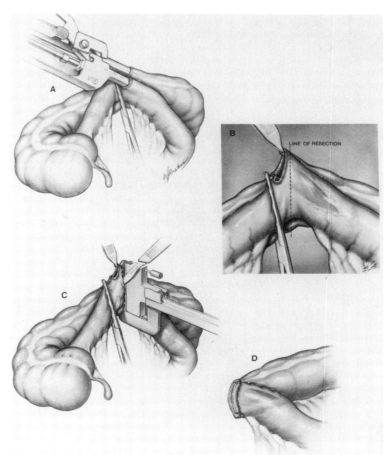

Fig. 3-12. Example of sequential anastomosis first, resection second in ileo-transverse colostomy with the specimen in continuity (*A*), followed by right hemi-colectomy (*B*, *C*). The design of this technique allows for a wide V-shape (*D*) (Barcelona technique of M.M. Ravitch, M.D.).

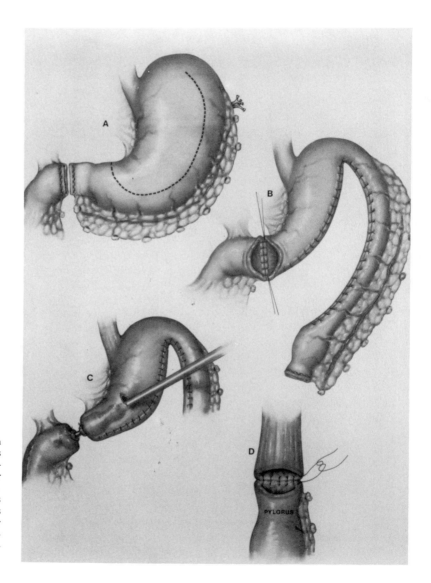

Fig. 3-13. *A, B.* Creation of an autologous substitute esophagus with stapling instruments by a reverse gastro-duodenal tube after pharyngo-laryngo-esophagectomy. The gastro-duodenostomy (*C*) is achieved by a circular anastomosis intersecting with the long linear gastric closure; the pharyngo-duodenal anastomosis is done manually (*D*).

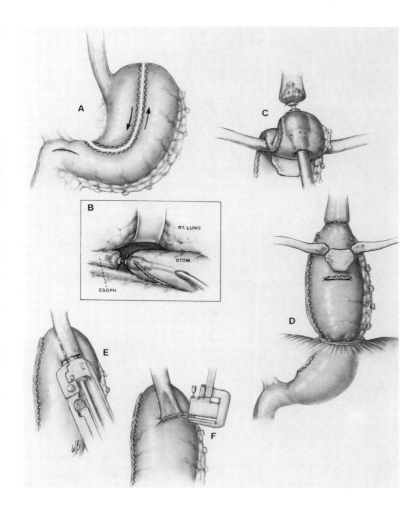

Fig. 3-14. *A.* Long isoperistaltic tube after esophago-gastrectomy (mostly lesser curvature). The tube can reach the base of the neck (*C, D*) or the apex of the chest (*B, E*).

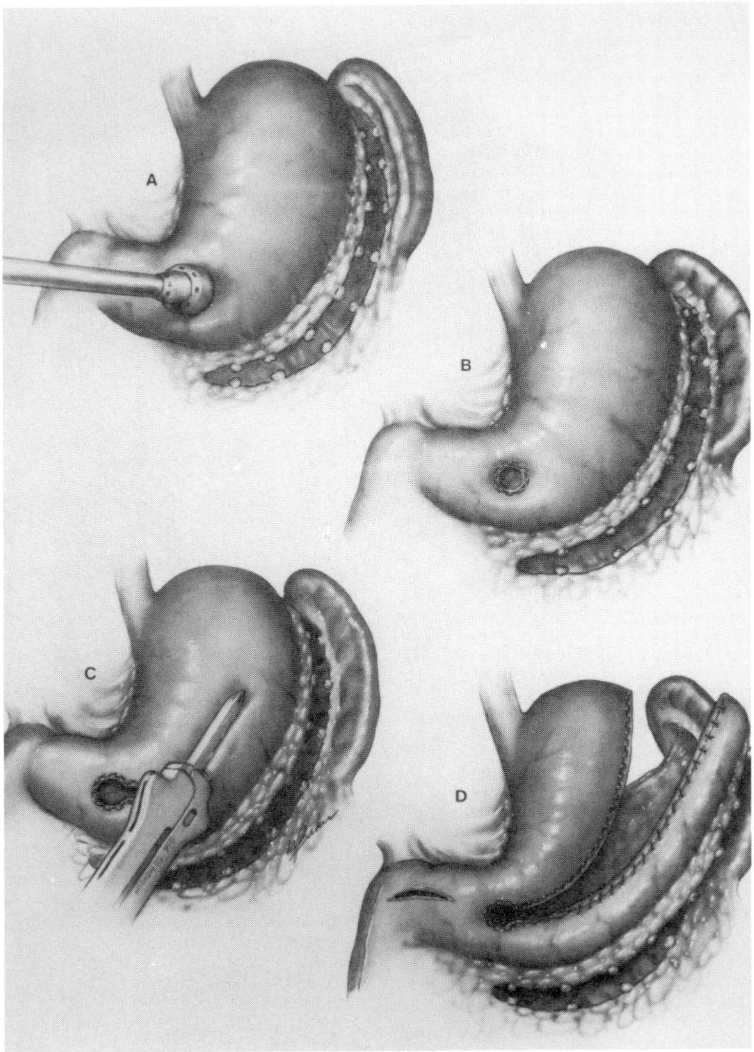

Fig. 3-15. Long isoperistaltic greater curvature tube, with esophago-gastric continuity (*A–C*), used mostly for retrosternal palliative bypass of the thoracic esophagus (*D*).

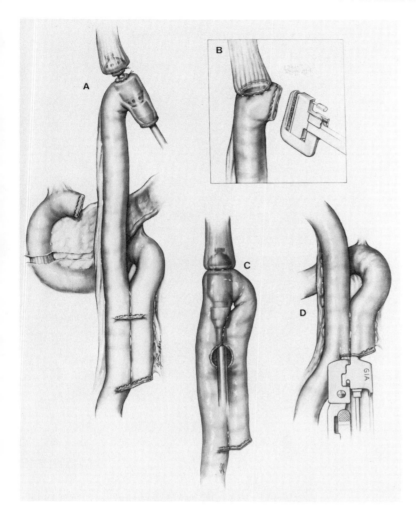

Fig. 3-16. Paulino (*A*, *B*) and Hunt-Lawrence (*C*) gastric substitutes after total gastrectomy. Circular anastomosing instrument is used through the open jejunum, left long for that purpose (A), or through the apex of the Hunt-Lawrence pouch (*C*). Roux-en-Y jejuno-jejunostomy is end-to-side (*D*).

even in simpler procedures, because staplers facilitate reconstruction at the end of an operation and eliminate the potential for needle punctures by members of the operating team.

If one had to predict the future, a reasonable basis for a gaze into the crystal ball would be to consider the conditions of successful anastomosis: technically simple and economical methods that are universally applicable, with minimal tissue trauma and reliable results at all levels of surgical competence. Of the three contenders, the sutureless, absorbable, and fragmentable compression rings of the future, placed with EEA- or SPTU-like delivery instruments, may well fulfill the goals of a successful bowel anastomosis or closure.

REFERENCES

1. Steichen FM, Ravitch MM: Stapling in Surgery. Chicago: Year Book, 1984.

2. Welter R, Patel J-Cl: Chirurgie Mécanique Digestive. Paris: Masson, 1985.

3. Ravitch MM, Steichen FM: Principles and Practice of Surgical Stapling. Chicago: Year Book, 1987.

4. Knight CD, Griffen FD: An improved technique for low anterior resection of the rectum using the EEA stapler. Surgery 88:710, 1980.

5. Lembert A: Mémoire sur l'entéroraphie. Rep Gén d'Anat et de Physiol Pathol II:101, 1826.

6. Tomoda M: Ein neuer Magen-Darmnähapparat. Zentrabl Chir 64:1455, 1937.

CHAPTER 4

"ANASTOMOSE-RÉSECTION INTÉGRÉE" (WITH INSPECTION ENTEROTOMY OR GASTROTOMY)

Roger Welter

Stapling instruments have changed the basic features of the various reconstructive techniques that follow excision of segments of the gastro-intestinal tract at different levels or of entire organs. These changes evolved progressively with the understanding that staple lines could be safely placed in ways that heretofore were not advisable or reliable with manual sutures. The concept of overlapping, crossing, and intersecting staple lines is basic to this development, together with the demonstration that mucosa-to-mucosa and serosa-to-serosa closures and anastomoses of the bowel heal reliably, albeit along different histologic patterns.[1–3]

Following the initial period, in which stapling instruments were modeled on manual sutures to reconstruct the gastro-intestinal tract after excision, it became apparent that the fully dissected specimen—left temporarily attached to the planned anastomotic site—could be used to facilitate exposure and creation of a linear anastomosis with the GIA instrument first. The anastomosis would then be completed by the simultaneous closure of both the GIA introduction site and the lumen of the specimen with the TA instrument, followed by resection of the specimen. These second and third steps make the resection an integral part of the anastomosis, which has preceded the resection.[2–12] This technique can be accomplished with the specimen kept intact temporarily[6] or with one anastomotic viscus transected and the opposite one left in continuity, to facilitate traction.[4,11,12] We used this second approach, which gives mobility to the specimen and facilitates the

technical steps of the anastomosis, in a subtotal distal gastrectomy in 1973 for the first time.

As experience with this technique grew, it became apparent that an enterotomy or gastrotomy on the specimen side—preceding the application of the TA instrument and resection of the specimen together with this enterotomy or gastrotomy—would allow inspection of the linear GIA lines and permit corrective steps, if necessary. Furthermore, this enterotomy or gastrotomy increases mobility at the open end of the GIA anastomosis and steers the TA closure of the separated GIA lines into the V-mode.[13] The V-mode assures the largest possible anastomotic cross-section.

BASIC TECHNIQUES

The principle of sequential anastomosis-resection with the GIA-TA instruments can be shown on two tubular structures that have been placed parallel to each other with their antimesenteric surfaces in apposition. The specimen has been transected at one end and is temporarily continuous with the opposite tube. The transected tube (viscus) had been stapled before severance of the specimen. The various arrangements possible at different levels of the GI tract will be shown in the specific techniques of partial and total gastrectomy, as well in anterior resection. In general, continuity of the specimen is maintained through that portion of the GIA tract that presents greater technical difficulty in the placement of the GI instrument (e.g., stomach for partial gastrectomy, esophagus for total gastrectomy, and rectum for anterior resection).

In the first step, the GIA instrument is placed through an excision of the antimesenteric corner of the closed segment of bowel, and through a stab wound in the antimesenteric wall of the bowel that is continuous with the specimen. This stab wound is situated in healthy tissues, at a safe distance from the planned margin of resection (Fig. 4-1).

After the creation of the linear side-to-side anastomosis, the GIA instrument is removed and the now common introduction site is delineated with stay sutures (Fig. 4-2A).

Next the TA-55 or -90 instrument is applied in the same plane as the previous bowel closure, across the segment that is continuous with the specimen and also across the common GIA opening. At the level of this opening, great care is taken to include its entire circumference within the jaws of the instrument. In this fashion, as the instrument is closed and fired, the GIA opening and the lumen of the bowel that is still attached to the specimen will be closed at the same time.

The specimen is then resected and this third step, an integral part of the anastomotic technique, completes the final design of this technical concept. The result is a functional end-to-end anastomosis with both GIA lines closed in the oval fashion (Fig. 4-2B, C).

If for various reasons a V-closure of the GIA lines is indicated or preferred, the TA instrument can be placed at a right angle to the linear staple lines. By separating the open ends of the linear GIA lines through traction in opposite directions, the result is a V-design. In addition, the medial tip of the linear staple line closing one bowel end is sutured to the mid-rim of the stab wound in the opposite bowel segment, so as to make for a safe closure of the common GIA introduction site (Fig. 4-3A).

The TA stapler is then applied at a right angle to the linear closure of the transected segment. It includes between its jaws the entire common GIA opening, as well as the walls of the segment that is continuous with the specimen (Fig. 4-3B). Following resection of the specimen, a functional end-to-end anastomosis of the V-mode is obtained with right-angle crossing of two staple lines, another step made possible by the use of staples.[1,8] Furthermore, the wide V-design of this anastomosis creates the largest possible anastomotic cross-section and is never complicated by anastomotic stricture.[14–16]

Inspection Enterotomy

This intermediate step takes place after the linear GIA side-to-side anastomosis has been accomplished and before closure of the bowel lumen and common GIA introduction site. It is designed to permit inspection of the GIA anastomotic lines ("quality control") and to give the surgeon an opportunity to correct any potential staple line insufficiencies.[13]

To demonstrate this inspection, enterotomy is shown following the linear GIA anastomosis of two bowel segments, with the specimen kept temporarily intact (Fig. 4-4). In this case the enterotomy is extended onto both loops of the specimen, as an extension of the GIA introduction site.

If the sequential anastomosis-resection mode with preliminary transection of the specimen at one end had been used, then inspection enterotomy would extend only into the loop of the specimen still attached to the anastomosis.

Besides allowing quality control of the anastomosis and corrective steps if indicated, this inspection enterotomy facilitates the wide V-closure of the now mobile, free ends of the linear GIA anastomosing staple lines. As the healthy side walls of the bowel are approximated and compressed by the linear TA stapler, a mucosa-to-mucosa closure is obtained. The posterior wall of the closure falls away from the anterior angle to create a wide V-shaped separation of

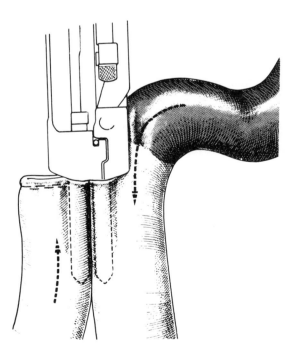

Fig. 4-1. Placement of the GIA instrument with one end of the specimen transected. The opposite viscus, left in continuity with the specimen, allows traction for easier anastomosis.

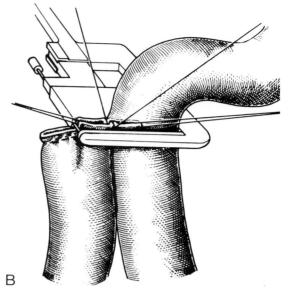

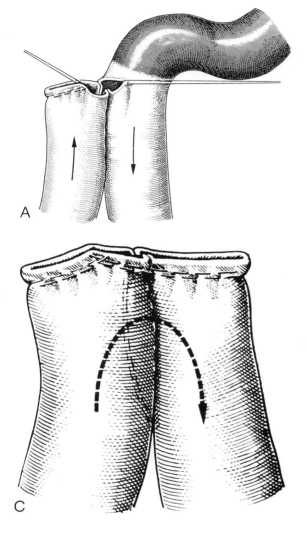

Fig. 4-2. *A.* Following side-to-side GIA anastomosis and removal of the instrument, the borders of the future closing are delineated with stay sutures. *B.* The GIA placement site and intact bowel are closed with one application of the TA stapler, in the same plane as the linear visceral closure of the transection site. *C.* The result is a functional end-to-end anastomosis with an oval cross-section.

the GIA lines and a closure that approximates one bowel wall to the other without interposition of a second layer (4-wall thickness), such as might be obtained if the V-separation is only partial.

Special Techniques

Sequential Gastro-Jejunostomy, Inspection Gastrotomy, and Distal Gastric Resection

Following complete liberation of the portion of stomach to be resected, the duodenum is transected proximal to a closure with the TA-55 instrument. The basic concept of this technique is to maintain gentle traction on the gastric specimen kept in continuity with the proximal stomach to facilitate the linear GIA

gastro-enterostomy along the posterior aspect of the greater curvature of the stomach (Fig. 4-5*A*).

The level of the gastric stab wound on the posterior wall is chosen somewhat proximal to the planned resection of the stomach. On the jejunal side the GIA is placed through a stab wound in the antimesenteric border of the appropriately chosen loop of jejunum. The anastomosis is accomplished in a proximal direction.

Following the linear GIA gastro-jejunostomy, the instrument is removed and an inspection gastrotomy is started on the posterior wall of the specimen and extended for some 3 to 5 cm (Fig. 4-5*B*). This gastrotomy will be included in the resection later on.

By gently retracting the enlarged orifice, it is pos-

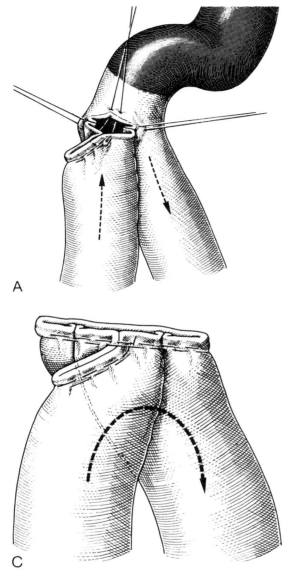

A

B

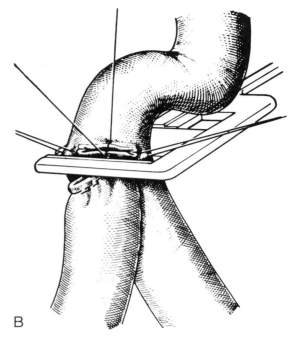

C

Fig. 4-3. *A.* Closure at right angle to the linear staple line of transected bowel. Free GIA ends are held apart in V-fashion. *B.* Closure of bowel and GIA sites. *C.* V-shaped cross-section.

sible to inspect the linear GIA lines, to complete hemostasis if needed, and to place a safety suture into the apical crotch of the GIA anastomosis from within (Fig. 4-5C).

After the surgeon has convinced himself that all is well with the linear gastrojejunostomy, the various anatomic relationships to assure a safe and patent anastomosis are re-established, and the TA-90 is placed from left to right (Fig. 4-5D). The instrument is placed in an oblique direction to the patient's right side, to ensure a gastric resection along the lesser curvature at some 2 finger-breadths below the gastro-esophageal junction. Furthermore, the free ends of the linear GIA staple lines are separated in a V-

fashion to create the largest possible anastomotic diameter.

In closing the TA-90 instrument and activating it, the inferior jejunal border is stapled against the anterior gastric wall along the greater curvature, and the posterior gastric wall is stapled to the anterior gastric wall in the center of the resection as well as along the lesser curvature. The specimen is then resected. With the single application of the TA-90 instrument, the final step of the anastomosis is achieved together with resection of the specimen containing the previously placed inspection gastrotomy.

This technique has multiple advantages. It results in a true end-to-side gastro-jejunostomy, along the

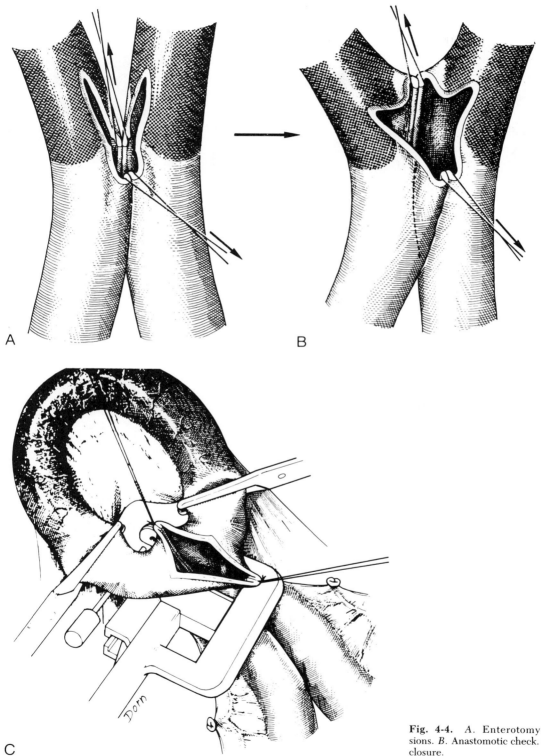

Fig. 4-4. A. Enterotomy incisions. B. Anastomotic check. C. V-closure.

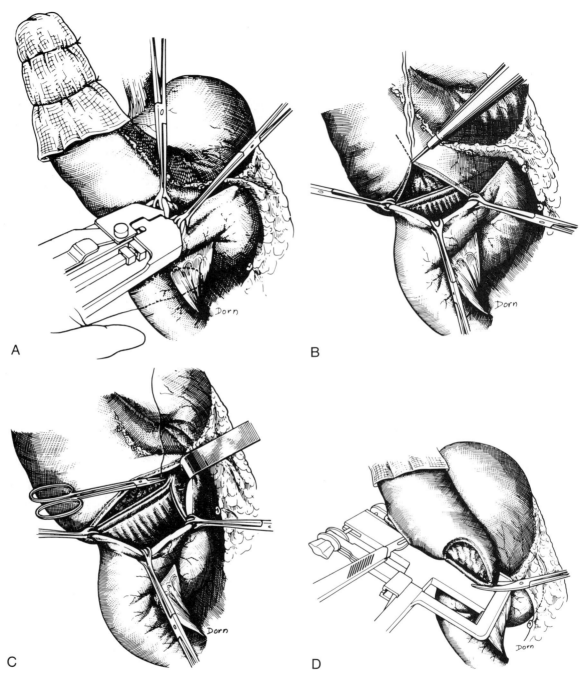

Fig. 4-5. *A.* Gastro-enterostomy along posterior wall of the greater curvature with specimen in place, used for traction. *B.* Inspection gastrotomy on specimen—posterior wall. *C.* Inspection of anastomosis, placement of apical safety suture. *D.* Closure of GIA placement opening and stomach with TA 90. Resection of specimen.

greater curvature of the stomach, at its most dependant aspect. Furthermore, the afferent loop of jejunum is suspended above the anastomosis to the greater curvature.

The temporary preservation of the specimen facilitates exposure and the technical steps of the anastomosis by allowing the surgeon to maintain gentle traction on the proximal stomach and the esophagus.

The inspection gastrotomy is made possible by this approach, which results in a saving of time and stapling cartridges. A reduction in contamination from the open stomach and jejunum, briefly only exposed to the operative site, is an important fringe benefit.

Sequential Esophago-Jejunostomy and Total Gastrectomy[12,17]

Following complete mobilization of the stomach, the specimen is elevated onto the anterior chest wall and gentle traction is maintained on the esophagus. Through a stab wound into the posterior wall of the esophagus just above the gastro-esophageal junction and a second stab wound into the antimesenteric wall of the jejunal loop, some 5 to 6 cm below its closed end, the GIA instrument is placed, closed, and activated (Fig. 4-6A).

Following removal of the GIA instrument, the free ends of the linear GIA anastomotic lines are grasped with Babcock clamps and are separated in a V-fashion. In addition, the posterior esophageal wall is sutured to the lower jejunal lip halfway between the Babcock clamps to assure complete apposition of the circumference of the GIA introduction site.

The TA-55 is then advanced again from the patient's left to his or her right. In placing the instrument, the surgeon has to take great care to incorporate between the jaws of the instrument the entire circumference of the now single GIA introduction site, as well as the circular esophageal wall overlying this opening anteriorly (Fig. 4-6B). After closing the instrument and activating it, the esophago-gastric specimen, together with the lower rim of jejunum, is resected with scissors.

It is of the utmost importance to exercise great caution in taking the various steps of this reconstruction, since the completed anastomosis ascends into the posterior mediastinum as soon as the TA instrument is removed. If the surgeon is not completely happy with the final result, corrective maneuvers can only be undertaken through a thoracotomy.

Sequential Colo-Rectal Anastomosis and Sigmoid Resection

Following proximal transection of the colon, the specimen is left in continuity with the rectum to exercise gentle traction to facilitate anastomosis. The proximal colon is curved back onto itself and placed alongside the upper rectum to achieve the final design of a functional end-to-end anastomosis.

The antimesenteric corner of the proximal colon closure is excised, and a stab wound is placed into the antero-lateral wall of the rectum just distal to the planned level of excision. A side-to-side GIA colorectal anastomosis is then performed. Following removal of the GIA instrument, the now single GIA

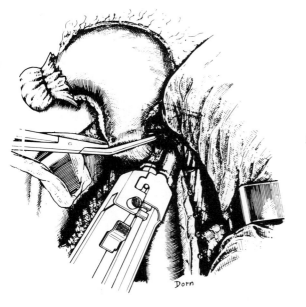
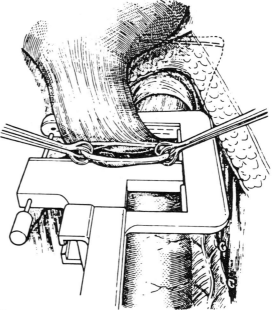

A   B

Fig. 4-6. *A.* Esophago-jejunostomy with the linear GIA instrument after gastric mobilization. *B.* Closure of esophagus and GIA site with the stapler. Total gastrectomy takes place thereafter by transecting the G-E junction on the edge of the instrument.

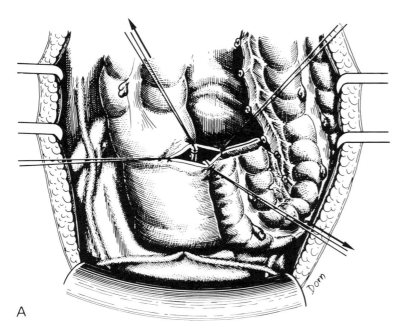

A

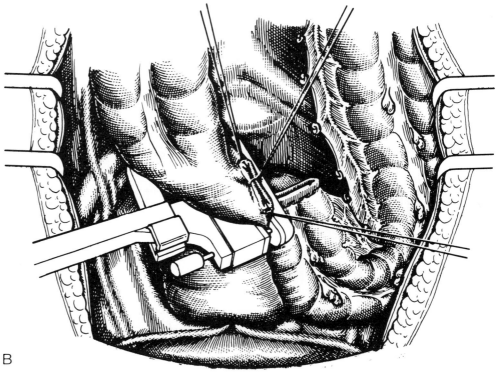

B

Fig. 4-7. *A.* Status after linear side-to-side colo-rectostomy. *B.* Closure of rectum and GIA opening with TA instrument.

introduction opening is separated in a V-fashion with stay sutures (Fig. 4-7A).

The single GIA opening, as well as the entire lumen of the rectum, are then closed with the TA instrument. With this maneuver the rim of colon is stapled to the anterior, lateral, and posterior walls of the rectum (Fig. 4-7B). Gentle traction on the specimen facilitates this step of the procedure. Finally, the specimen is excised on the superior edge of the instrument.

CONCLUSIONS

The sequential anastomosis-resection *(anastomose-résection intégrée)* facilitates dissection and liberation of the specimen, as well as all the steps of this special mode of anastomosis, by allowing traction on the specimen and better exposure, especially in difficult anatomic areas such as above and below the clavicle, above and below the diaphragm, and in the pelvis. This technique is possible only with the use of the GIA and TA instruments, and is the same at different levels of the GI tract: The first step consists of the use of the GIA instrument for side-to-side linear anastomosis that can be shaped into the wide-open V-design. The second step using the TA instrument consists of closing the now common GIA opening and the specimen, which is then removed in the third step.

It is quite obvious that this technique cannot be used in all circumstances. The combined application of the GIA and TA instruments has to be possible anatomically; otherwise, injudicious use of the GIA instrument without the possibility to complete the anastomosis with the TA instrument could lead to a near-disastrous intra-operative course. The use of this anastomotic mode therefore depends on the judgement and experience of the operating surgeon.

Translated from the French by F.M. Steichen, M.D.

REFERENCES

1. Ravitch MM: Principles of stapling, mucosa to mucosa suture and crossed staple lines. In: Ravitch MM, Steichen FM: Principles and Practice of Surgical Stapling. Chicago: Year Book, 1987:3–15.
2. Ravitch MM, Steichen FM: Symposium on surgical stapling techniques. Surg Clin North Am 64(3):429–433, 1984.
3. Steichen FM, Ravitch MM: Stapling in Surgery, Chicago: Year Book, 1984:192–193, 242, 280–281.
4. Charlier A: Gastrectomie avec anastomose gastro-jèjunale première intégrée, procédé mécanique original de Welter. Thèse de doctorat. Paris: Université René Descartes, 1981.
5. Gazzola LM: Les sutures mécaniques. Leur utilisation dans la résection-anastomose intestinale intégrée. Ed Médecine et Hygiène, Genève, 1976.
6. Ravitch MM, Ong TH, Gazzola LM: A new precise and rapid technique for intestinal resection and anastomosis with staples. Surg Gynecol Obstet 139:6, 1974.
7. Ravitch MM, Steichen FM: Staples in gastro-intestinal surgery. In: Maingot R, ed: Abdominal Operations.

New York: Appleton-Century-Crofts, 8th Ed. 1985: 1565–1568, 1575–1597.
8. Ravitch MM, Steichen FM: Principles and Practice of Surgical Stapling. Chicago: Year Book. 1987:3–46.
9. Rignault D, Champault G, Gautier-Benoit C, et al: Table ronde sur les sutures automatiques en chirurgie digestive. Actualités Chirurgicales. 78ème Congrès A.F.C., 1976. Tome 1. Paris: Masson, 1977:99–112.
10. Steichen FM, Richards V, Chassin JL, Weakley FL, Welter R. Staplers in intestinal surgery (Symposium). Contemp Surg 14:51, 1979.
11. Steichen FM: Sequential anastomosis and resection in operations on the gastrointestinal tract. In: Ravitch MM, Steichen FM: Principles and Practice of Surgical Stapling. Chicago: Year Book, 1987:31–46.
12. Welter R, Patel JCl: Chirurgie Mécanique Digestive-Techniques raisonnées. Paris: Masson, 1985:75–83, 172–180, 194–196, 210–216, 244–248, 259–264.
13. Psalmon F: Chirurgie du grêle. In: Welter R, Patel JCl: Chirurgie Mécanique Digestive—Techniques raisonnées. Paris: Masson, 1985:206–226.
14. Reys Ph, Frey G, Deereler JP, Rollin Cl. Anastomoses digestives par agrafes métalliques: choix de la meilleure procédure en vue de l'obtention du meilleur calibre anastomotique. J Méd Strasbourg 11:387, 1980.
15. Turbelin JM, Arnaud JP, Welter R, Adloff M: Etude comparative des surfaces anastomotiques obtenues par utilisation des sutures mécaniques en chirurgie digestive. J Chir (Paris) 117:541, 1980.
16. Welter R, Psalmon F: The geometry of functional end-to-end anastomosis and a comparative study of anastomotic surfaces using mechanical sutures in gastrointestinal surgery. In: Ravitch MM, Steichen FM: Principles and Practice of Surgical Stapling. Chicago: Year Book. 1987:16–30.
17. Moller E, Brun JG, Deliere Th, Patel JCl, Psalmon F, Welter R: Gastrectomie totale. Anastomose oeso-jejunale première pièce en place utilisant les pinces à suture mécanique linéaire. Presse Méd 12:41, 1983.

ADDITIONAL READING

Patel JCl, Fekete F, Breil PH, et al: Les sutures digestives mécaniques. Séance Thématisée, 85ème Congrès français de Chirurgie, 19–22 Sep., 1983.
Ravitch MM, Steichen FM: Technics of staple suturing in the gastrointestinal tract. Ann Surg 175:815, 1972.
Ravitch MM: Second thoughts of a Surgical Curmudgeon. Chicago: Year Book, 1987.
Reuter MJP: Les sutures mécaniques en chirurgie digestive et pulmonaire. Strasbourg: Thèse Université Louis Pasteur, 1982:132.
Turbelin JM: Les sutures mécaniques en chirurgie digestive. Thèse de doctorat, Université Louis Pasteur de Strasbourg, 1980:22, 32–34.
Welter R: Communication à la table ronde sur les sutures automatiques en chirurgie digestive. Actualités chirurgicales. 78ème Congrès A.F.C., 1976, Tome 1, Paris: Masson, 1977:99–112.
Welter R, Turbelin JM, Charlier A: Gastrectomie avec anastomose gastro-jéjunale "première." Technique originale d'emploi des procédés de chirurgie mécanique. Nouv Presse Méd 10:247, 1981.

CHAPTER 5

THE TEACHING AND LEARNING OF STAPLING

M. Adloff

Before using mechanical suture instruments, the surgeon should become thoroughly familiar with the various manual techniques of suturing and anastomosing bowel, since even today these techniques are the basis of visceral repair, regardless of the anatomic or operative circumstances in a given operation.

While using mechanical sutures, it is important to realize that staples are a particular modality of suturing live tissues. Like other suture procedures, stapling can be followed by complications that should not be automatically attributed to the instruments or to "fateful" mechanical failures of these instruments.

Furthermore, stapled anastomoses require the same respect for basic surgical principles as hand-sewn anastomoses do: gentle dissection that preserves tissue integrity at the bowel ends to be anastomosed, careful hemostasis, absence of abnormal traction on the anastomosis, and placement of sutures into healthy tissues supplied with normal blood vessels. If for various reasons a manual suture is considered unsafe, stapling cannot remedy these and result in a better, safer anastomosis or closure of bowel. Stapling is not a solution to technical inadequacy or operative deficiencies and cannot possibly allow a surgeon to perform above his or her level of competence.

Stapling alone is not synonymous with greater technical ease in the difficult anastomosis deep in a narrow pelvis or high at the apex of the chest, unless the surgeon has become familiar with the use of the various instruments through experience acquired in the laboratory and through progressive clinical experience, starting with easier operative procedures (Table 5-1).

PRINCIPLES

To suture live tissues with staples, the staples must penetrate through the entire tissue and be shaped into the (by now familiar) B-configuration. Compression of the tissues does not result in ischemia; in fact, experimental studies have shown that the vessels do penetrate through the oval opening of the B-shaped staples, to the line of resection. Because of this fundamental design, a first practical consequence is that inflamed, edematous, and thick tissues cannot be safely penetrated, even with the 4.8-mm staples. The compression of the tissues between the instrument jaws is difficult and can result in an incomplete formation of the staples as well as in laceration of the sero-muscular layer of the bowel. Conversely, tissues that are thinned out, such as a very distended ascending colon, may not offer enough substance for a fully aerostatic, leak-free staple line.

Minimal oozing of blood from the transected bowel circumference shows that the tissues beyond the staple lines are viable. However, in all gastro-intestinal anastomoses, especially at the level of the stomach, it is at times necessary to achieve a complementary hemostasis with a few manual sutures. Each anastomosis should be inspected to control bleeding beyond the level of a simple hemorrhagic blush (Table 5-2).

To achieve a successful application of stapling techniques, four basic steps have to be mastered:

1. Placement of the stapling instruments
2. Placement of purse-strings for the circular anastomosing instrument
3. Tissue compression by closing the cartridge

Table 5-1. Teaching and Learning Points of Surgical Stapling

Stapling is a mechanical method of suturing biologic tissues

This method is safe, but not foolproof

It requires traditional respect for sound surgical principles

It is not a solution to technical inadequacy or deficiency

It does not reduce the challenge of difficult or unfamiliar surgical steps

bearing portion of the instrument against the anvil

4. Removal of the stapling instrument

Placement of the Stapling Instruments

Linear Staple Lines

While using the TA or GIA instruments, the surgeon has to make sure that all tissues to be stapled are contained within the jaws, or forks, of the instruments. This prescription is easily followed with the TA instruments, since the tissue pin is specifically designed to maintain the open bowel within the confines of the instrument.

With the GIA instrument a conscious effort has to be made by the surgeon to ensure that the width of the bowel does not exceed the length of the instrument's forks. If, on the other hand, the GIA instrument is used for a linear anastomosis, it is important to place the instrument along the antimesenteric border of the bowel. If several applications of the GIA instrument are used, as in the creation of a gastric tube, the crossing and overlapping of a beginning staple line with the end of the previous one is important (Table 5-3).

Circular Staple Lines

The ease with which the circular instrument can be advanced into the bowel lumen depends on the cal-

Table 5-2. Surgical Principles and Safety Steps

The choice of suturing method depends on tissue quality and thickness

The method chosen should

Avoid ischemia

Insure hemostasis

Maintain healthy tissue viability

Lead to safe healing

Safety and ease of technique depend on

Instrument/operative-site interface

Need for purse-string with circular stapler

Degree of tissue compression

Prefer simple and test-proven techniques

Avoid "routine patterned" solutions

Table 5-3. Instrument/Operative-Site Interface

Linear Staple Lines

Include all tissues to be stapled

Avoid pitfalls while crossing and intersecting staple lines

Circular Staple Lines

Consider choice of instrument caliber, need for pre-placement dilatation, glucagon level

Separate anvil from cartridge and rotate instrument for removal

iber of the bowel and the choice of corresponding cartridge sizes. If there is a significant difference between the two, longitudinal lacerations of the various layers, especially the serosa, may occur and create a precarious anastomosis. This may not be obvious to the surgeon, since such lacerations can be masked by epiploic appendages. The choice of the cartridge is therefore of great importance; the cartridge should ideally fill the lumen of the gently dilated bowel without over-distending and lacerating the bowel walls.

In our experience, placement of a circular stapler is at times facilitated by the intravenous injection of glucagon (Table 5-3).

Placement of the Purse-String Suture

This is the most important single step in the creation of a circular anastomosis. Attention to all details of the purse-string suture will result in a reliable anastomosis. The purse-string should be accomplished with a monofilament suture that achieves the following objectives:

1. The individual bites should penetrate through all layers of the intestinal wall.

2. They should be equidistant from the line of transection and should contain sufficient tissue to ensure safety without invaginating excessive amounts of bowel wall that could not be accommodated between the anvil and the cartridge.

3. The separation between the individual needle penetrations and suture placements should be optimal, so as to avoid suture crowding on one hand and excessive laxity on the other, resulting in evasion of a portion of the bowel circumference from the instrument. The tying of the purse-string suture should bring the entire bowel circumference into comfortable and secure contact with the central rod. Several additional ties will prevent a slippage of the purse-string from the pressure of closing the anvil against the cartridge.

4. The suture beyond the tied knots should be cut appropriately so as to avoid loose ends protruding through the circular anastomosis.

The presently available purse-string instrument cannot be used routinely because of anatomic constraints of space or the presence of a thickened bowel wall, in which case the passage of the purse-string through the instrument may not traverse all layers of the bowel.

For this reason we prefer to use the method described by Charles Knight in low anterior colo-rectal anastomoses. With this technique, a circular anastomosis through a linear staple closure of the rectal stump is accomplished; therefore, the difficult step of the rectal purse-string suture is eliminated. The intersection of a linear staple line by a circular staple line is not a dangerous procedure and will at most require a more careful extraction of the instrument.

As a matter of fact, with the new EEA instrument—in which the anvil and the cartridge can be placed separately, one into each end of the bowel to be anastomosed—it is now possible to create an anastomosis that intersects with two linear lines, one at the rectal stump and the other one for closure of the proximal colon (Table 5-4).

Instrument Closure and Tissue Compression

For this purpose the intestinal ends to be anastomosed are prepared sufficiently to avoid the inclusion of mesentery and epiploic appendages between the cartridge and the anvil, thus avoiding anastomotic insufficiency or bleeding. This preparation of the bowel ends does not equal that necessary for a manual, double-layer suture. Hemostasis of vessels and fat around the proposed site of anastomosis should never be done with metallic clips, since they would interfere with the transection of tissues by the circular knife. Similarly, it is important to avoid the interposition, between the anvil and cartridge, of other tissues, organs, or foreign bodies such as the bladder or compresses. To eliminate all of these potential complications, a finger is passed around the deep posterior end of the anastomosis. The tightening of the stapling instrument should always be to the level that will result in a perfect B-formation (Table 5-5).

Removal of the Circular Stapling Instrument

The disengagement of a circular stapling instrument can only take place after complete separation of

Table 5-4. Criteria for Quality of Purse-String Suture

Running suture with monofilament; full-thickness bites with each needle passage
Regularly spaced sutures parallel to resection margin
Good tightening of purse-string
No suture tails left
Double and triple linear-circular stapling (these techniques eliminate the need for purse-string sutures)

Table 5-5. Tissue Compression by Stapling Instruments

Avoid inclusion of extraneous tissue, drapes, pads, compresses and metal clips
Use optimal compression for given tissue conditions
Avoid excessive circular anastomotic discrepancies

the anvil from the cartridge. This maneuver is difficult (if not impossible) if the circular transection of the purse-stringed bowel ends has been incomplete for whatever reason, most often an incomplete closure and compression of the anvil against the cartridge. If a double- or triple-stapling technique has been used with the intersection of linear and circular staple lines, the passage of the anvil may encounter more resistance than for a simple EEA extraction, for which two classic purse-string sutures are used. Rotation and gentle vertical or side-to-side movement of the instrument is all that should be needed to remove it from the anastomotic site. If force is required to extract the instrument from the anastomosis, damage will occur and the entire procedure should be reviewed to be sure that no technical mistakes were committed. If the anvil still resists extraction, it should be separated from the cartridge and removed through a separate proximal colotomy.

INTRA-OPERATIVE EXAMINATION OF THE ANASTOMOSIS

We are in the habit of examining the competency of each anastomosis, first by checking the completeness and thickness of the tissue rings obtained from the purse-strings. Next, the condition of the anastomosis can be examined by the injection of methylene blue into the bowel lumen or air, with the anastomotic site covered by saline.

These two controls are important but do not always allow judgement as to the overall quality of a given anastomosis. A minimal, localized area of leakage, or a break in the symmetry of the staple line or circle on postoperative x-ray examination, will lead to a redoubling of precautions next time, but may not always be in itself a sign of staple-line failure.

Repair of a Defective Anastomosis

The technical steps to be taken for the repair of a defective anastomosis depend on the importance of the defect. A minimal area of leakage in a complete anastomosis within healthy tissues is simply repaired with two or three inverting manual sutures.

If the defect is more important, an operation of proximal decompression may be indicated following manual repair. This can be done by temporary colostomy in the case of colo-rectal anastomosis.

Finally, an important disruption of the anastomosis requires excision and construction of a new anastomosis, using a similar technique or, if necessary, a different operative approach.

If the imperfect anastomosis is observed following anterior resection, two solutions can be considered. If the construction of a new anastomosis, especially by stapling, appears to be impossible, the patient should undergo an abdomino-perineal resection, or at the least a temporary rectal exclusion using the principle of Hartmann. At times, continuity can be re-established, most often by a transanal anastomosis, using the technique of Parks (Table 5-6).

The reasonable use of stapling techniques always imposes choices: the method of suturing or stapling should be simple and optimally adapted to a given anatomic situation. If there is a discrepancy of the lumina of both bowel ends, the end-to-end anastomosis may not be indicated and should be replaced by an end-to-side or even side-to-side anastomosis.

The decision for primary stapling (or suturing) should always be based on the presence of healthy tissues, of average thickness, with adequate blood supply. Circular anastomoses are especially helpful in anterior colo-rectal reconstructions, as well as in esophago-gastric anastomoses, where they represent a significant advance. In the more "routine" large and small bowel operations, the surgeon should be able to use manual techniques. To us, under these circumstances, the mechanical sutures do not represent an advantage in either technical application or improved reliability. We continue to favor the use of mechanical sutures for gastrectomy and right-sided colectomies, since their use yields a definite saving of operative time.

CONCLUSIONS

A good knowledge of all of the potential hazards and pitfalls of stapling procedures is the best means of prevention. It would be regrettable to let the ignorance of, or disrespect for, safety rules and sound surgical principles develop to the point where mechanical sutures could not be trusted, because staples are one of the most significant advances in the operative approach to visceral surgery. Such lack of respect for safety precautions is the result of:

1. A defective instrument that has not been checked before its use: this is an act of negligence.
2. Inappropriate or incorrect use of the various stapling instruments: this is act of inattention.
3. A poor indication in the use of the instruments: this is an act of inexperience.
4. Poor choice of suture procedure: this is an act of bad judgement.

Negligence, lack of attention and experience, poor judgment: all of these are unacceptable, as much in stapling as in all other areas of surgical endeavors.

Translated from the French by
F.M. Steichen, M.D.

Table 5-6. Quality Control and Remedial Actions

Examine tissue "doughnuts" in circular anastomosis and examine staple-line competence with intraluminal air or fluid injections
Check postoperative staple geometry by x ray

Tailor remedy to importance of defect:

Minimal	Local suture repair
Intermediate	Repair and proximal diversion
Major	Excision of anastomosis, creation of new anastomosis or diversion of both ends

Part II

Instruments and Methods:
Old, New and Different

CHAPTER 6

EXPERIENCE AND RESULTS WITH THE RUSSIAN CIRCULAR SPTU INSTRUMENT

M. Kantartzis, J. Lersmacher, J. Winter, and E. Hoffman

The use of stapling instruments is by now well established in abdominal and thoracic surgery. Although the Russian instruments preceded the development of the more recent generations of stapling instruments, they should not be relegated to mere ancestry, in spite of some of their (correctable) mechanical infirmities. In the course of this evolution in instrument design, the single-row circular stapling instrument was the precursor of the double-row instrument, which has now become available also as a disposable model. The Russian circular SPTU stapler, however, has not lost its usefulness. In 1980 and 1981 we accomplished 208 circular anastomoses in the GI tract with the American EEA stapler. This was our initial experience with stapling in abdominal surgery. Since 1982 we have used the SPTU circular stapling instrument exclusively in 866 anastomoses. Table 6-1 shows the breakdown of stapled anastomoses at the St. Josef Hospital since 1980. Except for the 140 Roux-en-Y anastomoses, all were done in end-to-end fashion. A second layer of manually placed sutures was only used in colo-rectal anastomoses, mostly extraperitoneal, if the intraluminal insufflation of air demonstrated bubbling through the single-row stapled anastomosis. All of the intraperitoneal anastomoses were covered with moderately spaced interrupted seromuscular sutures following the observation of bleeding in two Roux-en-Y anastomoses.

This second manual layer was also used to telescope the esophagus into the jejunum in the 51 patients undergoing esophago-jejunostomy. With this technique we observed no anastomotic leaks in this area. The anastomotic leak rate of the colo-rectal anastomoses was 7.9%; of the esophago-jejunostomies, 2.8%; and of the entero-enterostomies, 2%. In the two small bowel anastomotic leaks, the pa-

Table 6-1. Stapled Anastomoses from 1980 to 1987 at the St. Josef Hospital, Wuppertal

Type of Anastomosis	SPTU	EEA
Colorectal anastomosis	419	87
Ileo-transversostomy	59	9
Transverse-colocolostomy	21	2
Esophago-jejunostomy	71	56
Entero-enterostomy	98	7
Duodeno-jejunostomy	50	22
Roux-en-Y anastomosis	148	25
Total	866	208

Table 6-2. Number of Anastomotic Leaks in Stapled Anastomoses Performed from 1980 to 1987 at the St. Josef Hospital, Wuppertal

Type of Anastomosis	SPTU	EEA
Colorectal anastomosis	33 (7.9%)	16 (18.4%)
Ileotransversostomy	0	0
Transverse-colocolostomy	0	0
Esophago-jejunostomy	2 (2.8%)	2 (3.5%)
Entero-enterostomy	2 (2%)*	0
Duodeno-jejunostomy	0	0
Roux-en-Y anastomosis	0	0

* Following radiation therapy

Table 6-3. Literature Review of Esophago-Jejunostomy Results

Author	Year	Instrument	No.	Leakage Rate	Mortality Rate
Ulrich[1]	1986	EEA	110	5 (4.5%)	1 (0.9%)
Witte[2]	1984	EEA/ILS	75	11 (14.7%)	4 (5.3%)
		ILS	82	6 (7.3%)	4 (4.8%)
Gunther[3]	1986	ILS	211	19 (9.0%)	6 (2.8%)
Sugimachi[4]	1982	SPTU/EEA	17/11	1 (3.5%)	0
Kantarzis, Lersmacher,	1987	SPTU	71	2 (2.8%)	1 (1.4%)
Winter, Hoffman		EEA	56	2 (3.5%)	0
Collective results	—	Manual sutures	640	88 (13.8%)	45 (7.0%)
(ranges are given				6.5–21.4%	0–7.9%
with rates)					

tients had had previous radiation therapy to the abdomen. In all other small and large bowel anastomoses, no leak or fistula was observed (Table 6-2). The results obtained with the use of the circular SPTU instrument compared favorably with those published in the international literature (Tables 6-3 and 6-4). With sufficient experience in the handling of the instrument, we have come to recognize advantages that justify our preference in its present use. Since this is not a disposable instrument, however, it is of great importance to load and prepare the instrument for each application. Among the precautions to be taken are the following:

1. Expert responsible care and cleaning of the instrument after each application.
2. Inspection of staple loading and mechanical function of the instrument by the surgeon before each application, since the circular blade or pressure plate of the anvil can be left out during the preparation of the instrument.
3. If several instruments of the same size are available, cartridge and anvil are not exchangeable.
4. Careful control of the degree of compression indicated by the corresponding markings on the shaft of the instrument.
5. Replacement of the circular blade whenever indicated by repeated use of the instrument.

6. Following minimal separation of anvil from cartridge, a 180° turn along the axis of the instrument assures removal from the anastomotic site without any trouble.

The conical shape of the anvil facilitates a very smooth and atraumatic introduction into the bowel lumen, even when the larger instruments are used. The separation of the open instrument from the single-row circular suture is greatly facilitated by the minimal rim created by the single row. Furthermore, we have the clinical impression that the single-row staple line has reduced the incidence of postoperative strictures. It is important to consider the reduction in cost with the use of this instrument while the results are comparable to the ones obtained with other stapling instruments.

CONCLUSIONS

We have found that with sufficient experience in the preparation and use of the SPTU circular instrument, the results obtained in various anastomoses throughout the gastro-intestinal tract are comparable to those obtained with other instruments.

Translated from the German by F.M. Steichen, M.D.

Table 6-4. Literature Review of the Colorectal Anastomoses Results

Author	Year	Instrument	No.	Leakage Rate	Mortality
Heald[5]	1981	EEA	100	13 (13%)	1 (1.0%)
Leff[6]	1982	EEA	106	9 (8.5%)	4 (3.8%)
Kennedy[7]	1983	EEA	174	8 (4.6%)	2 (1.2%)
Overy[8]	1980	EEA	22	0	0
Beart[9]	1981	EEA	35	1 (2.9%)	1 (2.9%)
Brennan[10]	1982	EEA	50	7 (14%)	2 (4.0%)
Kantarzis, Lersmacher,	1987	EEA	87	16 (18.4%)	0
Winter, Hoffman		SPTU	419	33 (7.9%)	0

REFERENCES

1. Ulrich B, Kockel N: Maschinelle Ösophagus-anastomosen. *In* Ulrich, B (ed.): Chirurgische Gastroenterologie mit Interdisziplinären Gesprächen. Hameln: TM-Verlag, 1986:47–60.
2. Witte J, Günther B, Denecke H: Technik der zirkulären Stapleranastomose nach abdominaler Gastrektomie. *In* Häring, R (ed.): Therapie des Magenkarzinoms. Weinheim: Edition Medizin, 1984:313–323.
3. Günther B, Demmel N, Teichman R: Osophagojejunostomie nach Gastrektomie mit dem zirkulären Klammernachtgerät proximate ILS—operationstechnische Aspekte, Früh- und Späterergebuvose. *In* Ulrich, B (ed.): Chirurgische Gastroenterolgie mit Interdisziplinären Gesprächen. Hameln: TM-Verlag, 1986:61–65.
4. Sugimachi K, Ikeda M, Ueo H, Kai H, Okudaira Y, Inokuchi K: Clinical efficacy of the stapled anastomosis in esophageal reconstruction. Ann Thorac Surg 33(4): 374–378, 1989.
5. Heald RJ, Leicester RJ: The low stapled anastomosis. Br J Surg 68:333–337, 1981.
6. Leff E, Hoexter B, Labow SB, Eisenstadt TE, Rubin RS, Salvati EP: The EEA stapler in low colorectal anastomoses. Dis Colon Rectum 25:704–707, 1989.
7. Kennedy HL, Rothenberger DA, Goldberg SM, et al: Colocolostomy and coloproctostomy utilizing the circular intraluminal stapling devices. Dis Colon Rectum 26:145–148, 1983.
8. Overy RS, Godfrey PJ, Evans M, et al: Staples or sutures in the colon? A random controlled trial of three methods of colonic anastomosis. Br J Surg 67:363–364, 1980.
9. Beart RW, Kelly KA: Randomized prospective evaluation of the EEA stapler for colorectal anastomoses. Am J Surg 141:143–147, 1981.
10. Brennan SS, Pickford IR, Evans M, Pollock AV: Stapler or sutures for colonic anastomoses—A controlled clinical trial. Br J Surg 69:722–724, 1982.

CHAPTER 7

A STAPLING INSTRUMENT FOR EVERTING ANASTOMOSIS OF THE ESOPHAGUS: CLINICAL RESULTS

Amadeu P.A. Pimenta, Valdemar M.B. Cardoso, Joaquim Guimaraes, and
Eduardo O.P. Cernadas

A circular stapling instrument for end-to-end, end-to-side, or side-to-side everting anastomosis was used in operations on 72 patients with esophageal and gastric cancer. This device is applicable principally to esophago-gastric, esophago-jejunal, esophago-colic, or entero-enteric anastomoses. A total of 107 everting anastomoses with a double staggered circular row of stainless steel wire staples were performed.

Because of the fragility of the tissues involved and the complicated techniques required, suturing of the esophagus continues to be responsible for postoperative complications, of which dehiscence of the anastomosis is the most common and most serious.[1–13] Giuli,[14] in his retrospective analysis of 2400 patients who underwent operations for cancer of the esophagus and of the cardia by 22 surgeons from different countries, noted that the percentage of anastomotic leakage varied from 10 to 25%, depending on the location of the anastomosis.

Surgeons, dissatisfied by their results with manual suturing, explored techniques that would eliminate or significantly reduce operative trauma. The suture materials had to be strong, cause the least possible biologic reaction, avoid contributing to infection, and reduce the duration of operation. The importance of technical proficiency becomes apparent with the results of an esophageal anastomosis that concludes operations lasting up to 6 hours.[7] Fatigue is usually incompatible with technical quality. Thus, a rapid and safe technique that can be performed with equal perfection by surgeons with different degrees of experience is needed.

A few years ago, a careful analysis of the advantages and disadvantages of existing circular anastomotic devices inspired us to perfect an instrument that would facilitate a safe, economical, everting circular anastomosis, specially designed for esophageal surgery.[15–17] We will present the clinical results obtained with our instrument as it was used in operations for cancer of the esophagus and of the stomach.

METHODS

The instrument, made of stainless-steel, is 4 cm high and has an external diameter of 5 cm. It is composed of a circular cartridge and anvil. Each component is formed of two hinged halves held together by two lateral latches. A safety switch prevents premature firing of staples.

To achieve an anastomosis in the digestive tract, the ends of the visceral segments to be joined are placed, one inside the circular anvil and the other inside the cartridge. The bowel edges are turned outward and held in place by a few temporary sutures (Figs. 7-1 through 7-3). Anvil and cartridge, carrying the respective everted bowel ends, are joined and maintained in position by closing the lateral latches (Fig. 7-4). The safety switch is released with gentle compression of cartridge against anvil, using a pair of pliers (Fig. 7-5). As the cartridge moves into position, it places two alternating circular rows of staples

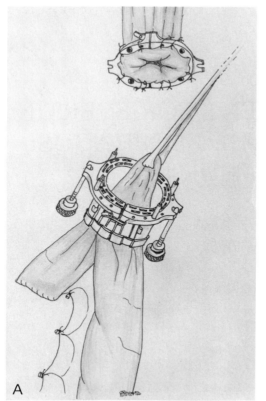

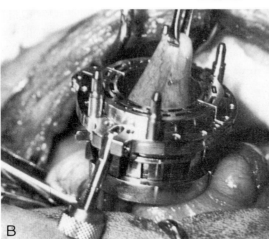

Fig. 7-1. *A, B.* The instrument is composed of a circular cartridge and anvil, each one formed of two hinged halves, held together by two lateral latches.

through both bowel ends. The temporary sutures are cut, the excess tissue is excised, and the latches are released (Fig. 7-6), liberating the two anvil and cartridge halves, which are then removed by gently rotating them around the anastomosed tract (Fig. 7-7).

To avoid traction on the anastomosis, some three to four widely spaced reinforcing sutures are placed. Whenever possible, the anastomosis is wrapped with gastro-epiploic omentum.[18–22] The esophageal anastomosis was studied radiologically in all patients on the seventh postoperative day (Fig. 7-8). Oral feeding was only reestablished if the contrast study confirmed the integrity of the anastomosis.

RESULTS

Between March 1980 and March 1988, 71 patients with cancer of the lower esophagus, cardia, gastric stump, gastric corpus, or fundus, and 1 patient with a gastric lymphoma, underwent operations with the new circular device (Table 7-1). The age of the 54 male and 18 female patients ranged from 26 to 76 (mean 59) years.

A total of 107 anastomoses were performed (Table 7-2). Two anastomoses, esophago-jejunostomy and jejuno-jejunostomy, were accomplished during the same operation in 35 patients for cancer of the cardia, gastric stump, stomach, and gastric lymphoma. One patient who had cancer of a gastric stump with invasion of the colon received an esophago-jejunal and a colo-colic anastomosis.

In patients with an esophageal lumen of normal caliber, we dilated the esophagus with progressively larger Hégar dilators (up to size 24) before attaching its open circumference to the annular instrument. In this manner we hoped to avoid the usual spasm of the sectioned esophagus and to make it easier to evert the edges.[23,24] No dilatation was necessary to anastomose segments of the small bowel or colon.

In the early postoperative period 3 patients developed an anastomotic leak; 2 patients died as a consequence of this. In the other 1 the ensuing blind fistula closed 3 weeks later (Table 7-3). Two other patients died, but as a result of acute respiratory failure; the first one died 3 weeks after operation, while he was still in the intensive care unit. By then he had been fed orally for 2 weeks, as the postoperative radiographic control had proven the integrity of the esophageal anastomosis. The other patient, a 72-year-old man, died within 12 hours of operation. Late postoperative complications (Table 7-4) of importance are represented by four cases of anastomotic stricture. Three patients began to complain of dysphagia 2 months post-operatively; the strictures were successfully dilated. The fourth patient began to complain of dysphagia 6 weeks after operation; his stricture, although more difficult to treat, was also dilated with success. Table 7-5 shows the percentage of complications more directly related to the anastomoses—leaks and stricture—and compares them with the results of

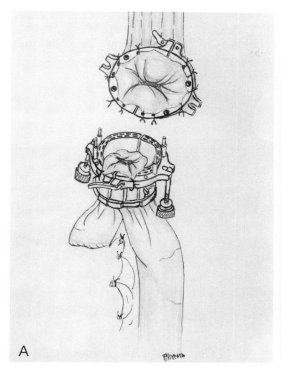

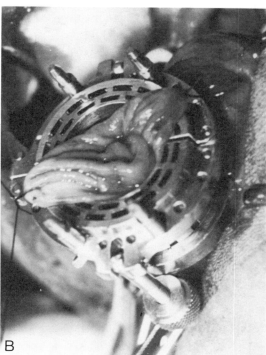

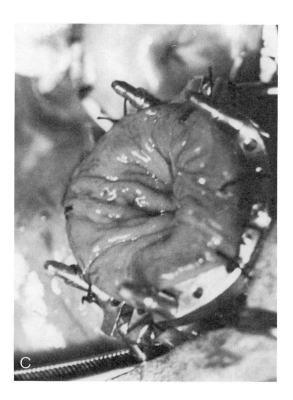

Fig. 7-2. The bowel edges are turned outward (*A*, *B*) and held in place by a few temporary stitches (*C*).

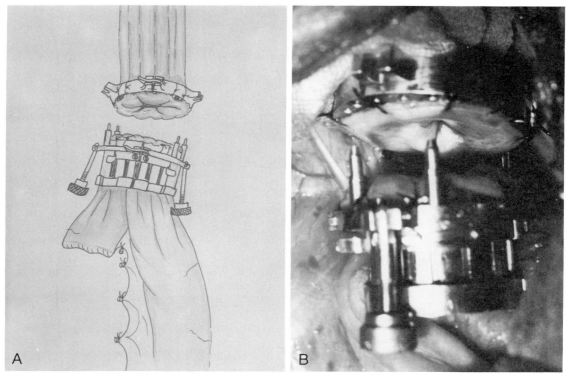

Fig. 7-3. *A, B*. The two instrument halves are then approximated.

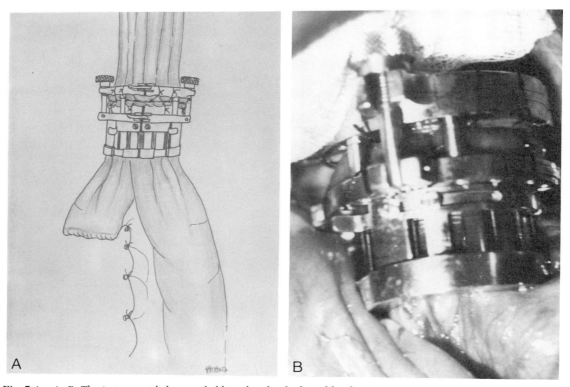

Fig. 7-4. *A, B*. The instrument halves are held in place by the lateral hatches.

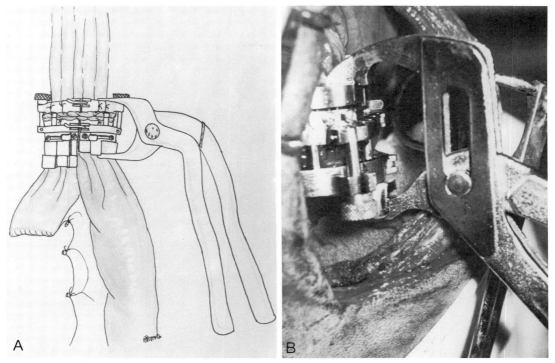

Fig. 7-5. *A, B.* The safety brake is released and gentle pressure is applied with forceps to release the cartridge and advance and shape the staples against the anvil.

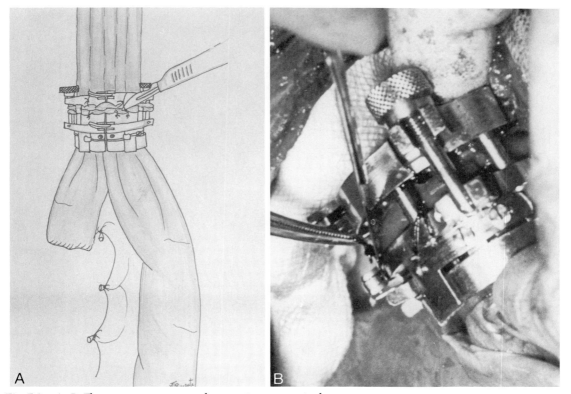

Fig. 7-6. *A, B.* The temporary sutures and excess tissue are excised.

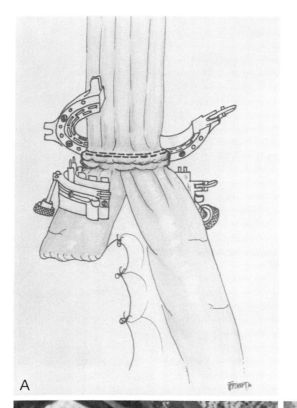

A

Fig. 7-7. The two instrument components are easily removed by releasing the latches that connect each half (*A, B*) and gently rotating the component halves around the anastomosed tract (*C*).

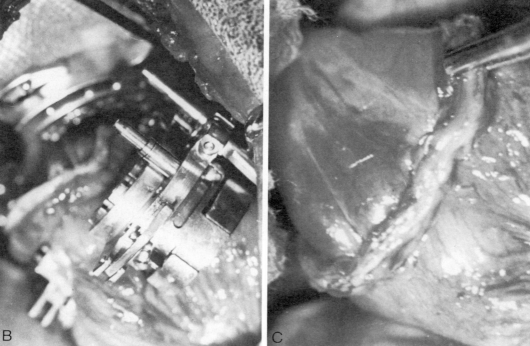

B

C

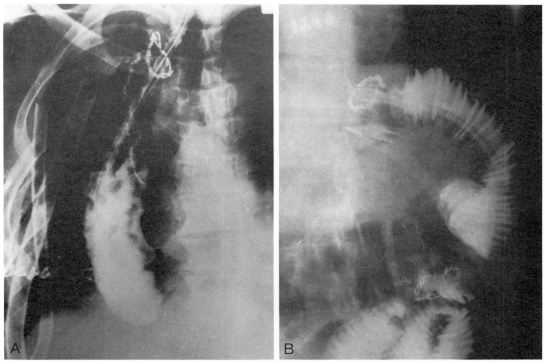

Fig. 7-8. Esophago-gastric (A) and esophago-jejunal and jejuno-jejunal (B) anastomoses, studied radiologically on the seventh postoperative day.

another group of patients who received manually sutured anastomoses by the same surgical team. Table 7-6 gives the mortality rate up to the sixtieth postoperative day.

DISCUSSION

There were no intra-operative technical complications either in performing the anastomosis or in removing the device. It was obviously easier to do the anastomosis in more accessible locations than deep in the upper abdomen, for instance. These more diffi-

cult infrahiatal anastomoses often required additional technical attention.

We had no opportunity to use our device for anastomosis in the neck. Although it would appear easy to create an anastomosis superficially in the neck, this can be difficult if the bowel segment to be anastomosed to the esophagus is not long enough to be brought out above the sternal notch. The new device has definite advantages over other models and over manual suturing. Its design enables the surgeon to

Table 7-1. Patients According to Their Diseases

Disease	No. of Patients
Carcinoma of the esophagus	22
Carcinoma of the cardia or gastric fundus	41
Carcinoma of the gastric stump	4
Carcinoma of the gastric stump with invasion of the colon	1
Carcinoma of the gastric corpus	3
Gastric lymphoma	1
Total	72

Table 7-2. Type and Number of Anastomoses Performed

Type of Anastamosis	No. Performed
Esophago-gastric End-to-side (after Sweet or Ivor-Lewis operation)	31
Esophago-jejunal End-to-side (after total gastrectomy)	41
Jejunal-jejunal End-to-side (after total gastrectomy)	34
Colo-colonic End-to-end (after colectomy)	1
Total	107

Table 7-3. Immediate Post-Operative Complications (up to 30 days)

Complication	No. of Patients
Respiratory failure	2
Pleural effusion	3
Sub-phrenic abscess	2
Mediastinal abscess	1
Pneumonia	1
Pulmonary abscess	1
Pyloric obstruction	1
Idiopathic jaundice	1
Anastomic fistula	3

Table 7-4. Delayed Post-Operative Complications

Complication	No. of Patients
Sub-phrenic abscess	1
Neoplasic fistula	1
Anastomotic stricture	4
Intestinal obstruction	1
Recurrence of the tumor	3
Vertebral metastasis	1

place and remove it without making an additional opening in the digestive tract. Since shorter operations result in fewer postoperative complications,[7,25,26] we had to determine if mechanical suturing reduced the duration of reconstructing bowel continuity.

The time required to perform an anastomosis varied according to the difficulty encountered in attaching both visceral segments to the device: approximately 15 minutes were necessary for simple anastomoses; the more complicated cases required about 30 minutes. Overall, we averaged 25 to 30 minutes per anastomosis, a definite improvement over esophageal manual suturing in our experience.

With everting staple lines, hemostasis and anastomotic competence are easily examined intraoperatively, and excess tissue can be trimmed before removing the instrument. Moreover, in an experimental study, we confirmed that the device neither crushes nor lacerates the bowel edges. In some instances the anastomosis was wrapped with gastro-

epiploic omentum to contribute to a more hermetic seal, limit the spread of infection, and isolate the esophagus from the aorta.[27–32] As the everting technique places the ridge of tissue to be sutured outside the bowel lumen, the caliber of both ends is the same, a significant advantage over an invaginating anastomosis that reduces the size of the digestive tract lumen in the area of the anastomosis in the initial phase of healing.

In 4 patients, dehiscence of the anastomosis could be partly attributed to tension. Also, the poor nutritional condition of 1 patient could well have been responsible for poor healing.

A detailed analysis of the more frequent complications directly related to the suturing technique, and comparison of the results obtained by mechanical and manual techniques by the same surgical team, showed that the mechanical technique gave better results.[17] Although this study was not prospective and the patients were not chosen at random, there were a great many similarities between both groups: esophageal pathology in comparable patient groups; same surgical teams providing the same preoperative and postoperative care; and identical surgical techniques, except for the type of suture. The integrity of the anastomosis was checked radiologically on the seventh postoperative day in both groups; the assessment of the results was done in the same manner.

This study showed that, in patients with esophagectomy or total gastrectomy, the incidence of leakage decreased when the mechanical device was used, both as it relates to the number of patients and as it relates to the number of anastomoses (Table 7-5). Stricture, a late postoperative complication, also decreased in frequency, but not as much. Regarding mortality (Table 7-6), once again the mechanical device proved to be better. A further comparison of these results to those obtained in 22 surgical centers confirmed the superiority of mechanical suturing.[14]

The results reported by authors who use a circular inverting mechanical device [23,24,29,33–37] show an incidence of anastomotic leaks that varies from 0 to 12%, of strictures that varies from 0 to 18.4%, of overall mortality that varies from 0 to 25%, and of mortality related to the suture that varies from 0 to 8.3%. Lagache et al.,[24] who in 75% of their cases used a double suture (they inverted the staple lines

Table 7-5. Complications Following Esophagectomy and Total Gastrectomy

Complication	Manual Suture		Mechanical Suture	
	Patients	Anastomoses	Patients	Anastomoses
Fistulae	13.3%	9.8%	4.2%	2.8%
Strictures	6.7%	4.9%	5.6%	3.7%

Table 7-6. Mortality Rate (up to the 60th day) Following Esophagectomy and Total Gastrectomy

Type	Manual Suture		Mechanical Suture	
	Patients	Anastomoses	Patients	Anastomoses
Overall	20%	14.6%	5.6%	3.7%
Related to the suture	10%	7.3%	2.8%	1.9%

with a manual suture), did not, however, specifically mention the overall mortality rate related to each type of technique. It appears that eversion reduces the rate of strictures, whereas the invaginating suture favors the narrowing of the digestive lumen in the area of anastomosis, although other factors—such as individual variations in the reaction to trauma, small tissue fissures, local infection, and ischemia in and beyond suture lines—may also contribute to the stenosis.[36–38] Our device can be used repeatedly during the same operation, both for esophageal and jejuno-jejunal anastomoses. Although manual loading is time-consuming, the unit price is much lower.

In conclusion, this new circular mechanical device can be used for all end-to-side and end-to-end anastomoses required in the surgical treatment of esophageal disease. Although its reduced size permits its application in both the chest and abdomen, it is difficult to use it in the cervical area. The device makes performing anastomoses easier, shortening the overall length of the operation. It is most economical, can be reloaded and used repeatedly during a single operation, and does not require an additional opening in the digestive tract to place or remove it. The evaginating suture created is easily examined intraoperatively.

REFERENCES

1. Buntain WL, Payne WS, Lynn HB: Esophageal reconstruction for benign disease: a long-term appraisal. Am Surg 46:67, 1980.
2. Franklin RH, Burn JI, Lynch G: Carcinoma of the esophagus. Review of 129 treated patients. Br J Surg 51:178, 1964.
3. Huang G, Zhang D, Wang G, et al: Traitement chirurgical du carcinome de l'oesophage. A propos de 1647 cas. Lyon Chir 77:349, 1981.
4. Inberg MV, Linna MI, Scheinin TM, Vänttinen E: Anastomotic leakage after excision of esophageal and high gastric carcinoma. Am J Surg 122:540, 1971.
5. Kasai M, Mori S, Watanable T: Follow-up results after resection of thoracic esophageal carcinoma. World J Surg 2:543, 1978.
6. Launois B, Paul JL, Lygidakis NJ, et al: Results of the surgical treatment of carcinoma of the esophagus. Surg Gynecol Obstet 156:753, 1983.
7. Maillard JN, Launois B, Lagausie Ph, Lellouch J, Lortat-Jacob JL: Cause of leakage at the site of anastomosis after esophagogastric resection for carcinoma. Surg Gynecol Obstet 129:1014, 1969.
8. Maillet P, Baulieux J, Boulez J, Benhaim R: Carcinoma of the thoracic esophagus. Results of one-stage surgery (271 cases). Am J Surg 143:629, 1982.
9. Miller C: Carcinoma of thoracic oesophagus and cardia. Br J Surg 49:507, 1961.
10. Papachristou DN, Fortner JG: Adenocarcinoma of the gastric cardia. The choice of gastrectomy. Ann Surg 192:58, 1980.
11. Papachristou DN, Fortner JG: Anastomotic failure complicating total gastrectomy and esophagogastrectomy for cancer of the stomach. Am J Surg 138:399, 1979.
12. Pimenta APA, Cardoso VMB, Rodrigues JS: A mechanical suturing method for the gastrointestinal tract: clinical experience with a new stapling instrument. Lisbon: 6th World Congress of the Collegium Internationale Chirurgiae Digestivae, 1980.
13. Saubier EC, Gouillat C, Janati R, Michaelides A: Le traitement chirurgical du cancer du cardia. Bilan de 86 observations. Lyon Chir 80:123, 1984.
14. Giuli R, Gignoux M: Treatment of carcinoma of the esophagus. Retrospective study of 2,400 patients. Ann Surg 192:44, 1980.
15. Pimenta APA, Cardoso VMB, Rodrigues JS: A mechanical suturing method for the gastrointestinal tract: clinical experience with a new stapling instrument. World J Surg 6:786, 1982.
16. Pimenta APA, Cardoso VMB, Rodrigues JS: Un nouvel instrument pour agrafage mécanique en chirurgie gastro-intestinale. Étude expérimentale préliminaire. Ann Chir 35:469, 1981.
17. Pimenta APA, Cardoso VMB, Rodrigues JS: Tratamento cirúrgico do carcinoma do esófago: sutura automática versus sutura manual. Arq Gastroenterol 19:113, 1982.
18. Lewis I: The surgical treatment of carcinoma of the esophagus. With special reference to a new operation for growths of the middle third. Br J Surg 34:18, 1946.
19. Lortat-Jacob JL: Chirurgie de l'oesophage. Paris: Editions Médicales Flammarion, 1951.
20. Lortat-Jacob JL: Voie d'abord de l'oesophage thoracique. Presse Med 57:453, 1949.
21. Sweet RH: Carcinoma of the esophagus and the cardiac end of the stomach. Immediate and late results of treatment by resection and primary esophagogastric anastomosis. JAMA 135:485, 1947.
22. Vankemmel M: Principales applications cliniques de la suture mécanique. Encycl Med-Chir, Paris. Techniques chirurgicales. Appareil digestif 40061, 4.5.10.
23. Fékété F, Breil Ph, Ronsse H: Anastomoses mécaniques à la pince EEA en chirurgie oesophagienne. Chirurgie 106:659, 1980.
24. Lagache G, Bourez J: La place des agrafeuses métalliques en chirurgie digestive. A propos d'une série de 970 sutures mécaniques comportant 358 anastomoses. Chirurgie 107:408, 1981.
25. Alexander JW: Nosocomial infections. In: Current

Problems in Surgery. Chicago: Year Book, August 1973:18.

26. Cruse JPE, Foord R: A five-year prospective study of 23,649 surgical wounds. Arch Surg 107:206, 1973.

27. Abbes MJ, Richelme H, Demard F: The greater omentum in repair of complications following surgery and radiotherapy for certain cancers. Int Surg 59:81, 1974.

28. Fékété F: Anastomoses mécaniques à la pince ILS dans la chirurgie de l'oesophage. Soixante-treize cas. Presse Med 13:39, 1984.

29. Fékété F, Breil Ph, Ronsse H, Tossen JC, Langonnet F: EEA stapler and omental graft in esophagogastrectomy. Experience with 30 intrathoracic anastomoses for cancer. Ann Surg 193:825, 1981.

30. Jurkiewicz MJ, Nahai F: The omentum. Its use as a free vascularized graft for reconstruction of the head and neck. Ann Surg 195:756, 1982.

31. Lau OJ: Acute aortogastric fistula following gastro-oesophageal anastomosis. Br J Surg 70:504, 1983.

32. McLachlin D, Denton W: Omental protection of intestinal anastomoses. Am J Surg 126:345, 1973.

33. Adloff M, Arnaud J-P, Ollier J-Cl: Les sutures mécaniques en chirurgie digestive. Premier bilan. J Chir (Paris) 117:231, 1980.

34. Berard Ph, Papillon M, Jacquemard R, Labrosse H, Bigay D, Guillemin G: Les anastomoses digestives à la E.E.A. A propos de cent quatre cas. Ann Chir 35:403, 1981.

35. Partensky C, Lescoeur N, Saubier EC: Anastomoses oesophagiennes mécaniques à l'EEA. Expérience de 25 cas. Lyon Chir 77:193, 1981.

36. Shahinian TK, Bowen JR, Dorman BA, Soderberg CH, Thompson WR: Experience with the EEA stapling device. Am J Surg 139:549, 1980.

37. West PN, Marbarger JP, Martz MN, Roper CL: Esophagogastrostomy with the EEA stapler. Ann Surg 193:76, 1981.

38. Smith LE: Anastomosis with EEA stapler after anterior colonic resection. Dis Colon Rectum 24:236, 1981.

CHAPTER 8

SUTURELESS COMPRESSION ANASTOMOSIS OF THE DISTAL COLON AND RECTUM

E. Gross and F.W. Eigler

Clinical and symptomatic leakage of colo-rectal anastomoses after low anterior resection occurs in 2 to 30% of patients if a protective colostomy is placed only in high-risk anastomoses and not routinely.[1-7] If anastomotic fistulae are looked for systematically in the early postoperative period, even higher rates of leakage are found. In colo-anal anastomoses, various authors regard protective colostomy as obligatory because of an even higher rate of fistulae (up to 50%).[8-11] Fistulae and leakage of colo-rectal anastomoses cause the major proportion of the morbidity and mortality after colon and rectum resections. Between 30 and 100% of deaths occurring after deep anterior resections are attributable to anastomotic leakage.[7,12,13]

Our animal experiments exploring the influence of anastomotic techniques on tissue healing have shown that anastomosis is possible without the use of sutures or staples that serve initially to join the bowel and then remain temporary or permanent foreign bodies. This "sutureless" anastomosis is markedly superior to conventionally sutured anastomoses, according to biomechanical and morphologic criteria as well as histologic features and micro-angiographic investigations (Fig. 8-1).

The absence of foreign material within the tissues, thus avoiding side effects such as localized vascular compromise and necrosis around sutures or staples, bacterial transport along the sutures or staples with channel infections, and foreign-body reactions, prompted the application of the sutureless compression technique (AKA-2) in a clinically prospective study on the distal colon and rectum.

THE AKA-2 INSTRUMENT

In its usable and spent configuration, the compression device is composed of three plastic rings. Two rings—base and intermediate—are placed into one bowel end. The third ring (circular anchor, shaped from the periphery of a plastic plate) is placed into the opposing bowel end. The flat base ring carries six blunt pins, each alternating with three ($6 \times 3 = 18$) fish-hook-shaped pins. Blunt and hooked pins pass freely through corresponding holes in the intermediate ring. The flat ends of the blunt pins, which are larger than the corresponding holes, keep base and intermediate rings from separating. However, the two rings are held apart by small metal springs surrounding the blunt pins between the two rings. The range of movement of the intermediate ring, along its common axis with the base ring, extends along the length of the blunt pins, minus the space occupied by compressed springs. Both rings can be pushed against each other, but because of the springs, the intrinsic force of the double ring assembly is one of separation and expansion of the intermediate from the base ring (Figs. 8-2, 8-3).

The anchor (third) ring is created in the actual process of anastomosis from a plate, fastened to the tip of the central rod of the AKA-2 instrument by a flat metal cone that fits within the circumference of the circular blade. The advancing blade stamps out both

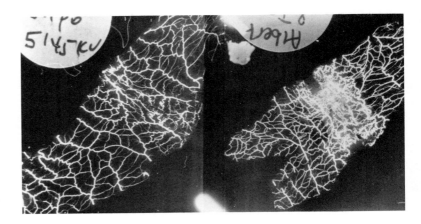

Fig. 8-1. Micro-angiographic aspect of a sutureless (*left*) and sutured (*right*) colon anastomosis in the rat on the eighth postoperative day.

purse-stringed bowel walls, contained between the double ring (base and intermediate) and the anchor plate, and then punches out the center of the anchor plate held by the metal cone. This leaves a third ring that serves as an anchoring berth for the hooked pins that advance through both bowel rims to penetrate and hold the anchor ring, slightly ahead of the circular blade (Figs. 8-4, 8-5).

With the distance between base and anchor rings held constant by the safely impaled hooked pins, the intermediate ring is pushed against the anchor (third) ring by the springs and compresses the inverted bowel margins between these two rings. As the union of both bowel ends takes place and their inner rims are sealed by compression necrosis, the entire assembly comes loose as a unit, and is eliminated through the anus.

The use of the AKA-2 instrument is similar to that of the circular stapling instruments (SPTU, EEA, ILS). The head of the instrument houses the double ring, the circular blade, and the advancing or retracting central rod, carrying at its tip the plastic plate (to become the anchor ring) and metal cone held by a

screw. The double ring and plastic plate (which is the future anchor ring) can be moved apart or closer together along the axis of the central rod. Preparation of bowel ends, placement of purse-string sutures, intraluminal introduction of the closed AKA-2, and all other details of a mechanical end-to-end inverting anastomosis are the same as with stapling instruments. The foreign material (the compression rings) remains only on or in the tissues for a few days. After spontaneous detachment of the rings, an anastomosis results without any permanent or temporary inclusion of foreign material.

Anastomosis by compression of the resection margins is an old principle,[14] first described by Denans.[15–18] The technical problems have only been recently solved, thanks to the development of mechanical anastomotic techniques and suitable materials.[19]

Method of Operation

The principle of compression anastomosis consists of the inverting union of the resection margins of the

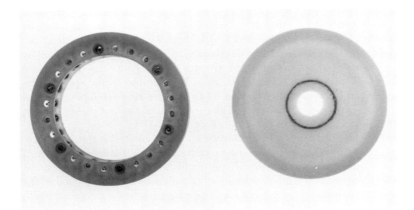

Fig. 8-2. The base and intermediate plastic rings (*left*) and the plastic plate later to become the third, or anchor, ring (*right*).

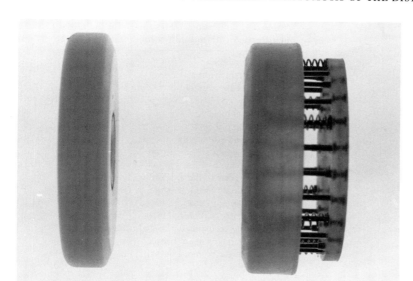

Fig. 8-3. The plastic base and intermediate rings (*right*) and plastic plate (*left*) are shown in profile.

distal and proximal intestinal ends to be anastomosed by transient compression.

In the restoration of continuity after Hartmann's operation, the instrument is introduced without the plastic plate. The rectal stump is opened over the central mandrel or rod. The plastic plate, or future anchor ring, and the flat metal cone holding it in place are screwed onto the mandrel. After lifting the proximal purse-stringed bowel over the plastic plate and bringing the two ends of the intestine together, the anastomosis is created. As with stapling instruments, extensive mobilization, wide opening of the rectal stump, and placement of a purse-string suture on the rectum can be dispensed with.

Clinical Study and Results

Our experience with compression anastomosis by the AKA-2 is so-far based on 115 operations on the sigmoid colon and rectum, mainly resections for carcinoma (Tables 8-1 and 8-2). The patients received an orthograde bowel lavage on the day preceding operation with 1 l of 20% mannitol solution and 3 l 0.9% NaCl solution. The rectosigmoid or rectal stump was irrigated before anastomosis with a polyvinyl-pyrollidone-iodine solution for disinfection and to kill shed tumor cells. Peri-operative antibiotic prophylaxis consisted of a single preoperative and two postoperative doses of 1 g of metronidazole and 5 g of cefotaxim.

The following investigations were carried out prospectively: Intra-operative testing of the anastomosis with a polyvinyl-pyrollidone-iodine solution, Gastrografin-enema between the twelfth and fourteenth

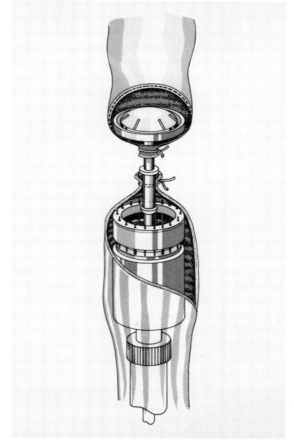

Fig. 8-4. Plate and base-intermediate rings with the mounted, purse-stringed bowel ends before approximation of the bowel ends.

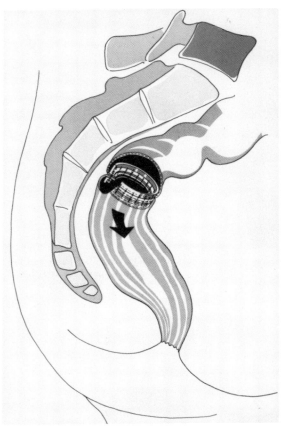

Fig. 8-5. Completed compression anastomosis holding inverted bowel margins between the intermediate and anchor plates within a correctly assembled device.

postoperative day in patients with a clinically normal course, and endoscopy between the second and fourth week after operation with measurement of the level of anastomosis. Besides this, major complications (e.g., disorders of wound healing) were registered.

In 12 patients, a protective colostomy was done, primarily during the pilot phase of the study, which comprised 15 patients. Five patients received protective colostomy because of an extended resection for advanced tumors, 1 patient because of simultaneous implantation of a Port-A-Cath catheter for chemotherapy of diffuse liver metastases, and 1 patient because of immunosuppression after kidney transplantation. In 1 patient a pre-existing colostomy was left in place after descending-colon-to-rectal anastomosis (Table 8-3).

Surgical Mortality

Two of the 115 patients died during the hospital stay. One female patient died on the third postoper-

Table 8-1. Indications for Resection of the Distal Colon and Rectum with Sutureless Anastomosis (AKA-2)

Sigmoidcarcinoma	34
Sigmoid-diverticulitis	12
Affection of the sigmoid or rectum by carcinoma of the ovary	6
Rectal carcinoma	39
Rectal carcinoid	1
Rectosigmoid carcinoma	4
Villous adenoma of the rectum	1
Villous adenoma of the sigmoid	1
Benign stenosis of the sigmoid (radiogenic?)	1
Crohn's disease of the sigmoid or rectum	4
Plastic enlargement of the bladder	1
Endometriosis of the rectum	1
Anastomotic recurrence of rectal carcinoma	2
Radiogenic rectovaginal fistula	2
Affection of the sigmoid by MFH	1
Angiodysplasia	1
Segmental polyposis	2
Total	115

ative day of a fulminant pulmonary embolism, and the second patient died of an advanced tumor condition 14 days after rectum resection and protective colostomy and simultaneous implantation of a Port-A-Cath into the gastro-duodenal artery for treatment of diffuse liver metastases.

Anastomotic Leakage

Anastomotic failure occurred in 7 of the 115 patients (6%). Of the 58 patients with anastomosis at or below 10 cm, 5 patients developed an anastomotic leak (8.6%). If the patients who did not receive a protective colostomy are considered, the rate of insufficiency at an anastomosis level of up to 10 cm is 10% (5/50) (Table 8-4).

Table 8-2. Indications for Protective Colostomy in 12 Patients with Resection of the Distal Colon or Rectum

Pilot period of the study	4
Extended resection for advanced rectal cancer	2
Extended resection for advanced cancer of the ovary	2
Rectal carcinoma in a patient with immunosuppression	1
Implantation of Port-A-Cath in the hepatic artery for advanced rectal carcinoma and liver metastasis	1
Extended resection for local pelvic recurrence	1
Colostomy was performed before descendo-rectostomy	1
Total	12

Table 8-3. Operative Procedures (AKA-2)

Procedure	No. of Patients	Protective Colostomy	Tube Colostomy
Sigmoid-resection	43	4 (2)*	1
High anterior resection	17	2	
Low anterior resection	45	11 (5)	1
Descendo-rectostomy following			
Hartmann procedure	7	2	
Total	115	19 (7)	2

* Numbers in parentheses refer to colostomies performed because of anastomotic leakage

The anastomotic leaks occurred mostly on the fourth and fifth postoperative day. One female patient developed a leak on the fourteenth postoperative day. This complication had not been visible on the twelfth postoperative day with gastrografin enema, and the patient was then without symptoms. This patient had received high preoperative doses of corticosteroid because of idiopathic thrombocytopenia (ITP), which had led to recurrent hemorrhage from an advanced rectal carcinoma. Anastomotic leaks occurred only in patients with carcinoma (including 4 patients with advanced carcinoma) (Table 8-5).

Apart from 3 patients who underwent colostomy secondarily because of an anastomotic fistula, and who have since died because of their advanced tumor condition, primary or secondary colostomies were closed in all other patients.

The gastrografin investigation revealed an asymptomatic fistula in 1 of the 108 patients in whom the clinical features did not provide any indication of an anastomotic leak. Endoscopy in the second or fourth week after the operation showed a delicate line of anastomosis without noteworthy epithelial defects in the vast majority of patients. Occasionally, the anastomotic line could be identified only from the different folding of the colon mucosa compared to the rectal mucosa.

An anastomotic stricture was observed in 1 female patient after rectosigmoid resection and application of a protective colostomy because of Crohn's disease. The high-grade stricture was cured by transanal dilatation.

In 3 patients with very deep anastomoses situated in front of the sphincters, the ring had to be detached digitally from the bowel wall on the twelfth day. The remaining patients excreted the rings between the sixth and twelfth postoperative days.

DISCUSSION

Compression anastomosis has advantages over hand-sutured and stapled anastomoses because of the absence of any foreign material in the postoperative period within 6 to 12 days. The endoscopic observation of early complete epithelialization indicates minimal inflammatory reaction during the healing of the anastomosis. The fact that only one clinically asymptomatic fistula could be demonstrated may also be regarded as a sign of minimal tissue reaction during the healing phase as compared to other anastomotic techniques. Such clinically nonapparent fistulae occurring at a rate of up to 50% have been described[7] mostly with manual and also stapling techniques.

The absence of permanent or temporary persistent foreign material in compression anastomosis makes

Table 8-4. Level of Anastomosis and Rate of Leakage (AKA-2)*

Level	No. of Patients	Rate of Leakage
5 cm	33	4
5–10 cm	25	1
>10 cm	57	2
Total	115	7

Endoscopy between the second and third postoperative week: no epithelial defects

* Results from the Dept. of Surgery, University Clinics of Essen

Table 8-5. Conditions of 7 Patients with Leakages of AKA-2 Anastomosis

Condition	No. of Patients
Normal (sigmoid and rectal carcinoma)	2
Advanced rectal cancer (multiple liver and lung metastases)	3
Advanced sigmoid cancer (multiple liver metastases)	1
Emergency rectal resection for rectal carcinoma with massive bleeding due to ITP (Werlhoff)	1

this technique appear more suitable for patients with Crohn's disease. An additional manifest advantage of compression anastomosis is the protection of the anastomotic line from the bowel contents by rings in the early postoperative phase, maintaining a patent lumen and splinting the narrow rims of the bowel union at the same time. The anastomosis is not exposed to traction or torsion while the device separates from it.

The width of compression anastomosis exceeds that of stapled anastomoses, since the external diameter of the compression ring determines the final width of the anastomoses which, for comparable cartridge values, is decided by the internal diameter of stapled anastomoses.

However, the rate of complications is crucial in the evaluation of a surgical technique—in this case in particular, the rate of anastomotic fistulae or leaks after low anterior resections. The rate of 10% (5/50) for clinically apparent anastomotic leaks after resection of the rectum is in the middle range of the 2 to 20% rate for clinically symptomatic leaks or fistulae with stapled anastomoses. The factors that influence anastomotic healing, such as level of anastomosis and protective measures (cecostomy and colostomy), are to be considered. The consequences of anastomotic leaks under the protection of a colostomy are more bland than those without anastomotic protection, so that a higher rate of clinically symptomatic fistulae is to be expected with the latter approach. If the literature is analyzed in terms of these criteria, the rate of anastomotic leak after low anterior resection without anastomotic protection is 10 to 30%.

Morphological and functional criteria are arguments for sutureless compression anastomosis of the colon and rectum. Disadvantages associated with suture technique or the use of foreign material are not present.

REFERENCES

1. Beart WRW, Kelly KA: Randomized prospective evaluation of the EEA stapler for colorectal anastomoses. Am J Surg 141:143–147, 1981.
2. Blamey SL, Lee PWR: A comparison of circular stapling devices in colorectal anastomoses. Br J Surg 69:19–22, 1982.
3. Denecke H, Wirsching R: Colorectale Anastomosen. Chirurg 55:638–644, 1984.
4. Everett WG, Friend PJ, Forty J: Comparison of stapling and handsuture for left-sided large bowel anastomosis. Br J Surg 73:345–348, 1986.
5. Kirkegaard P, Christiansen J, Jhortrup A: Anterior resection for mid-rectal cancer with EEA stapling instrument. Am J Surg 140:312–314, 1980.
6. McGinn FP, Gartell PC, Clifford PC, Brunton FJ: Staples or sutures for low colorectal anastomoses: a prospective randomized trial. Br J Surg 72:603–605, 1985.
7. Thiede A, Jostarndt L, Hamelmann H: Interpretation der Ergebnisse klinischer Studien für die praktische Kolon- und Rektumchirurgie. Zentralbl Chir 110:539–557, 1985.
8. Enker WE, Stearns MW, Janov AJ: Peranal coloanal anastomosis following low anterior resection for rectal carcinoma. Dis Colon Rectum 28:576–581, 1985.
9. Gross E, Eigler FW: Komplikationen der Anastomosenheilung nach tiefer Rectumresektion mit peranaler und maschineller Anastomosierung. Langenbecks Arch Chir (Kongreßber) 366:623, 1985.
10. Parks AG, Percy JP: Resection and sutured coloanal anastomosis for rectal carcinoma. Br J Surg 69:301–304, 1982.
11. Wunderlich M, Karner-Hanusch J, Schiessel R: Results of coloanal anastomosis. A prospective study. Int J Color Dis 1:157–161, 1986.
12. Adloff M, Arnaud J-P, Soomeswear B: Stapled vs. sutured colorectal anastomosis. Arch Surg 155:1436–1438, 1980.
13. Brennan SS, Pickford IR, Evans M, Pollock AV: Staples or sutures for colonic anastomosis—a controlled trial. Br J Surg 69:722–724, 1982.
14. Senn N: Enterorrhaphy: its history, technique, and present status. JAMA 21:217, 1893.
15. Csiky M, Gál S, Fekete Gy: Experience with MaSa-2 Anastomotic Apparatus in Rectal Surgery. 2nd Biennial Congress of the European Council of Coloproctology—Advances in Coloproctology, 5–7 May 1988, Genève, Switzerland.
16. Hallenbeck GA, Judd ES, David C: An instrument for colorectal anastomosis without sutures. Dis Colon Rectum 6:98–101, 1963.
17. Hardy TG Jr, Pace WG, Maney JW, Katz AR, Kaganov AL: A biofragmentable ring for sutureless bowel anastomosis. An experimental study. Dis Colon Rectum 28:484–490, 1985.
18. Rosati R, Rebuffat C, Pezzuoli G: A new mechanical device for circular compression anastomosis. Ann Surg 207:245–252, 1988.
19. Kanschin NN, Lytkin MI, Knysch VI, et al. Pervyi opyt nalozheniia kompressionnykh anasromozov apparatom AKA-2 pri operatsiiakh na tolstoi kishke. Vestn Khir 132:52–57, 1984.

ADDITIONAL READING

Eigler FW, Gross E: Die maschinelle Kompressionsanastomose (AKA-2) an Colon und Rectum. Ergebnisse einer prospektiven klinischen Studie. Chir Surg 57:230–235, 1986.
Gross E, Schaarschmidt K, Donhuijsen K, Beyer M, Weidauer T, Eigler FW: Die nahtlose Anastomose: histologische, biomechanische und mikroangiographische Untersuchungen am Kolon der Ratte. Langenbecks Archir Suppl Chir Forum (S):277–281, 1986.
Tanos G und Gewalt R: Colon-Anastomose ohne Naht- und Fremdmaterial. Chirurg 56:284–289, 1985.

CHAPTER 9

CLINICAL USE OF A NEW COMPRESSION DEVICE IN COLO-RECTAL SURGERY

Giuseppe Pezzuoli, Carlo Rebuffat, and Riccardo Rosati

With the aim of improving the quality of anastomoses obtained with suturing and stapling, we returned to the idea of compression popularized by Murphy who introduced his "anastomotic button" into clinical practice in 1892.[1] These devices cause compression of the intestinal ends and act as temporary support for the tissues, allowing "natural" healing to take place immediately outside the area of compression. After this goal is achieved, the whole compression apparatus becomes detached from the anastomosis, falls into the intestinal lumen, and is evacuated.

The main advantages of compression anastomoses are: impermeability (because of the circumferential coaptation of bowel ends produced by the device); immobility (the intraluminal apparatus protects the anastomosis from distension by gas and feces); and absence of foreign bodies at the anastomotic site, which lessens the likelihood of stenosis and perianastomotic adhesions.[1,2,3] However, technical problems related to the inadequacy of mechanical compression devices such as the Murphy "button" and its many modifications limited acceptance, study, and development of sutureless anastomosis.[4]

At the First Department of Surgery of the University of Milan we developed and tested a new mechanical device that achieves compression anastomosis by intraluminal placement of an apparatus consisting of three polypropylene rings (Fig. 9-1). Our experimental results were sufficiently encouraging for us to proceed to the use of the device in humans, as reported in our preliminary publication.[5] This chapter describes surgical technique and further clinical experience in colo-rectal surgery with this anastomotic device.

MATERIALS AND METHODS

The anastomotic device developed consists of three interlocking polypropylene rings, already described in our preliminary publication[5] (Fig. 9-1). Fifty-six patients underwent large bowel compression anastomosis with this device in our institution from May 1986 through December 1988 (Table 9-1). The operations were all performed by the same team and all the patients gave their informed consent to the procedures. The followup program of the patients after hospital discharge was very strict: all patients were controlled endoscopically 1 and 3 months after operation, then at 6-month intervals, and radiologically with double contrast enema once in the first year.

RESULTS

Results are summarized in Table 9-2.

One patient (1.8%) died of myocardial infarction on the third postoperative day. At autopsy the gross appearance of the anastomosis was very good: the rings were firmly in place and were gently removed after longitudinal opening of the bowel by cutting the intestinal walls compressed between the buttons. The anastomosis was studied histologically and was at an advanced stage of healing.

As for postoperative anastomotic complications, we observed one subclinical (1.8%) and one clinical (1.8%) anastomotic leak. They involved a very low colo-rectal anastomosis and a total colectomy with extraperitoneal ileo-rectal anastomosis, early in our experience. No hemorrhages or other anastomotic complications were observed.

As for extra-anastomotic complications, one patient (1.8%) with intraperitoneal colo-rectal anastomosis

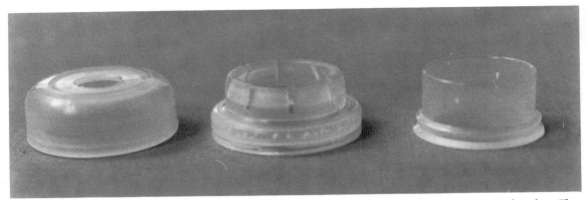

Fig. 9-1. The anastomotic apparatus consists of three molded plastic rings that lock together as anastomosis takes place. The outer ring, shown on the left, is mounted on a central rod and placed into the purse-stringed proximal bowel end (like an EEA anvil). The intermediate ring (*middle*) is placed within the purse-stringed distal bowel, held by the placement instrument (like the EEA cartridge). After advancing the distal, intermediate ring into the proximal outer ring and thus invaginating the purse-stringed bowel ends, the instrument is activated and the inner ring (*right*) and a circular blade within it are advanced. With this maneuver the purse-stringed bowel ends are excised like rings (doughnuts), the intermediate ring flanges (*middle*) are opened like a tulip petal and press against the outer ring (*left*), and the central plate of the outer ring is cored out. The locked rings (*left, middle, right*) stay in place, and the carrying instrument becomes free and can be extracted.

had pulmonary embolism, and one (1.8%) had severe antibiotic-associated pseudomembranous colitis (AAPMC): they both recovered with medical therapy without developing any anastomotic complication.

Endoscopic long-term controls showed wide anastomoses without any evidence of strictures. Even the patients who complained of leaks and those with diverting colostomies all had wide, non-stenotic anas-

Table 9-1. Clinical Experience with Compression Anastomoses in Surgery of the Large Bowel: May 1986–December 1988

Patients (N = 56)	
Males	38
Females	18
Mean age and range (years)	59.6 (40–82)
Indications for Surgery	
Adenocarcinoma	39
Diverticulosis	8
Crohn's disease	3
Miscellaneous	6
Operations Performed	
Right hemicolectomy	7
Left colon resection	7
Left hemicolectomy/anterior resection of the rectum	40
Total colectomy	2
Distance of Rectal Anastomosis from the Anal Verge	
<4 cm	7 (16.6%)
4–8 cm	9 (21.5%)
>8 cm	26 (61.9%)
Intra-operative colostomies	5 (8.9%)

tomoses. The anastomotic line was often difficult to detect, even by video-endoscopy. Radiologically, the anastomoses were wide and difficult to locate.

COMMENT

Sutureless compression anastomoses have been known since the early nineteenth century. The Murphy anastomotic button and other devices introduced later[1,2,3] created very good intestinal anastomoses, but they never gained widespread acceptance, mainly because of the difficulties of mechanical placement.[4,6] Currently there is a renewal of interest in compression devices,[7] and the Russians have in-

Table 9-2. Clinical Experience with Compression Anastomosis in Surgery of the Large Bowel: May 1986–December 1988

Evacuation of the rings (mean and range, in days)	11.3 (5–23)
Postoperative hospital stay (mean, in days)	14.3
Operative mortality (myocardial infarction)	1 (1.8%)
Anastomotic Complications	
Sub-clinical leak	1 (1.8%)
Clinical leak	1 (1.8%)
Hemorrhage	0
Stenosis	0
Extra-Anastomotic Complications	
Pulmonary embolism	1 (1.8%)
AAMPC	1 (1.8%)
Diarrhea	6 (10.9%)
Urinary infections	4 (7.3%)

troduced an instrument for compression anastomosis, the AKA-2, that has elicited favorable comments in the Soviet Union and in Europe.[8,9,10] This instrument is reusable and needs to be assembled and loaded at the time of operation; it places a series of plastic rings kept together by a complicated mechanism of metal pins and coaxial springs. Another sutureless anastomotic apparatus, called the "Bowel Anastomosis Ring" (BAR), was recently described, and animal trials were reported.[11,12] This is a biofragmentable ring made of polyglycolic acid that holds the two intestinal ends to be anastomosed in contact. It becomes detached from the anastomosis by fragmentation and then passes out in the feces. The initial clinical experience with this instrument was favorable,[13] but the lack of an applicator precludes its use for low and very low colo-rectal anastomoses.

A sutureless anastomosis is certainly the "ideal anastomosis,"[1,4,6] so we tried to combine the old principle of compression with the most recent technological improvements. The anastomotic apparatus we describe here consists of an instrument that assembles three molded plastic rings that simply lock together (Fig. 9-1). The metal prototype we employed for this trial was easy to use and reliable (Fig. 9-2), but only the completely disposable device,

which will be available shortly, will satisfy the need for an always properly functioning instrument.

The initial animal trial was very encouraging and confirmed the biologic concept of good quick healing.[5] The surgical technique for the anastomosis is even easier than the one usually employed with staplers. The particular shape of the outer ring allows its easy introduction into the proximal bowel lumen; the rings themselves must be smaller than the bowel circumference, so this makes it even easier to introduce the instrument. The instrument is extracted on completion of the anastomosis with greater ease than with a stapling instrument of comparable size. The circular blade first cuts the bowel edges held by the two purse-string sutures, then cuts the central part of the outer ring, automatically separating the locked rings from the carrying instrument.

As with staplers, the tissue doughnuts cut by the circular blade must always be carefully inspected. They must be complete to ensure that intact tissue ends are compressed between the rings.

Regular stool evacuation was not impaired by the presence of the rings. Even when the smaller rings were still in place at the anastomotic site, evacuation of solid stool was normal. Occurrence of severe diarrhea in some patients, such as the patient with AAPMC, is good evidence of the impermeability of

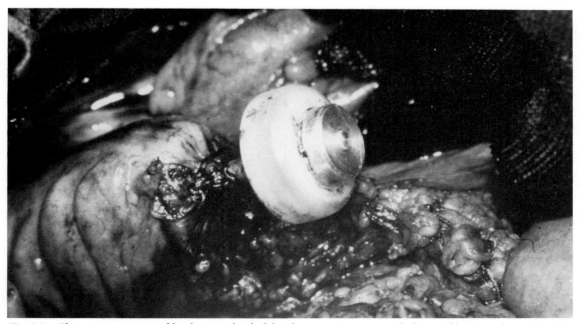

Fig. 9-2. The outer ring is carried by the central rod of the placement instrument, which resembles a circular stapler. The outer ring will be placed into one bowel and the purse-string will be tied around the central rod. The placement instrument, carrying intermediate and inner rings, has been placed through a colotomy into the opposite bowel end, with its purse-string tied around the central rod.

the system, because none of them experienced any anastomotic complications.

The rings were evacuated postoperatively at very different intervals (between 5 and 23 days). Since no complication arose in the patient who evacuated the rings on the fifth day (in dogs, ring detachment does not depend on the amount of compression), we believe that rings detach only when healing of the anastomosis is complete.[5] Evacuation of the rings did not cause any problems in any of the patients with regular fecal transit, who often did not even feel their passage.

Long-term controls have all confirmed the good quality of the anastomoses, which were often difficult to identify even endoscopically. Radiologically, they all appeared very good. The fact of not having foreign bodies such as staples or sutures at the anastomotic site was considered a definite advantage if CAT scans or Magnetic Resonance Imaging (MRI) are required for these patients in the future.

In conclusion, we believe that this series confirms the preliminary results already reported and is undoubtedly encouraging. It is even easier to operate this device than to operate stapling instruments. The incidence of protective diverting colostomies is low, and postoperative complications are few.

Mechanically, the anastomotic apparatus confirmed its reliability. The steel prototype performed well, but only when the disposable instrument is available for clinical use in the near future will an always properly functioning tool be obtained.

REFERENCES

1. Murphy JB: Cholecysto-intestinal, gastro-intestinal, entero-intestinal anastomosis and approximation without sutures (original research). Medical Record, New York 42:665, 1892.
2. Juvara E: Un nouveau modèle du bouton anastomotique intestinal avec une nouvelle technique. Arch Sci Méd (Bucarest), Paris I:253, 1896.
3. Boerema I: The technique of our method of transabdominal total gastrectomy in cases of gastric cancer. Arch Chir Neerl 6:95, 1954.
4. Ballantyne GH: The experimental basis of intestinal suturing. Dis Colon Rect 27:61–71, 1984.
5. Rosati R, Rebuffat C, Pezzuoli G: A new mechanical device for circular compression anastomosis. Preliminary results of animal and clinical experimentation. Ann Surg 207:15–22, 1988.
6. Hogstrom H, Haglund U: Postoperative decrease in sutures holding capacity in laparotomy wounds and anastomoses. Acta Chir Scand 151:533–535, 1985.
7. Jansen A, Brummelkamp WH, Davies GS, Klopper PJ, Keeman, JM: Clinical application of magnetic rings in colorectal anastomosis. Surg Gynecol Obstet 153:537–545, 1981.
8. Knys BI, Capjuk VF, Guskov IA, Sackov AE: Primenenie anastomose "s/pod davleniem" v kirurgieskom lacenii raka tolstoj kiski. Kirurgija, Zurnal imeni N.I. Pirogova. Moskva Meditzina 3:107–114, 1984.
9. Liboni A, Mari C, Tartari V, et al: AKA-2: una nuova suturatrice meccanica circolare introflettente nella chirurgia colorettale. Acta Chir Italica 41:536–538, 1985.
10. Gross E: Sutureless compression anastomosis of the distal colon and rectum. 2nd International Symposium on Stapling, 1ér Congrès Européen de Viscéro-Synthèse, Luxembourg 2-4 June 1988:25.
11. Hardy TG, Pace WG, Maney JW, Katz AR, Kaganov AL: A biofragmentable ring for sutureless bowel anastomosis: an experimental study. Dis Colon Rectum 28:484–490, 1985.
12. Maney JW, Katz AR, Pace WG, Hardy TG: Biofragmentable bowel anastomosis ring: comparative efficacy studies in dogs. Surgery 103:56–62, 1988.
13. Hardy GT, Aguilar PS, Stewart WRC, et al: Initial clinical experience with a biofragmentable ring for sutureless anastomosis. Dis Colon Rectum 30:55–61, 1987.

CHAPTER 10

ANASTOMOSIS WITH BIOLOGIC GLUE

Bruno S. Walther, Olof Jansson, and Thomas Zilling

Foreign material penetrating the intestinal wall undeniably causes some form of inflammatory reaction. Consequently, many attempts to join bowel ends with glue have been made but without great clinical success, presumably because of technical circumstances, which involve applying and compressing the glue while it is hardening. In an attempt to eliminate these drawbacks, we developed and investigated the following approach.

EXPERIMENTAL DESIGN

Four pigs had their mid-jejunums divided under pentobarbital induction, and general anesthesia with nitrous oxide-oxygen and endotracheal intubation used for ventilation. The EEA stapler (size 21) was introduced through one cut bowel end, and anastomosis was performed at a distance of 15 cm from this jejunal end. The used stapler, with its cartridge spent but circular blade intact, was then introduced through the opposite bowel end to the 15-cm level. The anvil was separated from the cartridge and the resulting indentation in the bowel wall was tightened around the central rod with a circular thread and tied. The glue (Tisseel) was applied between the anvil separated from the spent cartridge, and the instrument was closed. The bowel ends and sandwiched glue were compressed for 5 minutes. The EEA instrument was then activated, advancing only the circular blade to core out the two bowel rings. After withdrawal of the instrument, the two jejunal ends of the original transection were anastomosed with 4-0 Maxon (running, single-layer). In conclusion, a prototype of a "glue stapler" was developed for inverting, end-to-end anastomoses (Fig. 10-1A).

Before sacrificing the animals 4 days postoperatively, microspheres were injected into their left ventricles. The jejunal specimens were removed and examined by radiologic contrast studies, followed by tensile tests and blood flow measurements.

Radiologic examinations were performed in two perpendicular planes with a 10% contrast solution. An anastomotic index, using the ratio between the two perpendicular planes by crossing inner diameters of the anastomoses and the same ratios 5 cm above and below the anastomoses, was calculated (Fig. 10-1B).

Tensile Tests

The breaking strength was tested according to Löwenhielm, using a piezoelectric force transducer and a transient recorder.[1]

Measurement of Blood Flow in the Anastomotic Area

Specific organ blood flow was calculated by means of the reference organ method, described by Hafström et al.[2] (Fig. 10-2). According to this method, arterial blood flow f_1 (ml $\times$ min^{-1}) in an organ (1) can be calculated using the equation:

$$f_1 = \frac{q_1}{q_r} \times f_r$$

Where f_r is the known blood flow in a reference organ (r); q_1 and q_r are the amount of radioactivity (Bq) in the organ (1) and the reference organ (r), respectively.

In the present study we used 15 ± 3 pre-labeled, non-biodegradable ^{141}Ce-microspheres in isotonic saline. After the syringe was vigorously shaken, the spheres were injected into the left ventricle within 10 seconds. The collection of blood in the reference or-

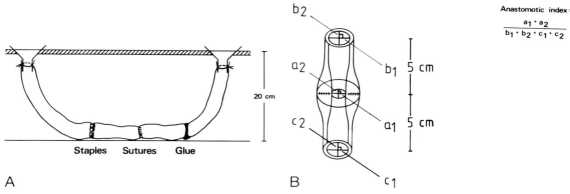

Fig. 10-1. *A.* Standard model used for radiologic examination of the anastomosis. *B.* Calculation of the anastomotic index.

gan was started immediately prior to and terminated 2 minutes after the injection of the microspheres. Samples from both kidneys were taken for testing of even distribution of the microspheres, which is a requirement for the reliability of this method. Blood flow in the samples is expressed as a percentage of cardiac output.

Results

During the 4 postoperative days, the animals (Swedish domestic female pigs) lost a median of 1 kg

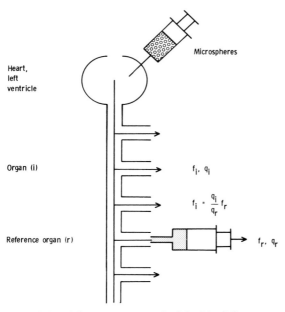

Fig. 10-2. Reference organ method for blood flow measurements: f_i and f_r = blood flows to the organs i and r; q_i and q_r = activities in the same organs. Fifteen-micrometer-sized [141]Ce-labeled microspheres in isotonic saline are injected into left ventricle.

in weight from a preoperative weight of 15 to 20 kg. No anastomotic leaks were observed; preoperatively, food but not water had been withheld for 24 hours. Postoperatively the pigs received a normal diet.

Radiologic Findings

As seen from Figure 10-3, there were no strictures and no differences in the anastomotic width. Figure 10-4 shows a typical x-ray study of the three anastomoses.

Tensile Tests

The glued anastomoses had about half the breaking strength of the stapled ones. The strength of the sutured anastomosis was in between these two (Fig. 10-5).

Blood Flow Measurement

From Figure 10-6 it becomes obvious that the two anastomoses created with the EEA instrument (glue

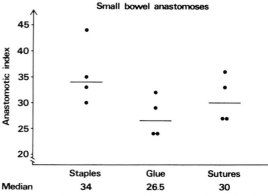

Fig. 10-3. The anastomotic width in 4 pigs that underwent operations with the approach described in the experimental design.

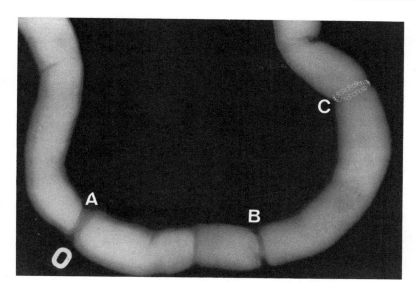

Fig. 10-4. X-ray picture of a glued (*A*), a sutured (*B*), and a stapled (*C*) jejunal anastomosis in the pig 4 days after the operation. The specimen is mounted according to Figure 10-1.

and staples) are underperfused, in contrast to the highly perfused manually sutured anastomoses.

DISCUSSION

Foreign material penetrating all bowel layers may be an important factor in the cause of infected anastomoses and in anastomotic breakdown.[3] The breaking strength of sutureless, fibrin-sealed anastomoses of the colon and the small intestine is similar to that of a two-layer, manually created anastomosis.[4,5] With the tensile tests performed on the seventh postoperative day, it is shown that the weakest period has passed.[6] In our study the fibrin-adhesive anastomoses had only half the breaking strength of the stapled ones. The difference may be explained by the fact that our animals were sacrificed on the fourth postoperative day. Many studies deal with breaking strength of the anastomosis, but very few deal with the anastomotic circulation,[6] even though in 1929 Saint and Mann had already pointed out the importance of good anastomotic circulation.[7] Chung showed that tight stapling reduces the suture-line blood flow significantly, peri-operatively. We found a

reduced circulation on the fourth postoperative day in the EEA-compressed group, whether glue or staples were used, with a stapling device where adjustment for bowel wall thickness is not possible. The pig, however, has a very thin intestinal wall: the instruments were closed without any form of resistance.

Experimentally, we have shown that after 1 week there is a hyperemia in experimentally performed esophago-jejunal anastomoses after total gastrectomy in the pig. This hyperemia is the same in both stapled and sutured anastomoses. It can be speculated that the compression of the stapling instruments increases the length of the initial hypo-perfusion in the anasto-

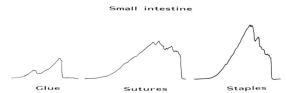

Fig. 10-5. The median breaking strength in 4 pigs that underwent operations with three different jejunal anastomoses.

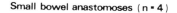
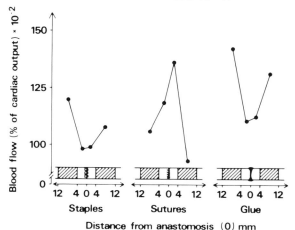

Fig. 10-6. Blood flow distribution around the small bowel anastomoses after 4 days. The values are expressed as medians.

moses. Further experimental studies will clarify this. The anastomotic width obtained with the glue technique is, after 4 days, equal to that of the manually sutured and stapled anastomoses. Long-term studies are necessary to see what will happen to the glued anastomotic ring. Will it be absorbed?—will there be widening?—invasion by vessels?

REFERENCES

1. Löwenhielm P: Dynamic strain tolerance of blood vessels at different postmortem conditions. Journal of Bioengineering 2:509–515, 1978.
2. Hafström LO, Persson B, Sundquist K: Measurements of cardiac ouput and organ blood flow in rats using 99 Tc^m-labelled microspheres. Acta Physiol Scand 106: 123–128, 1979.
3. Goligher JC, Graham NG, De Dombal FT: Anastomotic dehiscence after anterior resection of rectum and sigmoid. Br J Surg 57:109–118, 1970.
4. Hjortrup A, Nordkild P, Kjaergaard J, Sjöntoft E, Olesen HP: Fibrin adhesive versus sutured anastomosis: A comparative intraindividual study in the small intestine of pigs. Br J Surg 73:760–761, 1986.
5. Kjaergaard J, Nordkild P, Sjöntoft E, Hjortrup A: Non-sutured fibrin adhesive vs. sutured anastomosis. A comparative intra-individual study in dog colon. Acta Chir Scand 153:599–601, 1987.
6. Jiborn H, Ahonen J, Zederfeldt B: Healing of experimental colonic anastomoses. I. Bursting strength of the colon following left colon resection and anastomosis. Am J Surg 136:587–594, 1978.
7. Saint JH, Mann F: Experimental surgery of the esophagus. Arch Surg 18:2324–2358, 1929.
8. Chung RS: Blood flow in colonic anastomoses. Effect of stapling and suturing. Ann Surg 204:335–338, 1986.

Part III

Healing of Stapled Tissues: Comparison with Manual Techniques

CHAPTER 11

HEALING AND LONG-TERM FATE OF STAPLED ANASTOMOSES

Bruno S. Walther

In this experimental study we compare manual and stapled circular esophago-jejunal and colo-rectal anastomoses, as well as esophageal transection and anastomosis done by hand or with a stapling device. The time required to perform the anastomosis, as well as its resistance to breaking, rate of leakage, anastomotic width, and vascular integrity, were studied and measured. All other parameters being equal, the stapled esophago-jejunostomy was faster to perform (20 minutes) than the manually sutured one (28 minutes) ($p < 0.05$). During the healing process of colonic anastomoses, stapling techniques ensure anastomotic width and preserve vessels in a manner comparable to the single-layer manual anastomosis. Stapling is faster than with the two-layer hand-sewn technique, which narrows the lumen much more than both previous techniques ($p < 0.05$). In 40 patients with stapled esophago-jejunal anastomoses after total gastrectomy, we have measured the anastomotic width every third month, using an endoscopically placed balloon. After 9 or 10 months, the diameter of the anastomosis ceases to increase and stabilizes at about twice the initial size. Not a single patient ended up with anastomotic narrowing. Experimental esophageal transection and anastomosis is associated with a high stricture rate, irrespective of the technique used.

Leakage from esophageal, colic, and rectal anastomoses is still a cause for postoperative morbidity and mortality.[1] The introduction of mechanical stapling devices presents an alternative method of achieving anastomosis. So far, few randomized controlled trials have compared manually and mechanically sutured colo-rectal anastomoses, and not a single study compares stapled and hand-sutured esophago-jejunal

anastomoses.[2,3] Clinical studies may not be valid in evaluating different anastomotic techniques if many surgeons are involved, because the ability of the surgeon is a better predictor of results than the anastomotic technique used. This may explain the contradictory results obtained in comparing anastomotic operative time and dehiscence rates for manual and mechanical techniques.[2–5]

The aim of this study is the short-term healing of stapled and manually sutured intestinal anastomoses, in a highly standardized experimental model where all animals underwent operations by the same surgeon. The long-term fate of stapled anastomoses was studied in patients; the element of variable surgical ability was eliminated by comparably high levels of competence in the operating surgeons.

MATERIALS AND METHODS

Experimental Esophagojejunal Anastomoses

Animals

Using the same protocol for all animals, 30 Swedish domestic female pigs, weighing 15 to 20 kg at the time of operation, were used (Fig. 11-1). The pigs were randomized to hand-sewn or stapled end-to-side esophago-jejunal anastomoses after total gastrectomy. The anastomotic techniques used were 3-0 Dexon, two layers, interrupted manual sutures, and mechanical anastomosis using the 25-mm EEA stapler (US Surgical Corporation).

Experimental Design

One week postoperatively, half of the pigs in each group were randomly killed. The rest were observed

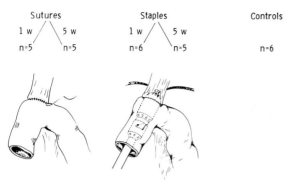

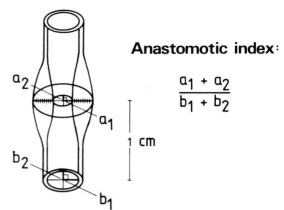

Fig. 11-1. After total gastrectomy and Roux-en-Y preparation, the pigs were randomized to hand-sewn or stapled end-to-side esophago-jejunal anastomoses. The animals were killed 1 or 5 weeks after their operations. Controls (n = 6).

Fig. 11-3. The esophago-jejunostomy region showing the calculation of the anastomotic index: $(a_1 + a_2)/(b_1 + b_2)$.

for another 4 weeks and weighed once weekly. Microspheres were injected before the animals were killed. The esophago-jejunal specimen was removed and examined by radiographic studies, tensile tests, and blood flow measurements.

Radiologic Examinations

Radiologic examinations were performed in two perpendicular planes using 10% contrast solution (Mixobar Ventrikel, Astra-Meditec AB, Mölndal, Sweden) (Fig. 11-2). An anastomotic index, using the ratio between two perpendicular inner diameters of the anastomosis and the same diameters 5 cm above, was calculated (Fig. 11-3). In this way, differences in diameter of the anastomosis and that of the normal esophagus were observed. By using an index, every animal served as its own control, and differences in size between animals were eliminated. The wall thickness was calculated and compared in the same way.

Tensile Tests

The breaking strength was tested according to Löwenhielm, using a piezoelectric force transducer and a transient recorder.[6]

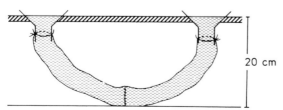

Fig. 11-2. The standard set-up used for radiologic examinations of the anastomoses.

Measurement of Blood Flow in the Anastomotic Area

Specific organ blood flow was calculated by means of the reference organ method, described by Hafström et al.[7] According to this method, arterial blood flow f_i (ml $\times$ min^{-1}) in an organ (1) can be calculated using the equation:

$$f_1 = \frac{q_i}{q_r} \times f_r$$

where f_r is the known blood flow in a reference organ (r); q_i and q_r are the amount of radioactivity (Bq) in the organ (1) and in the reference organ (r), respectively.

In the present study we used 15 ± 3 μm prelabelled non-biodegradable ^{141}Ce microspheres in isotonic saline. After the syringe was vigorously shaken, the spheres were injected into the left ventricle within 10 seconds. The collection of blood in the reference organ was started immediately prior to and terminated 2 minutes after the injection of the microspheres (Fig. 11-4). Samples from both kidneys were taken for testing of even distribution of the microspheres, which is a requirement for the reliability of this method. Blood flow in the samples is expressed as a percentage of cardiac output.

Histologic Examination

From the anastomotic area, a longitudinal strip of tissue was taken for histologic examination and stained with hematoxylin-eosine and the van Gieson and McManus techniques.

Esophago-Jejunal Anastomoses in Patients

Since 1984, all patients operated by total gastrectomy have been evaluated to measure esophago-

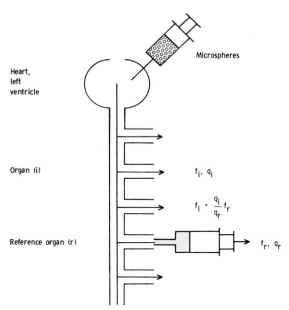

Fig. 11-4. Reference-organ method for blood flow measurements (f_i and f_r = blood flow to the organs i and r, respectively; q_i and q_r = activities in the same organs). Fifteen-micrometer-sized ^{141}Ce-labeled microspheres in isotonic saline are injected into the left ventricle.

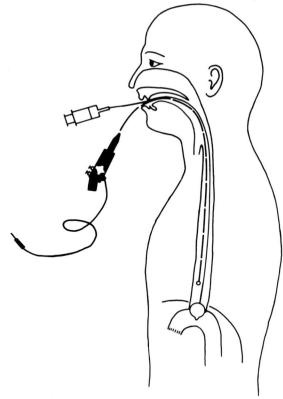

Fig. 11-5. The method used for measuring the anastomotic width in 40 patients who underwent total gastrectomy and esophago-jejunal anastomoses in the abdomen or the left or right chest. For details, see the text.

jejunal anastomotic width every third month. The esophagus was intubated with a fiberoptic endoscope carrying a balloon catheter connected to a syringe. The balloon was insufflated under endoscopic vision until it completely filled the lumen of the anastomosis, without getting caught when it was pulled up and down through the anastomosis (Fig. 11-5). This was repeated three times; the average volume of filling was noted. After these measurements, the air was aspirated and the catheter with the syringe withdrawn without disconnection. The balloon was now filled again by the volume of air contained in the syringe, and its diameter was measured with a caliper.

Anastomoses of the Colon

Experimental Design

In 18 animals, a 5-cm segment of colon was resected 10 cm above the peritoneal reflection. Three types of anastomoses were performed. The first two involved either single-layer Gambee-sutures (n = 6) or conventional interrupted two-layer sutures (n = 6); the material was Vicryl 4-0 in both. The third type was an ILS (Ethicon Inc., Somerville, NJ) stapled anastomosis (n = 6), with which the disposable purse-string tissue-measuring devices were used.

The animals were killed in 7 days, after an overnight fast.

Radiologic Examinations

The anastomotic index was calculated as in the esophago-jejunal anastomosis, but here a third measuring point 3 cm distal to the anastomosis was added, giving an ideal anastomotic index of 0.5. This type of anastomotic index was used because it was the same type of intestine on both sides of the anastomosis, which was not the case for the esophagojejunal anastomosis.

Tensile tests and measurements of anastomotic blood flow and histological examinations were the same as used for the study of esophagojejunal anastomoses.

Esophageal Transection

Surgical Procedures

Twelve animals were operated after a 24 hour fast undergoing esophageal transection in a standardized manner. The transection and reanastomosis were performed 2 cm above the cardia either by stapler (ILS—Ethicon) or manually, by resection of 0.5 cm of the esophagus and end-to-end anastomosis with a continuous one-layer suture line (Dexon 4-o, N = 6) (Fig. 11-6).

Radiological Examinations

The anastomotic index was calculated by comparing the 2 perpendicular planes in the anastomotic area to 2 perpendicular planes 1 cm distally, giving an optimal index of 1.0. Tensile test and blood flow measurements were studied as for the experimental esophagojejunal anastomoses.

Statistical Methods

To evaluate differences between the three groups, the Kruskal-Wallis one-way analysis of variance by ranks was applied. Whenever a significant difference was noted, the Mann-Whitney U-test was used to determine the groups between which this significance was valid. In testing two groups, the Mann-Whitney U-test was used directly. The Pearson product moment correlation coefficient was used to test the association between two variables.

RESULTS

Experimental Esophago-Jejunal Anastomoses

Animals

Three animals from different groups died during the first postoperative week because of incarceration of the small intestine through a para-esophageal hiatal hernia.

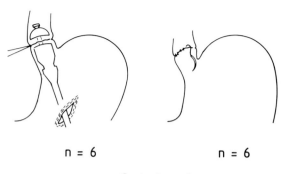

n = 6   n = 6

Controls = 6

Fig. 11-6. After laparotomy the pigs were randomized to manually or stapled esophageal transection. The animals were killed after 4½ months.

Radiologic Findings

No leakage was found. No differences were observed between the stapled and manually sutured groups concerning anastomotic indices or wall thickness (Table 11-1).

Tensile Tests

The stapled anastomoses were slightly but insignificantly stronger than the manually sutured ones, both 1 and 5 weeks after operation (Table 11-2). However, from the first to the fifth week, the anastomotic strength increased significantly for both techniques.

Blood Flow Measurements

The blood flow was lower in the esophagus than in the Roux-en-Y jejunal loop, both 1 and 5 weeks after operation. These differences were also observed in the control animals (Fig. 11-7). After 1 week there is a significantly higher blood flow ($p < 0.05$) in the esophageal part immediately proximal to the anastomosis, regardless of technique used, as compared to the controls. The anastomotic circulation decreased 5 weeks after resection, as compared to the 1-week level in the controls—especially in the jejunal limb ($p < 0.05$).

Microscopic Appearance

The mucosal gap seen in the 1-week group was covered after 5 weeks with proliferating stratified squamous epithelium. No differences between stapled and manually performed anastomoses were seen.

Esophago-Jejunal Anastomoses in Patients

The anastomotic diameter increases during the first 10 months, after which the anastomotic width stabilizes at about twice its initial size. Not a single patient ended up with a narrowing (Fig. 11-8).

Anastomoses of the Colon

No intra-operative or postoperative mortality or morbidity was experienced. The time to complete the two-layer anastomosis was significantly longer (21 minutes, Inter Quartile (IQ) range 20 to 24 minutes) than the time to perform the stapled anastomosis (13 minutes, IQ range 12 to 14 minutes) ($p < 0.05$). The time for the single-layer anastomosis was in between these two techniques (16 minutes, IQ range 15 to 20 minutes).

Table 11-1. Anastomotic Index* and Wall Thickness* (Median and IQ** Range) 1 and 5 Weeks after Total Gastrectomy in the Pig

Period after Gastrectomy	Anastomotic Index	Wall Thickness (mm)
1 week		
Sutures (n = 5)	0.59 (0.49–0.63) (n = 5)	0.42 (0.37–0.49) (n = 5)
Staples (n = 6)	0.60 (0.56–0.65)	0.38 (0.35–0.47)
5 weeks		
Sutures (n = 5)	0.51 (0.41–0.66) (n = 5)	0.38 (0.38–0.46) (n = 5)
Staples (n = 5)	0.48 (0.35–0.65)	0.41 (0.40–0.65)

* No differences were seen within groups from 1 to 5 weeks. Test for differences: Mann-Whitney U-test.
** IQ = Inter Quartile.

Radiologic Examinations

The anastomotic index was highest for the single-layer manual anastomosis (0.38) and the stapled anastomosis (0.37). Both anastomoses have better anastomotic indices than the two-layer hand-sewn technique (0.24) ($p < 0.05$). The narrowing was due to a thicker wall in the two-layer anastomoses (two-layer = 8 mm, single-layer = 5 mm, stapler = 4.5 mm) (Table 11-3).

Tensile Tests

As seen from Table 11-4, no differences were found in breaking strength among the three groups.

Blood Flow Measurements

The two-layer technique had a lower median blood flow (0.79) than the other two groups (1.44 for the single-layer, 1.09 for the stapler) immediately distal to the anastomoses. In all groups, as in the esophagojejunal group, there was a higher flow in the anastomotic area compared to areas 8 cm distal or proximal ($p < 0.05$). A significant correlation exists between wall thickness and circulation; i.e., with a thicker wall comes a decreased blood flow (Fig. 11-9).

Esophageal Transection

One animal in each group died during the first week because of intestinal obstruction due to adhesions. No leakage was encountered.

Radiologic Findings

The anastomotic index was equal in the two groups (Fig. 11-10). Three animals in the manually sutured group and two in the stapled group showed an anastomotic index lower than 0.5, indicating a stricture.

Tensile Tests

All specimens ruptured outside the anastomotic area and showed the same breaking strength as the controls.

Blood Flow Measurements

The anastomotic circulation was the same in all three groups (Fig. 11-11).

DISCUSSION

Technically, the most demanding sites for anastomosis are at the upper and lower ends of the gastro-

Table 11-2. Ultimate Breaking Force (Median and IQ Range) for Sutured or Stapled Esophago-Jejunal Anastomoses at Different Time Intervals after Total Gastrectomy in the Pig

Anastomosis Type	Breaking Force (kp)		
	1 week		5 weeks
Sutures (n = 5)	13.0 (11.9–17.4) (n = 5)	p < 0.05	37.0 (27.4–50.7) (n = 5)
Staples (n = 615)	19.4 (16.5–23.0) (n = 6)	p < 0.01	50.1 (42.0–60.8) (n = 5)

Test for differences: Mann-Whitney U-test

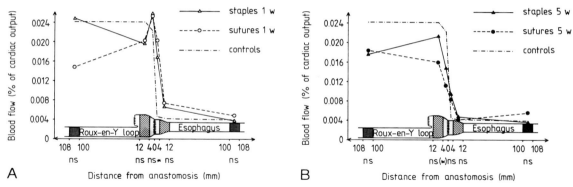

Fig. 11-7. Blood flow distribution (percent of cardiac output) around the esophago-jejunostomy after 1 week (*A*) and 5 weeks (*B*). Samples were taken at different distances from the anastomosis and at corresponding sites in controls with a two-blade cutter.

intestinal tract. Stapling instruments have facilitated the construction of low rectal anastomoses. The use of mechanical suture devices has become increasingly popular for other parts of the gastro-intestinal tract. The only way of evaluating new anastomotic techniques in detail is by experimental scrutiny of a highly standardized model. We have used pigs be-

cause their intestinal tract is large enough to permit the use of standard stapling devices. To eliminate the influence of surgeon experience, the operations should be done by one surgeon, which is easy to arrange in the experimental setting. Clinically, however, multi-surgeon trials, with very large patient cohorts, are necessary to completely eliminate the

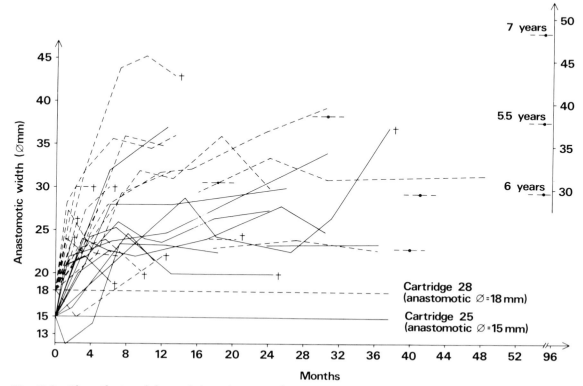

Fig. 11-8. The widening of the stapled esophago-jejunal anastomoses in 40 patients undergoing operations with total gastrectomy. After 1 month there was a slight narrowing of the anastomosis, which spontaneously widened in a couple of months.

Table 11-3. Anastomotic Index and Thickness of Bowel Wall (Median and IQ Range)

Anastomosis Type	Anastomotic Index	Wall Thickness (mm)
One-layer	0.38 (0.34–0.42)	5 (4–6)
Two layer	0.24 (0.23–0.27)	8 (7–9.5)
Stapled	0.37 (0.34–0.42)	4.5 (3.5–7)

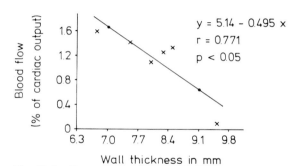

Fig. 11-9. Regression analysis of blood flow (percent of cardiac output) vs. wall thickness (mm); r = 0.89, p < 0.05.

influence of surgeon experience, at least in smaller countries.

Since the introduction of the EEA instrument in 1977, many reports of the results obtained with its use have been published. In this study of esophago-jejunal and low colo-rectal anastomoses, the stapled procedure was performed faster than the double-layer manual suture technique. This is confirmed by other authors.[3,4] In comparing one-layer with stapled colo-rectal anastomosis, there was no time difference.

In a clinical series of total gastrectomy and end-to-side esophago-jejunostomy with the EEA stapler performed by one surgeon, there was not a single anastomotic leak.[8]

In a review of our complete series representing the work of 23 surgeons, the leakage rate is 14% and the mortality rate is 5.6%, indicating the various levels of surgical competence. The study of leakage rates in colo-rectal anastomoses cannot demonstrate any difference between manual and stapled techniques in most series.[2–5] However, routine radiologic studies conducted postoperatively are not a part of all published series. In a review of cumulative results from seven uncontrolled studies, Waxman showed a lower incidence of leakage following stapled colo-rectal anastomosis.[10] Viste prospectively studied the incidence and cause of esophago-jejunal anastomotic leakage in 350 patients who underwent operations within the Norwegian Multicenter Stomach Cancer Trial.[11] The odds for leakage were 2.37 times higher in patients with hand-sutured anastomoses than in those with stapled anastomoses. Wong, in comparing EEA- and ILS-stapled anastomoses with manually sutured esophago-gastrostomies after esophagectomy, demonstrated no difference in leakage frequency.[12]

After total gastrectomy and esophago-jejunostomy, not a single patient ended up with a stricture. After 1

Table 11-4. Ultimate Breaking Force in Tensile Testing of Various Anastomotic Techniques (Mean ± SD)

Technique	Breaking Force (kp)
Single-layer	4.6 (±1.3)
Double-layer	4.6 (±0.9)
ILS	4.8 (±1.0)

month, however, two patients were seen with narrowing of the anastomosis, which subsequently widened spontaneously. All the esophago-jejunostomy patients underwent operations with a 50-cm-long Roux-en-Y loop to prevent regurgitation.

With esophago-gastrostomy, however, there is always severe regurgitation of gastric contents, which might be an explanation of the more common stricture formation. In studies by Wong and West, a higher incidence of strictures was seen when the smallest cartridge was used.[12,13] By comparing the different circular staplers to hand-sutured anastomosis, however, there was no difference in stricture formation in esophageal transection and re-anastomosis. The stricture frequency is high regardless of the technique used. Spontaneous widening of colo-rectal anastomoses is seen with time.[14] In the experimental colo-rectal series, the width of the stapled and one-layer hand-sewn anastomoses was superior to that of the double-layer technique. Not a single patient series compares the width of stapled and hand-sewn colo-rectal anastomosis.

In 1929 Saint and Mann pointed out poor blood supply as an important reason for leakage of esopha-

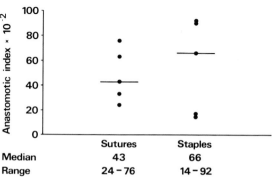

Fig. 11-10. The anastomotic indexes in the two groups of pigs that underwent operations with sutured or stapled esophageal transection were equal.

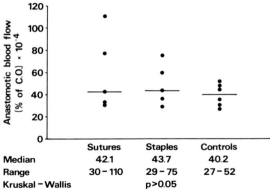

	Sutures	Staples	Controls
Median	42.1	43.7	40.2
Range	30 – 110	29 – 75	27 – 52
Kruskal – Wallis		$p > 0.05$	

Fig. 11-11. The blood flow distribution (percent of cardiac output) in the esophageal transection was, after 4½ months, equal to that of the controls.

geal anastomoses.[15] This has been confirmed many times. The esophagus and rectum have low blood flows: this might be one explanation why anastomoses in this area are encumbered with a high frequency of leakage and stricture formation. Both in the colo-rectal and esophago-jejunal anastomoses, there was hyperemia on the seventh postoperative day. This hyperemia diminished after 5 weeks in the esophago-jejunal anastomoses. Studies on esophageal transection after 4½ months showed no hyperemia at all, indicating the end of the healing process. There was, however, no difference in the stapled and manually sutured groups. To evaluate anastomotic circulation during the most important time—directly postoperatively—further experimental studies are needed.

CONCLUSIONS

Except for being faster, the stapled esophago-jejunostomy after total gastrectomy in pigs is equal to the manually sutured procedure with reference to leakage frequency, anastomotic index, breaking strength, and blood flow 1 and 5 weeks after resection. In colo-rectal anastomoses, one-layer and stapled anastomoses are equal; both are superior to the two-layer technique. In esophageal transection, there is a high frequency of strictures with all methods. The risk of narrowing, therefore, seems to depend more on the organ anastomosed than on the anastomotic method used.

ACKNOWLEDGEMENTS

This article is based on our clinical and experimental work in the field of gastro-intestinal anastomoses, and was in part previously published.[8,16,17] I am indebted to all patients, co-authors, and experimental animals.

REFERENCES

1. Lygidakis NJ: Total gastrectomy for gastric carcinoma: a retrospective study of different procedures and assessment of a new technique of gastric reconstruction. Br J Surg 68:649–655, 1981.
2. Brennan SS, Pickford IR, Evans M, Pollock AV: Staples or sutures for colonic anastomoses—a controlled clinical trial. Br J Surg 69:722–724, 1982.
3. Beart RW, Kelly KA: Randomized prospective evaluation of the EEA stapler for colo-rectal anastomoses. Am J Surg 141:143–146, 1981.
4. Everett WG, Friend PJ, Forty J. Comparison of stapling and hand-suture for left-sided large bowel anastomosis. Br J Surg 73:345–348, 1986.
5. McGinn FP, Gartell PC, Clifford PC, Brunton FJ: Staples or sutures for low colo-rectal anastomosis: a prospective randomized trial. Br J Surg 72:603–605, 1985.
6. Löwenhielm P: Dynamic stain tolerance of blood vessel at different postmortem conditions. Journal of Bioengineering 2:509–515, 1978.
7. Hafström LO, Persson B, Sundqvist K: Measurements of cardiac output and organ blood flow in rats using 99Tcm-labelled microspheres. Acta Physiol Scand 106:123–128, 1979.
8. Walther B, Oscarson J, Graffner H, Vallgren S, Evander A: Esophago-jejunostomy with the EEA stapler. Surgery 99:598–603, 1986.
9. Scher KS, Scott-Conner C, Jones CW, Leach M: A comparison of stapled and sutured anastomoses in colonic operations. Surg Gynecol Obstet 155:489–493, 1982.
10. Waxman BP: Large bowel anastomoses II The circular stapler. Br J Surg 70:64–67, 1983.
11. Viste A, Eide GE, Söreide O: Stomach cancer: a prospective study of anastomotic failure following total gastrectomy. Acta Chir Scand 153:303–306, 1987.
12. Wong J, Cheung H, Lui R, Fan YW, Smith A, Siu KF: Esophagogastric anastomosis performed with a stapler: the occurrence of leakage and stricture. Surgery 101:408–415, 1987.
13. West PN, Marbarger JP, Martz MN, Roper GL: Esophagogastrostomy with the EEA stapler. Ann Surg 193:76–81, 1981.
14. Fasth S, Hedlund H, Svaninger G, Hultén L: Autosuture of low colo-rectal anastomosis. Acta Chir Scand 148:535–539, 1982.
15. Saint JH, Mann F: Experimental surgery of the esophagus. Arch Surg 18:2324–2358, 1929.
16. Walther B, Löwenhielm P, Strand S-E, et al: Healing of esophago-jejunal anastomoses after experimental total gastrectomy. A comparative study using manually sutured or stapled anastomoses. Ann Surg 203:439–446, 1986.
17. Graffner H, Andersson L, Löwenhielm P, Walther B: The healing process of anastomoses of the colon. A comparative study using single, double-layer of stapled anastomosis. Dis Colon Rectum 27:767–771, 1984.

CHAPTER 12

SUTURES VS. STAPLES IN GASTRO-INTESTINAL ANASTOMOSES

Jacqueline Ritchie, J. McGregor, D.J. Galloway, W.D. George, I. Morrice, B. Sugden, A. Munro, G. Bell, and J. Logie

Despite the wide availability of surgical stapling instruments, their use for gastro-intestinal anastomoses is still surrounded by controversy for some surgeons who doubt that staples are as safe as hand-suturing methods, question the possible savings in operating time, and refuse to accept that the additional cost is balanced by other benefits that reduce overall hospital costs.

This report presents the interim findings of a prospective, randomized, controlled comparison of the two methods in both elective and emergency operations. Five-hundred-and-ninety-eight patients from four surgical units were randomized in the operative theater to have either manually sutured (301) or stapled (297) gastro-intestinal anastomoses. Both groups were comparable with regard to age and sex.

Preoperatively, various data were collected as they related to the patients' nutritional status. Details of weight loss, hemogram, albumin, transferrin, and leucocyte ascorbic acid were all recorded. Bowel preparation was standardized. All patients were given the same anti-microbial prophylaxis unless contra-indicated by, for instance, allergic reactions or poor renal function. The randomization process took place in the operating room, once the surgeon was satisfied that either suturing or stapling would be suitable.

The techniques and materials used for sutured anastomoses were as follows:

Esophagus: single-layer, interrupted, non-absorbable suture material

Upper gastro-intestinal tract: two layers, both of absorbable material

Small bowel: one or two layers, depending on the surgeon's preference

Large bowel: single-layer, interrupted, non-absorbable sutures

During the operation, a record was kept of the total operating time, the anastomosis time, the site and type of anastomosis, and the materials used to construct it. Any surgical complications during the operation were noted. Postoperatively, the patients were monitored until discharge and various data were collected with regard to recovery. Blood counts and bilirubin were regularly checked; a note was made of the number of days it took for oral intake to first exceed 1 l, as well as of the day of each patient's first bowel movement. Many patients (244) underwent radiologic examination of their anastomosis, and any evidence of a clinical leak was recorded. Details were kept of chest, wound, and urinary tract infections, as well as of other indicators of sepsis.

RESULTS

A total of 598 patients were randomized, 301 with manual sutures and 297 with staples. These two groups were further subdivided according to the site of the anastomosis, as shown in Table 12-1.

Differences in operating times were statistically significant in the gastric/esophageal and colonic groups ($p < 0.01$) and in the colo-rectal group ($p < 0.05$). The anastomosis time was also significantly reduced in all stapled groups, but the differences in the clinical leak rates, which favored staples, failed to

Table 12-1. Results in 598 Patients Undergoing Either Stapled or Sutured Anastomosis, By Operative Site

Site and Patient Breakdown	Anastomosis Time (min)	Operating Time (min)	Clinical Leaks	X-Ray Leaks
Esophageal				
Staples 10	25.9 ± 3.4	210.3 ± 13.9	0	0
Sutures 11	49.5 ± 3.9*	219.3 ± 13.3	0	1
Gastric/enteric				
Staples 98	7.1 ± 0.6	81.3 ± 3.4	6	0
Sutures 107	19.5 ± 1.3†	99.6 ± 5.4**	3	0
Colonic				
Staples 115	8.4 ± 0.5	89.4 ± 3.1	2	2
Sutures 116	20.5 ± 0.9†	104.6 ± 3.4*	8	0
Colo-rectal				
Staples 65	18.6 ± 1.3	124.2 ± 5.2	2	2
Sutures 76	30.6 ± 1.7†	139.8 ± 5.2**	6	8

* $p < 0.01$
† $p < 0.001$ (Mann-Whitney test)
** $p < 0.05$

Table 12-2. Leakage, by Clinical and Radiologic Detectability

Detectability	Elective Surgery	Semi-Elective and Emergency Surgery
Clinical		
Stapled	8	2
Sutured	12	5
Radiologic		
Stapled	4	0
Sutured	8	1

reach statistical significance ($p < 0.07$). There were no significant differences in duration of hospital stay.

COMPLICATIONS

Of the 40 anastomotic leaks recorded, 27 were clinically evident and 13 were seen by x-ray examination only. A total of 244 radiologic investigations were carried out, as shown in Table 12-2. There were 3 significant upper GI hemorrhages, all occurring from stapled anastomoses, and 41 deaths in the immediate

Table 12-3. Results in 123 Emergency or Semi-Elective Anastomoses, By Operative Site

Site and Patient Breakdown	Anastomosis Time (min)	Operating Time (min)	Clinical Leaks	X-Ray Leaks
Gastric				
Sutured 11	17.4 ± 2.8*	73.4 ± 10.1	0	0
Stapled 7	5.7 ± 1.3	59.8 ± 9.6	0	0
Small bowel				
Sutured 18	27.3 ± 6.6†	106.7 ± 9.3*	1	0
Stapled 14	7.9 ± 1.8	85.1 ± 13.0	1	0
Large bowel				
Sutured 38	22.2 ± 1.8†	113.2 ± 7.7	3	1
Stapled 35	7.9 ± 0.7	100.9 ± 5.9	1	0

* $p < 0.05$
† $p < 0.001$ (Mann-Whitney test)

postoperative period, 6 of which were associated with clinical leaks and 1 with a radiologic leak.

CONCLUSIONS

The results of this study show significant differences in the anastomosis times between the two groups, a significantly reduced total operating time at certain sites using staples, and fewer clinical leaks in the stapled colonic/colo-rectal group, although this is not statistically significant.

STAPLING IN EMERGENCY GASTRO-INTESTINAL SURGERY

The following results are separately considered within the broader prospectively randomized, controlled study. One-hundred-and-five patients undergoing emergency (64) or semi-elective (41) gastro-intestinal resections were randomized in the operating room to have either a sutured (60) or stapled (45) anastomosis. There were 123 anastomoses constructed: 18 gastric, 32 small bowel, and 73 large bowel anastomoses. At operation the anastomosis time, site, and type were recorded, as were the materials used and the total operating time (Table 12-3).

Our results indicate that anastomosis times at all sites are significantly reduced with staples, but despite a reduction in overall time this is only statistically significant in the small bowel group (using the Mann-Whitney test). There were a total of 6 clinical leaks (5.7%), 4 in the sutured group and 2 in the stapled group.

Seventy-four of the anastomoses were carried out or supervised by consultants; the remaining 49 were done by registrars. Of the 6 clinical leaks, 3 occurred in procedures performed by consultants and 3 in procedures performed by registrars.

In conclusion, staples may be safely employed in emergency gastro-intestinal surgery with a significant reduction in anastomosis time and no obvious risk of complications (Table 12-3).

CHAPTER 13

A CONTROLLED RANDOMIZED STUDY TO COMPARE STAPLING AND MANUAL TECHNIQUES OF ESOPHAGO-JEJUNOSTOMY AFTER TOTAL GASTRECTOMY

Andreas Schmidt-Matthiesen, Rainer M. Seufert, and Peter A. Beyer

In operations on the stomach, small intestine, and large bowel, stapling instruments have found increasing acceptance, such as in esophago-jejunostomy after total gastrectomy for cancer. While a significant body of studies comparing manual and mechanical anastomoses in the GI tract has become available, to date no prospective randomized study has been accomplished that compares manual and mechanical suture techniques in esophago-jejunostomy after radical gastrectomy.

METHODS AND CLINICAL EXPERIENCE

All surgeons participating in the study had gained equal expertise in the use of the circular anastomosing EEA instrument and were established experts in manual suturing techniques. Since the start of this study, 80 patients who had consecutively undergone total gastrectomy for carcinoma have been entered into a preplanned, blind, randomized clinical trial. At the time of this writing, several patients are still hospitalized; the study therefore includes only the first 60 patients, randomly divided into two groups of 30 patients each. These patients were comparable in age, associated diseases, tumor histology, and staging, as well as in sex distribution (Tables 13-1, 13-2). The operative procedure was similar in both groups and consisted of a total gastrectomy with lymph node dissection of compartment 2 and portions (hepato-duodenal ligament and liver hilus) of compartment 3. In addition, the lesser and greater omenta were resected and splenectomy was performed, with the exception of operations for distal prepyloric carcinoma of the intestinal type.

Depending on local spread of the tumor to adjacent organs, extended operations were performed that are comparable in numbers and importance in both groups (Table 13-3). The esophagus was anastomosed to a Roux-en-Y jejunal loop in one layer with resorbable (polyglyconate) monofilament sutures or with the use of the curved EEA-25 stapler. All other sutures employed in the construction of the Roux-en-Y loop were accomplished with the use of the TA-55-3.5 and GIA instruments. Factors specifically monitored during the study were duration of the operation, technical intra-operative problems, and postoperative course. The results were statistically analyzed using the Median-Quartil system, the U-test of Wilcoxen, and the chi^2 test analysis.

The median duration of operation of 172 minutes in the staple group was shorter than that in the manual group (median 190 minutes). However, this difference was not statistically significant, mainly because of a slightly higher frequency of extended operations in the manual suture group. Sample probing of the duration of anastomosis showed only a minimal saving of time with the use of the staplers. In three patients

Table 13-1. Patient Groups

Patient Characteristic	Stapling Group	Manual Group	Totals
Males	18 (60%)	14 (46.7%)	32 (53%)
Females	12 (40%)	15 (26.7%)	28 (47%)
Median age	59 (25–78)	60 (42–74)	59.5 (25–78)
Non-related preoperative disease	10 (33.3%)	10 (33.3%)	20 (33.3%)
History of previous operations	7 (23.3%)	10 (33.3%)	17 (28.3%)
Previous operations in stapled group		*Previous operations in manual group*	
Appendectomy		Appendectomy	
Cholecystectomy		Cholecystectomy	
Colon-resection (Ca)		Hysterectomy	
Ovarian (Ca)		Billroth-II (ulcer)	
Billroth II (Ca/benign)			
Cysto-jejunostomy (pancreas)			

with stapled anastomosis, untoward events occurred. On two occasions, the examination of anastomotic integrity showed a small leak that had to be oversewn by hand. In a third patient, a technical deficiency of the special purse-string instrument produced a longitudinal split in the esophageal stump; the surgeon decided to resect the esophagus proximally to a safe level and accomplish a hand-sewn anastomosis. Postoperatively, these three patients did not suffer any consequences related to these intra-operative complications. In the manual suture group, no intraoperative technical problems were noted. Again, this difference between anastomotic techniques during the operation was not statistically significant (Table 13-4).

Postoperative complications were also not statistically significant between the two groups. In 1 patient (1.66%) of the stapling group an anastomotic leak was noticed on the fifth postoperative day. This leak healed completely, without the need for reoperation. In 1 patient (1.66%) in the manually sutured group, a temporary anastomotic stricture regressed spontaneously 5 weeks after operation. One patient (1.66%) in the staple group died 1 week after operation from a postoperative myocardial infarction. At the time of autopsy, the anastomosis was intact. A total of 4 pa-

tients (6.7%) required re-laparotomy. In 2 patients in the stapling group, re-laparotomy became necessary to achieve hemostasis of the operative field; 1 patient had to undergo operation for intestinal obstruction. One patient in the hand-sewn group required three operations for drainage of intra-abdominal abscess. None of these complications appeared to be directly related to the individual anastomotic technique (Table 13-4).

All other complications ranged from thrombophlebitis to lymphatic fistula to pure pulmonary complications, which were all brought under control with non-operative means.

The median postoperative hospital stay was 16 days in the stapled group and 17 days in the manually sutured group, with a range of 8 to 92 days.

DISCUSSION

The purported advantage of stapling techniques (e.g., speed, safety, and diminished incidence of

Table 13-2. Histology

Condition	Stapled Group	Manual Group	Totals
Lymphoma	3 (10%)	2 (6.7%)	5 (8.3%)
Carcinoma	27 (90%)	28 (93.3%)	55 (91.7%)
Intestinal	10 (33.3%)	13 (43.3%)	23 (38.3%)
Diffuse	15 (50%)	14 (46.7%)	29 (48.3%)
Mixed	2 (6.7%)	1 (3.3%)	3 (5%)

Table 13-3. Operations

Operation	Stapled Group	Manual Group	Totals
Potentially curative	23 (76.6%)	15 (50%)	38 (63.3%)
Splenectomy operation	20 (66.6%)	20 (66.6%)	40 (66.6%)
Extended	5 (16.7%)	7 (20%)	11 (18.3%)

In Stapled Group	*In Manual Group*
Pancreatic capsule (2×)	Pancreatic capsule (2×)
Mesocolon	Tail of pancreas
Tail of pancreas	Liver
Small bowel	Diaphragm
	Mesocolon
	Adrenal gland

Table 13-4. Clinical Study Comparing Stapling and Manual Techniques in Esophago-jejunostomy

INTRA-OPERATIVE OBSERVATIONS			POSTOPERATIVE OBSERVATIONS		
Recorded Data	Stapled (n = 30)	Manual (n = 30)	Recorded Data	Stapled (n = 30)	Manual (n = 30)
Total operation time (min)	172	190	Anastomotic leak	1	0
Detected primary leakage (oversewn)	2	0	Death (cardiac infarction)	1	0
			Anastomotic bleeding	0	0
Defective suture with ASP-50 (purse-string) suture	1	N/A	Anastomotic stricture	0	1 (transient)
Anastomotic bleeding	0	0	General complications	16	15
Extension of operation	5	7	Re-laparotomy	3	1
			Hospital stay (days)	16	17
No statistically significant differences			*No statistically significant differences*		

complication with a reduced hospital stay) were not confirmed in a statistically significant manner by this study. For surgeons equally well trained and competent in stapling and manual techniques in the creation of an esophago-jejunostomy, both methods offer a comparable level of satisfaction to the surgeon and safety to the patient. From this study it appears that the incidence of postoperative complications relates more to the extensive lymph-adenectomy required by the treatment of carcinoma of the stomach than to the specific technique of anastomosis. Although we were unable to confirm the premise that the use of stapling instruments resulted in a superior esophago-jejunostomy, the use of these instruments does result in a much higher cost (DM 600.00) to the patient.

In spite of this it does not appear sinful to us to continue the use of stapling in well defined instances: increasing experience in the handling of these instruments, and of the anastomoses that can be accomplished with them, allows the surgeon to extend the operative procedure in the upper GI tract and to facilitate preservation of bowel continuity in operations for low rectal carcinoma. The EEA instrument helps the experienced surgeon to perform an intrathoracic esophago-jejunostomy through an abdominal approach without the need for thoracotomy. This appears to us to be a real advance in treating patients with carcinoma of the stomach that extends into the lower esophagus.

Translated from the German by F.M. Steichen, M.D.

BIBLIOGRAPHY

1. Bittner R, Butters M, Roscher R, Beger HG: Oesophago-Jejunostomie—wie sicher ist die Handnaht heute? Chirurg 58:43–45, 1987.
2. Eigler FW, Albrecht KH: Einhüllende Oesophago-Jejunostomie im Rahmen der Gastrektomie. Chirurg 58:47–49, 1987.
3. Günther B, Koller J: Indikation und Stellenwert maschineller Anastomosen am oberen Gastrointestinaltrakt. Chirurg 56:216–219, 1985.
4. Hansen, Sommer HJ, Eichelkraut W: Die Durchblutung handgenähter und geklammerter Colonanastomosen. Langenbecks Arch Chir 370:141–151, 1987.
5. Hollender LF, Meyer Ch, Keller D: Magenersatzbildung in Frankreich. Med Welt 33:254–260, 1982.
6. Junginger Th, Walgenbach S, Pichlmaier H: Die zirkuläre Klammeranastomose (EEA) nach Gastrektomie. Chirurg 54:161–165, 1983.
7. Junginger Th: Kommentar zu Bittner R et al. (siehe Literaturzitat 1). Chirurg 58:46, 1987.
8. Peiper HJ, Siewert R: Magenersatz. Chirurg 49:81–87, 1978.
9. Siewert R, Meyer H, Peiper HJ: Klinische Ergebnisse der Oesophago-Jejunoplicatio. Langenbecks Arch Chir 343:45–52, 1976.
10. Thiede A, Fuchs KH, Hamelmann H: Klammernahtgeräte zur Rekonstruktion eines Ersatzmagens. Chir Gastroenterol 2:67–75, 1986.
11. Thiede A, Schubert G, Poser HL, Jostarndt L, Hamelmann H: Ergebnisse einer kontrollierten Studie maschineller und manueller Rektumanastomosen nach Rektumresektion. In: Ulrich B, Winter J (Hrsg): Klammernahttechnik in Thorax und Abdomen. Stuttgart: Enke, 1986:159–175.
12. Ulrich B, Kochel N: Maschinelle Oesophagusanastomosen. Chir Gastroenterol 2:47–60, 1986.
13. Walther B, Löwenhjelm P, Strand ST, et al: Healing of esophago-jejunal anastomoses after experimental total gastrectomy. Ann Surg 203:439–444, 1986.

CHAPTER 14

ANTERIOR RESECTION WITH EEA STAPLER AND MANUAL SUTURES: COMPARISON OF TWO PATIENT GROUPS

Yu Dehong, Tu Yue, Chen Qinglan, Jin Guoxiang, Meng Ronggui, and Chen Libing

From 1959 to 1986, we treated 137 patients with rectal cancer by anterior resection. Fifty-three anastomoses were accomplished by manual sutures (suture group), and 84 with the EEA stapling instrument (EEA group).

PATIENTS' CHARACTERISTICS

The age of the patients ranged from 18 to 81 years, most being between 40 and 50 years old. In the EEA group, there were 49 male and 35 female patients; in the suture group, 32 were male and 21 were female patients. Table 14-1 shows the location of the rectal carcinomas; in Tables 14-2 and 14-3, Dukes' classification and pathologic features of each group have been listed. In 47 patients, the anastomotic site was located above the peritoneal reflection; in the remaining 90 cases it was extraperitoneal.

RESULTS

There were no operative deaths in either group. In the EEA group, 31 patients survived over 5 years. Fifteen were still alive in 1988, including an 80-year-old man who has survived for 6 years. Twelve patients died within 5 years, 4 of whom had palliative resection because of hepatic metastases. One patient in this group was lost to follow-up. In the suture group, 32 patients have survived 5 years. Twenty of these were alive in 1988. Eleven died, including 1 who died 7 years after operation. One patient is lost to follow-up.

Forty-one patients in the EEA group and 21 patients in the manually sutured group died of various causes (including cancer within 5 years for the sutured group) in the follow-up period. The total 5-year survival rate of the group of patients receiving radical resection for cure is 65% (39/60). There is no significant difference between the two groups (EEA group: 66.7%, suture group: 63.6%; p > 0.05).

Tumor cells were found at the end of the resected rectum in 12 patients. All of these patients belonged to the suture group. Eight of them had a palliative resection because of tumor spread to the liver or to the abdominal cavity: they all died within the first year after operation. The remaining 4 had radical anterior resection. A completion Miles' abdomino-perineal resection was applied to 2 of the 4 patients within 2 months of the initial operation: they have survived for 16 and 2 years respectively. No recurrence was found during these periods. One patient underwent radiotherapy and has survived for 5 years. The fourth patient was lost to follow-up.

Anastomotic leakage was found in 5 patients, 4 in the EEA group and 1 in the suture group. Three of them responded to non-operative therapy, while the remaining 2 had to undergo temporary colostomy. Five patients experienced local recurrence (3.65%). The recurrence was usually found in the first or second year postoperatively.

In the EEA group of 3 patients with recurrence, Miles' operation was performed in 1 patient, who survived for 15 months. The remaining 2 patients died in

Table 14-1. Distance from Lower Margin of Tumor to Ano-Cutaneous Junction

Distance (cm)	EEA Group		Suture Group	
	No. of Patients	Percentage	No. of Patients	Percentage
6	8	5.84	0	0
7	8	5.84	1	0.73
8	16	11.68	13	9.49
9	7	5.11	6	4.38
10	11	8.03	3	2.19
11	2	1.46	6	4.38
12	10	7.30	4	2.92
12	22	16.06	20	14.60

the first year following palliative colostomy. In the suture group, 1 patient underwent Miles' operation; in the second patient, repeat low anterior resection was possible. They were both alive over a short period of follow-up (2 months and 15 months, respectively).

DISCUSSION

Anterior resection is an acceptable operation for patients with rectal cancer because it maintains normal bowel passage and continence, while satisfactory control of cancer is obtained. With the increasing use of the EEA stapler, rectal cancer at lower sites has become an indication for the operation; the length of the distal margin has become as short as 3 cm.[1] At the same time, however, surgeons have also begun to pay more and more attention to the complications of this procedure.

The 5-year survival rate of the anterior resection may be influenced by many factors: local recurrence is no doubt the most important of these. In the 3 patients with recurrence of the EEA group, 2 had a tumor margin 6 and 3 cm above the anal verge, of the Dukes B type. The other patient had a Dukes D lesion and underwent local resection of the tumor.

In the suture group, one patient with a high rectal cancer was found to have a malignant nodule at the anastomotic site in follow-up. This patient underwent another anterior resection with the EEA stapler. Another patient with a tumor of the middle part of the rectum had a recurrence 2 years after low anterior resection had been performed. He was treated with Miles' abdomino-perineal resection and radiotherapy. Both of these patients are alive and continue to be followed. According to these present data, we conclude that there were at least two patients whose recurrence may relate to insufficient resection of the distal rectum, but the numbers are too small to hold responsible a particular technique or the rationale that led to its use.

Anastomotic leakage is another serious complication. Because there is no peritoneal covering over the distal rectum, leakage after extraperitoneal resection is relatively common. As Dorricott reported, clinical leakage may develop in 6% of patients, and radiologic leakage rates may be as high as 20%.[2] In our series, there were four leaks in the EEA group and one in the suture group. All of these patients did not have peritonitis or sepsis and responded to non-operative therapy. The reason that the EEA group seems to be associated with a higher incidence of leakage is that it involved relatively lower anastomoses performed when we were still learning about stapling techniques, for all four leaks developed in the early stages of our using the stapler.

Two patients had incomplete dissection of the rectal stump involved in the staple line, and two had loss of vascular supply at the transected end of the colon.

Table 14-2. Dukes' Classification of 135 Patients*

Lesion	EEA Group		Suture Group	
	No. of Patients*	Percentage	No. of Patients	Percentage
Dukes A	14	10.37	10	7.41
Dukes B	28	20.74	21	15.56
Dukes C	35	25.93	20	14.81
Dukes D	5	3.70	2	1.48

* Two specimens were free of tumor: one following irradiation, and one after positive biopsy excision.

Table 14-3. Pathological Features in 137 Patients

Type	EEA Group		Suture Group	
	No. of Patients	Percentage	No. of Patients	Percentage
Adenocarcinoma	74	54.01	49	35.77
Muco-adenocarcinoma	9	6.57	4	2.92
Carcinoid	1	0.73	0	0.00

Preoperative radiotherapy in one of the four cases may also have played a detrimental role. To avoid anastomotic leakage, it is necessary to fully understand the functioning and use of the instrument. Precise dissection of the tumor, preservation of the vascular supply to the bowel ends involved in the staple lines, and careful check of the completed anastomosis[3] are of great value. We do not use air inflation or sigmoidoscopy as proposed by Smith after stapling,[4] as they may result in tearing of the anastomosis.

We think the distal margin must be at least 3 cm, and that it should be measured under slight tension during operation.[5] The use of the EEA stapler makes this easier than it is with manual sutures, especially in the very low anterior resection. Seventeen patients in our series had tumors 6 to 7 cm from the anal verge. Sixteen of them had the anastomosis made with the stapler placing the anastomotic site some 2 to 3 cm from the anal verge. On the other hand, four patients who had radical anterior resection with manually sutured anastomoses were not tumor-free at the resected end of the rectum. Adloff compared the use of EEA stapler and manual sutures in colo-rectal anastomosis.[6] He believes that the EEA stapler can accomplish a secure anastomosis and that leakage, should it occur, can be treated non-operatively in most instances.

In the constant follow-up of our patients, we found that stapled anastomotic sites were generally smooth, with minimal inflammation around them. It can therefore be expected that fewer complications will be associated with the stapling procedure as experience in using the EEA stapler is accumulated.

We conclude from our experience that the location of the tumor should be carefully evaluated to reduce the rate of complications. It is also important to measure tumor size, its depth of penetration, and the size of the patient's pelvis. Only if anterior resection (either with the EEA stapler or with manual sutures) is properly employed can we expect better survival rates and improved quality of life for our patients.

REFERENCES

1. Heberer G, Denecke H, Pratschke E, Teichman R: Anterior and low anterior resection. World J Surg 6:517, 1982.
2. Dorricott NJ, Braddley RM, Keighly MRB, et al: Complications of rectal anastomoses with end-to-end anastomosis (EEA) stapling instrument. Ann R Coll Surg Eng 64:171, 1982.
3. Yu Dehong, Tu Yue, Jin Guoxiang, Meng Ronggiu: Anterior resection with GF-1 stapler for rectal carcinoma. Surgical Rounds 10(9):73–85, 1987.
4. Smith LE: Anastomosis with EEA stapler after anterior colonic resection. Dis Colon Rectum 24:236–242, 1981.
5. Knight CD, Griffen FD: Techniques of low rectal reconstruction. Curr Probl Surg 20:391–456, 1983.
6. Adloff M, Arnaud J-P, Belarry S: Stapled vs. sutured colorectal anastomosis. Arch Surg 115:1436, 1980.

Part IV

Healing of Irradiated and Stapled Tissues of Rectum and Anus

THE EFFECT OF STAPLING RECONSTRUCTION OF THE RADIATED RECTUM ON SPHINCTER PRESERVATION

Scott D. Goldstein, Stefano Valabrega, Luca Pecchioli, and Maryalice Cheney

Sphincter preservation surgery for cancer of the distal rectum is recognized as being associated with a high incidence of local recurrence. By conventional standards, abdomino-perineal resection and permanent colostomy appear to be the only prudent choice. High-dose preoperative radiation therapy is being utilized with a variety of new surgical techniques in an attempt to widen the scope of sphincter preservation and to reduce the incidence of local recurrence in selected patients with cancer of the distal rectum. The objective of this study was to test the ability of radiated tissue to handle surgical staples in the distal rectum. A double-staple technique of anastomosis, as reported by Knight and Griffen in 1980,[1] was utilized.

MATERIALS AND METHODS

Patients

There were 16 patients ranging in age from 40 to 76 years, with a mean age of 60. Eight were men and 8 were women. All received full-dose preoperative radiation therapy. A minimum dose of 4000 to 4500 cGy was delivered over approximately 41½ weeks, using 180 to 250 cGy per fraction. Patients with tumor fixation were given an additional boost of 1000 to 1500 cGy.

Operative intervention was carried out 4½ to 8 weeks following the completion of radiation therapy. Mean level of tumor from dentate line was 9 cm (range: 3 to 25 cm).

Surgical Technique

A standard operative approach was used by a single surgical team. Patients were positioned in the lithotomy position with the aid of Lloyd-Davies stirrups, providing access to the perineum. The abdomen was then entered. The rectum was mobilized, along with the left colon and splenic flexure. Only the proximal colon, which was not in the radiated field, was used for anastomosis. It should be noted that the proximal descending or distal transverse colon more easily accepts the largest (31-mm) EEA instrument.

It is our policy to "wash out" residual fecal debris or exfoliated tumor cells prior to transecting the rectum distal to the tumor. The newer roticulating TA instrument facilitates this procedure when working deep in the pelvis (Fig. 15-1). Following this, another roticulating TA is placed most distally, and the bowel is then transected (Fig. 15-2). A 31-mm EEA stapling instrument is next inserted transanally and the shaft is "poked through" the rectal wall adjacent to the TA staple line at its midpoint (Fig. 15-3). The head of the EEA instrument is attached and placed in the proximal bowel, the purse-strings are secured, and the EEA is fired. Gently rotating the stapling device after unwinding the approximating screw for two turns allows the instrument to be removed. The proximal and distal "doughnuts" were inspected in all cases. All anastomoses were checked for gross leakage by the instillation of sterile water, darkened with Betadine, instilled trans-anally. Fifteen patients underwent protective loop stomas created prior to closure of the abdominal wall.

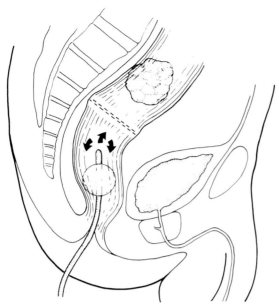

Fig. 15-1. Washing and flushing the rectum of residual fecal debris, by transanal catheter irrigation, after closing the rectum distal to the tumor with the roticulator.

RESULTS

Intra-operatively, complete proximal and distal doughnuts were retrieved in all patients. All anastomoses were evaluated approximately 5 weeks postop-

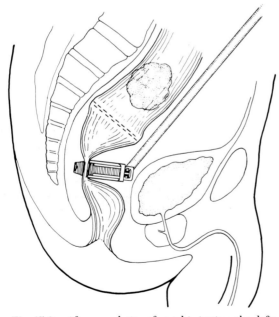

Fig. 15-2. After completion of rectal irrigation, the definitive rectal staple closure is placed as distally as is possible and required. The bowel is transected, proximal to this instrument.

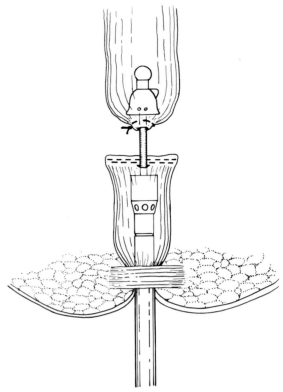

Fig. 15-3. Colo-rectal anastomosis, using the "double" stapling technique of Knight-Griffen, with intersection of the linear staple line by a circular anastomosing staple ring.

eratively. Water soluble contrast material was utilized for radiographic imaging, and sigmoidoscopic visualization was performed routinely. Neither extravasation of contrast material nor evidence of intraluminal purulence or fixed anastomotic strictures was observed. The 15 patients with diverting stomas underwent closure without incident.

DISCUSSION

With increasing interest in adjuvant preoperative radiation therapy and sphincter preservation, new techniques of anastomosis must be explored. The safety of performing very distal anastomoses in the rectum with surgical staples following radiation therapy has been questioned. Experimental animal models revealed high anastomotic leak rates following preoperative radiation. Schauer et al.[2] experienced a 10% clinical leak rate in dogs following 2000 cGy; Blake et al.[3] report a 25% leak rate after 6000 cGy; and Morgenstern et al.[4] found a 66% leak rate after 4000 cGy. Morgenstern concluded that "stapled anastomoses in irradiated colons are at severe risk of anastomotic dehiscence and, therefore, should be protected with a proximal colostomy." In human clinical trials, Roberson et al.[5] found no anastomotic complications following 4500 cGy preoperatively with EEA colo-rectal anastomosis in 17 patients. Feinberg et al.[6] utilized a double-staple technique of anastomosis following 3500 cGy without incident in 14 patients.

Our interest in testing a double-staple anastomosis stems from the problems inherent to the radiated bowel. Radiation injury results in a progressive endarteritis, with ischemia as the hallmark in the chronic stage of the process. The ideal suture material has yet to be determined, although stainless steel remains the least reactive material available. The B-formation of the staples results in less tissue ischemia and trauma. Uniform suture placement should be an advantage as well. The discouraging anastomotic results found in animal models would appear to be a clear deterrent to the use of surgical staples in patients following radiation therapy.

However, based upon the 31 patients found in the literature and the additional 16 presented herein, a total of 47 stapled anastomoses in the distal rectum following full-dose preoperative radiation therapy were achieved without anastomotic complications. Armed with this information, we feel that we have the ethical license to continue utilizing and promoting this form of anastomosis.

CONCLUSIONS

As a result of this preliminary study, we conclude that a double-stapled anastomosis should be considered a safe and reasonable option. The question of the necessity for protective colostomy remains unanswered.

REFERENCES

1. Knight D, Griffen FD: An improved technique for low anterior resection of the rectum using the EEA stapler. Surgery 88:710–714, 1980.
2. Schauer RM, Bubrick MP, et al: Effects of low-dose preoperative irradiation on low anterior anastomosis in dogs. Dis Colon Rectum 25(5):401–405, 1982.
3. Blake DP, Bubrick MP, et al: Low anterior anastomotic dehiscence following preoperative irradiation with 6000 rads. Dis Colon Rectum 27(3):176–181, 1984.
4. Morgenstern L, Sanders G, et al: Effect of preoperative irridation on healing of low colorectal anastomoses. Am J Surg 147:245–249, 1984.
5. Roberson SH, Heron HC, et al: Is anterior resection of the rectosigmoid safe after preoperative radiation? Dis Colon Rectum 28(4):254–259, 1985.
6. Feinberg SM, Parker F, Cohen Z, et al: The double stapling technique for low anterior resection of rectal carcinoma. Dis Colon Rectum 23(12):885–890, 1985.

CHAPTER 16

STAPLED COLO-ANAL ANASTOMOSIS AFTER RESECTION OF THE IRRADIATED RECTUM

C. Gouillat, Ph. Bérard, and F.M.D. Gaujoux

Colo-anal anastomosis will cautiously find an increasing field of application in the management of rectal carcinoma. Preoperative radiation therapy has merit in reducing bulky tumors and sterilizing surrounding dissection planes, and therefore diminishes the incidence of local tumor recurrence.

However, many surgeons have been reluctant to perform restorative operations after preoperative radiation; so far, stapling has been rarely used in the construction of colo-anal anastomoses.

The aim of this study is to evaluate the feasibility, safety, and functional results of circular stapled colo-anal anastomosis in patients with preoperative radiation therapy.

PATIENTS AND METHODS

Operative Technique

The patient is placed in the combined lithotomy-Trendelenburg position. The pelvic and rectal dissection is carried down to the levator muscles in the usual way for low rectal carcinoma. The rectum is pulled sharply upward and incised anteriorly at the level of the pelvic diaphragm.

From above, a hand-sewn purse-string suture is started over the anterior edge of the ano-rectal stump and continued laterally and posteriorly as circumferential transection of the stump progresses. The index finger held in the anal canal from below facilitates a good view of the whole wall of the ano-rectal remnant (Fig. 16-1). A lightening retractor is very helpful in assessing the distal margin of tumor clearance.

The left colon and the splenic flexure must usually be mobilized. If suitable, a colon reservoir is fashioned after resection of the specimen, and the EEA stapler without the anvil is introduced from above through the open colon (side-to-end anastomosis) or through a proximal colotomy (end-to-end anastomosis). In the case of side-to-end anastomosis, the central rod is brought through the anti-mesocolic wall, some 12 cm proximal to the open colon end. For an end-to-end anastomosis, a purse-string suture is placed over the rim of the proximal colon end. The loose ends of the distal purse-string suture and the rod of the stapler are placed into a rubber cuff to facilitate their downward progress in the anal canal (Fig. 16-2). The assistant removes the rubber cuff, ties the distal purse-string suture from below, and attaches the anvil. After tying the proximal purse-string, the stapler is closed and fired (Fig. 16-3). Thus is performed a safe anastomosis joining the colon to the whole wall of the anal canal, including the top of the internal and external sphincters (Figs. 16-3, 16-4). The anvil is detached from below, through the anus, by the assistant, and the EEA is removed from above. The double ring of tissue doughnut and the anastomosis are carefully inspected. A diverting colostomy is not mandatory. The pelvis is drained using two closed suction catheters.

Patients

From May 1984 to April 1988, this procedure was performed in 20 patients, 17 of them since October

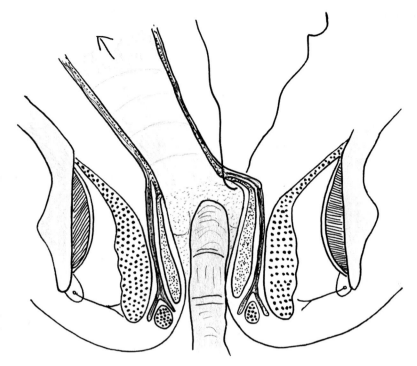

Fig. 16-1. Following dissection of the rectum to the level of the pelvic floor, the ano-rectal junction is exposed by pulling on the rectum. The ano-rectal segment is incised anteriorly, and a purse-string suture is started at this point and continued circumferentially as the ano-rectal ring is progressively transected. The index finger, placed from below and moved around the rim of the ano-rectal stump, facilitates the exposure of the bowel walls and placement of the purse-string stitches from above.

1986. Patients (16 men, 4 women) ranged in age from 31 to 78 years (m ± 1 SD = 62 ± 13). Seven patients were over 70 years old. All patients had a biopsy-proven adeno-carcinoma not suitable for local excision. The tumor was always palpable per anus and the mean distance from its lower border to the anal margin was 5.7 ± 1.2 cm (range: 4 to 8 cm). The tumor was adherent to the pelvic walls in 5 patients. All patients were first treated with preoperative radiation therapy (3000 to 3500 cGy) administered in 10 fractions over a 12-day period through a sacral field. Operation was performed 2 months later, when the reduction in tumor bulk is optimal.

RESULTS

Operative Course

The operative procedure was never disturbed by preoperative radiation. The mean duration of operation was 3 hours and 15 minutes (range: 2 to 5 hours), including additional procedures in some patients: cholecystectomy in 3, hysterectomy in 2, right colectomy in 1, and vagotomy-antrectomy in 1. A reservoir was made in 7 patients and a diverting colostomy in 11.

Postoperative Course

There was no hospital mortality. A diverting colostomy was performed in the early postoperative period in four patients. Three of them were thought to have a minor anastomotic leak. The third patient, who was 78 years old, had severe postoperative diarrhea with disturbing fecal incontinence. Two patients had prolonged urinary retention that responded to intermittent self-catheter-drainage. No pelvic sepsis was observed. The average postoperative hospital stay was 17 days (range: 11 to 27).

Pathological Findings

No evidence of residual tumor was demonstrated in seven operative specimens. According to Dukes' classification, the other specimens were tabulated as follows: stage A3, stage B6, and stage C4. The average length of normal rectum below the lower border of the resected tumors, measured on the fresh excised specimens was 2.5 ± 1.1 cm (range: 1.0 to 5.5 cm). Ano-rectal ring specimens of the circular staple device were free of tumor involvement in all patients and demonstrated anal squamous epithelium.

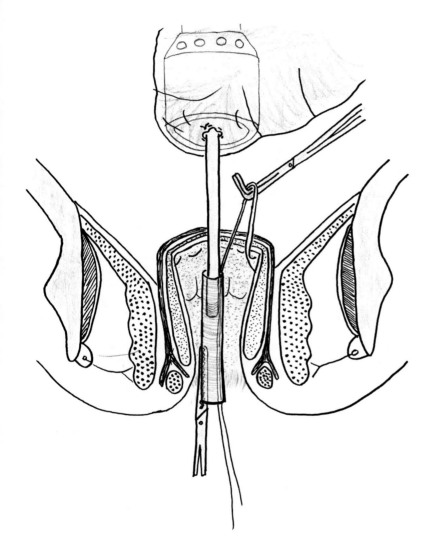

Fig. 16-2. Placement of the circular instrument into the proximal colon without anvil and tying of the proximal purse-string suture. The bare central rod and loose ends of the distal (ano-rectal) purse-string suture are then sheathed by a rubber cuff that facilitates the downward transanal progress of both. The assistant removes the protecting sheath.

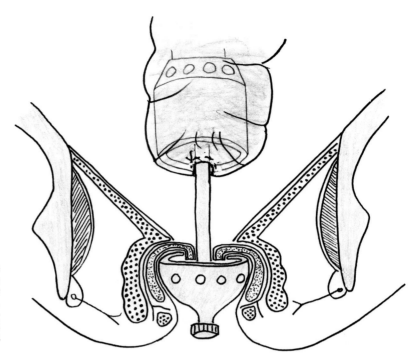

Fig. 16-3. The assistant ties the ano-rectal purse-string suture around the central rod transanally and attaches the anvil from below. The instrument is closed, approximating the proximal colon and anus, and is activated, creating a colo-anal anastomosis.

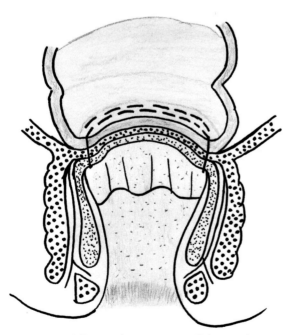

Fig. 16-4. Following disengagement of the circular stapling instrument, the anastomosis joining the colon to the entire wall of anal canal, including the top of the sphincter muscles, is inspected. The two tissue rings are examined to insure circular integrity.

Functional Results

Colostomy, if performed, was closed at an average of 3 ± 2 months (range: 1.5 to 7.5 months) after operation.

Functional results were assessed 2 months following resumption of bowel function.

Nineteen patients had a good result with an average of 2.5 ± 1.3 bowel movements per day (range: 1 to 5) without any particular diet or drugs. Defecation and continence were normal or near normal. Five of the 19 patients experienced incomplete evacuations.

Occasional gas leaks occurred in 11 patients, and occasional minor soiling in 9. These results were usually established at the time of hospital discharge. Only 3 patients needed an adaptive period of some weeks. At the late assessment, with a mean followup of 15 months, the functional result was maintained or improved in the 19 patients. No anastomotic stenosis occurred.

One patient, 78 years old, had a bad result. He had undergone a vagotomy-antrectomy for peptic ulcer in the same operation. After closure of the colostomy, he experienced an average of 8 bowel movements per day with major soiling. No improvement occurred. An anastomotic stenosis and several minor leaks were demonstrated and a permanent colostomy had to be performed 12 months after closure of the first colostomy.

CONCLUSIONS

Modifications in the mechanical anastomosing technique adapted to the ano-rectal and low pelvic anatomy facilitate circular stapling in the construction of a colo-anal anastomosis. The procedure is safe. Diverting colostomy is not mandatory and functional results are good.

Preoperative radiation therapy does not disturb the peri-operative course and is of value in reducing tumor bulk and risk of local recurrence in the overall management of low rectal carcinoma. So far, with a mean followup of 18 months (range: 6 to 48 months), no local recurrence has been observed in our series.

Part V

Morbidity and Mortality Associated with Stapling Procedures

STRICTURES IN ESOPHAGEAL ANASTOMOSES WITH MECHANICAL AND MANUAL SUTURES: A COMPARATIVE EXPERIMENTAL STUDY

P.A. Lehur and F. Gaillard

Anastomotic strictures following stapled circular esophageal anastomoses are a vexing complication.[1-5] Like those found in circular stapled colo-rectal anastomoses,[6] strictures occurring in the esophagus have no satisfactory explanation as to their physiologic cause and pathologic features.

CONTEMPORARY CLINICAL EXPERIENCE

The circular anastomosing instrument has found a wide field of application in esophageal surgery because of its reliability and its technical advantages in achieving a difficult anastomosis, which is at times impossible to accomplish by manual techniques.[2,5,7] The stapling method, however, is not free of complications: anastomotic strictures are among these. The incidence of strictures ranges from 1 to 15%, depending on the authors. These variations are explained by the following:

1. The anatomic conditions at the level of anastomosis (abdominal, thoracic, or cervical) and the organ that is anastomosed to the esophagus (stomach, jejunum, or colon). Each of these factors probably carries a specific risk of stricture.[4]
2. The modalities of diagnosis in the followup period: routine endoscopic or radiologic examinations (or both) as compared to a more selective approach, in which these examinations are only performed if clinical dysphagia appears.

In a recent study by Wong and his associates of their results in a series of 133 patients with esophageal resection and esophago-gastrostomy, a total of 18 patients developed an anastomotic stricture. These 133 patients were those who left the hospital with a patent anastomosis. Excluded from a large overall series were those patients who died in the early postoperative period or developed anastomotic leaks, fistulae, or both. Most strictures were observed before the fourth postoperative month, but some occurred as late as 1 year after the operation. Strictures were found in 8.7% of the 23 hand-sewn anastomoses, in 10% of the 60 patients in whom an ILS instrument was used, and in 20% of the 50 patients in whom the EEA was used (Table 17-1). The late occurrence of these strictures suggests excessive scar formation in those patients in whom cancer recurrence has been excluded. Wong also analysed the incidence of strictures as it relates to the caliber of the anastomosis and the type of circular instrument used (Table 17-2). Smaller cartridge sizes were found to have a higher incidence of stricture. With the use of the ILS instrument, the incidence of stricture was progressively reduced or eliminated as larger cartridges were employed, if the size of the esophagus permitted the placement of the 29- or 33-mm instruments.[5]

The incidence of esophageal strictures increases significantly—from 25 to 40%—in abdominal operations for control of bleeding esophageal varices with the use of the circular anastomosing instrument.[8,9] Structural changes due to the esophageal varices and

Table 17-1. Anastomotic Strictures in Intrathoracic Esophago-Gastrostomies Using Circular Anastomosing Instruments: Clinical Experience by Wong and Associates[5]

Measure	Total	Hand	ILS	EEA
Number	18/133	2/23	6/60	10/50
Percent	13.5	8.7	10	20

(174 patients underwent operation; 133 were discharged)

sclerotherapy may play an important role in the development of these strictures.

Whatever their cause, most if not all of these strictures are easy to treat by simple esophageal dilation. Usually, two dilatations at various time intervals are required to return the esophageal lumen to a normal caliber.[5,10]

FACTORS INFLUENCING ANASTOMOTIC HEALING

The type of suture material used is not the only factor responsible for the accounts of anastomotic stricture in esophageal surgery. Anastomotic leakage with formation of a fistula, collections of blood or lymph around the anastomosis, and gastro-esophageal reflux of acid or, more often, bilious-pancreatic secretions, most frequently observed in low intrathoracic anastomoses, are often equally responsible. Delayed strictures are also observed with postoperative radiotherapy or with enhancing chemotherapy.[2,3]

Factors more closely related to the anastomotic technique may be excessive dissection of the visceral ends, impairment of vascular supply to the longitudinal esophagus, and the substitute organ. This impairment can be arterial or can be caused by diminished venous drainage. Tension on the anastomotic line and local tissue trauma due to excessive manipulations are other factors.[4] In this respect, compression of tissues with the stapling instrument and forceful dilatation of the esophagus by a circular stapler of excessive caliber, with hidden lacerations of the submucosa, are all factors more specifically related to stapling techniques in general. To define the role played by circular stapling techniques only in the occurrence of anastomotic strictures, we undertook the following study.

EXPERIMENTAL DESIGN

Materials and Methods

Ten mongrel dogs, weighing 25 ± 4 kg, were prepared with a liquid diet for 48 hours and with prophylactic antibiotic therapy of penicillin (three doses). They underwent operation under general anesthesia and in sterile conditions. The cervical esophagus was exposed on the left, preserving the thyroid gland and recurrent laryngeal nerve. In five dogs (group I, 1–5), transection and circular anastomosis of the cervical esophagus was accomplished with the EEA-31 placed transorally and easily accepted by the canine esophageal caliber (Fig. 17-1). The single esophageal tissue doughnut was found to be complete in all cases. In a second group of five dogs (group II, A–E), the exposed cervical esophagus was transected and re-anastomosed by two running sutures of 3-0 polyglycolic acid in one layer. The cervical incisions were closed without drainage.

Following a postoperative recovery of 48 hours with intravenous hydration, the dogs were returned to their cages and given their normal diet by oral intake. The anastomoses were excised at 41 ± 6 days after the operation and were examined by direct inspection, radiologic contrast, and histologic studies. All gross specimens were photographed.[11]

Results

Postoperative Course and Radiologic Examination

The average weight loss in group I was 2.7 ± 0.2 kg, as compared to 0.4 ± 0.2 kg in group II. No anastomotic leaks were observed. A localized cervical abscess was found in dog II-B. Dysphagia with important regurgitation was observed in four dogs in group I, as compared to one dog in group II. These clinical findings correlated well with the radiologic examination demonstrating four strictures, two of which were advanced, in group I, as compared to two strictures (one advanced) in group II (Fig. 17-2). In four of the five stapled anastomoses, the double circle of staples was complete at the time of the excision of the anastomosis.

Anatomic and Histologic Examinations

The gross appearance of the two types of anastomosis was quite different. In the stapled group, the

Table 17-2. Clinical Study by Wong and Associates[5] Correlating Circular Stapler Size with Incidence of Strictures

Measure	EEA-25	EEA-28	EEA-31	ILS-25	ILS-29	ILS-33
Number	3/13	5/27	2/10	4/14	2/38	0/9
Percent	23	18	20	26	5	0

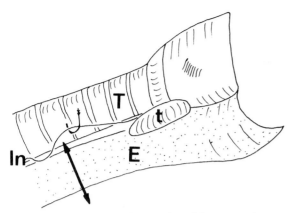

Fig. 17-1. Experimental surgical model. **T** = trachea, **E** = esophagus, **Ln** = recurrent laryngeal nerve, **t** = thyroid.

edges of the anastomosis protruded into the lumen with hypertrophy of the esophageal walls and with a variable number of staples visible in the esophageal lumen. The area of the manually sutured anastomoses was usually somewhat excavated or depressed, with a thinning of the esophageal wall. Inflammatory pseudo-polyps were observed at the borders of the scar in dogs I-4 and I-5 and in dogs II-A and II-D.

Squamous mucosa covered the anastomosis completely in three of the five dogs of group I, and large ulcers were observed in the two remaining dogs (I-2 and I-3). In group II, the coverage of the anastomosis

with regenerated mucosa was complete in all cases, although it was of uneven thickness. The healing and scar formation (Table 17-3) was different in each of the two types of anastomosis. The wider, fibrotic scar of the manual sutures showed minimal inflammation and joined the various constituent layers of the esophageal wall (Fig. 17-3A). The scar resulting from the stapled anastomosis was narrow and less uniform in its histologic architecture. Towards the open lumen, areas of inflammation and newly formed vessels were seen that created a type of protruding granulation. In-depth fibrosis was quite regular, containing but a few muscular fibers (Fig. 17-3B). Staples were recovered in 4 of the five dogs in group I. The staples were surrounded by a histiocytic reaction without macrophages, except in dog I-4, where a true abscess was observed (Fig. 17-4A). In group II, sutures were found in only two dogs, which confirms the rapid absorption of the suture material used. In these two animals the sutures were surrounded by a histiocytic reaction, with macrophages representing a classic foreign-body reaction (Fig. 17-4B).

DISCUSSION

Up to now, the experimental exploration of the long-term fate of stapled anastomosis is incomplete, since only two such studies concerned with the healing of colic and rectal anastomoses have been

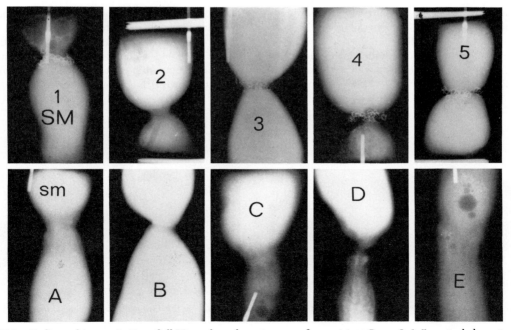

Fig. 17-2. Radiographic examination of all 10 esophageal anastomoses after excision. Group I, 1–5 = stapled anastomoses, group II, A–E = sutured anastomosis.

Table 17-3. Relative Degrees of Concentration and Duration of Histologic Findings

Finding	Group I: Circular EEA Stapled					Group II: Resorbable Hand-Sutured				
	1	2	3	4	5	A	B	C	D	E
Inflammatory reaction	+ +	+ +	+ +	+ + +	−	−	−	−	+	−
Neo-vascularity	+ +	+ +	+	+ + +	+	−	−	−	+	−
Muscular layers	−	−	+	+	−	−	−	−	−	+

Plus signs (+) indicate the relative degree of concentration and duration of the histologic finding; a negative sign (−) indicates average-to-low concentration and duration of the histologic finding

published.[10,11] No such study has been made of mechanical esophageal anastomoses. The development of a simple and reliable experimental model will allow the continued study of the physiology and pathology of healing in stapled anastomoses of the esophagus or colon and rectum.

The original experimental model described by us has several advantages:

1. It is technically simple, since the cervical approach avoids a thoracotomy.
2. The stapling instrument is easily placed through the mouth under direct laryngoscopic control.
3. The handling of the esophagus and the clearing of vessels from the anastomotic borders are minimal for both the stapling and manual techniques.
4. Anatomically, the canine esophagus is comparable to that of the human, although the caliber of the dog's esophagus is quite superior to the human's and, hence, the physiology of the swallowing act is also different.[12,13]
5. Preliminary anatomic studies have shown that the arterial supply to the dog's esophagus is similar to that in man[12,14]

6. The clear delineation of the operative procedure to a circular anastomosis only allows for the study of the healing process, at the exclusion of any other process that could be inherent in a more extensive operative procedure
7. The results obtained with this model demonstrate that anastomotic experimental strictures are observed after a postoperative period comparable to the one in man; this has so far not been possible at the level of the colon, where the only differences between stapling and manual sutures have been observed in the histologic examinations
8. The fact that the strictures were observed after the placement of manual sutures is in agreement with the observations made in the human group (2 to 10%)[1,3]

For these reasons we recommend this experimental model in the study of healing and scar formation after circular stapling anastomosis.

One objection could be the loss of a ring of tissue, albeit a small one, with the use of the circular instrument, as compared to the simple transection and reanastomosis with the manual sutures (which could

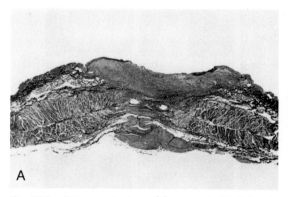 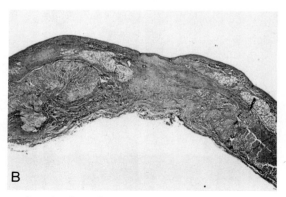

Fig. 17-3. Microscopic views of the scars. *A.* Stapled anastomosis in dog 3 (on the 48th postoperative day). There is mucosal ulceration opposite the site of a staple. In addition, the muscular layer is completely interrupted by a fibrotic cicatrix. *B.* Manual anastomosis in dog A (on the 41st postoperative day). The mucosal epithelium is completely regenerated. There is, however, the same complete interruption of the muscular layer by a fibrotic cicatrix.

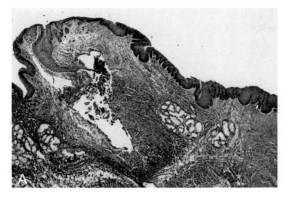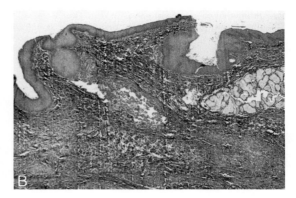

Fig. 17-4. Inflammatory reaction to the suture material. *A.* Stapled anastomosis on dog 4 (on the 48th postoperative day). A nonspecific inflammatory reaction with abscess formation is observed surrounding the passage of a staple. *B.* In a manual anastomosis in dog A (on the 41st postoperative day), there is a histiocytic reaction with macrophages of the foreign-body type surrounding a suture.

explain the greater incidence of strictures with the staplers). This loosely parallels the results observed in human operations.[8,9] Because of the small number of animal experiments, our results do not reach any statistical significance.

The histologic examination comparing scars of stapled anastomoses with those performed manually is important, since it allows a better understanding of the causes for postoperative strictures. The invagination of the esophageal walls with stapling was found to persist even at 40 days postoperatively, and distinguishes this technique from that of the manual suture, where the different layers of the esophageal wall are simply joined. This invagination of the wall rims at the level of the anastomosis is probably exaggerated by the usual healing and scar formation. It can therefore lead to a narrowing that forms a diaphragm at the level of the anastomoses, as has been observed in some of the low rectal anastomoses. Furthermore, the persistent delay in mucosal healing seen in two of our dogs could be implicated in the overall hypertrophy of the circumferential scar. Graffner and his associates have observed the same phenomenon in circular sutures of the colon examined 8 days postoperatively.[15]

Furthermore, the inflammatory reaction surrounding individual staples that we observed has already been described in a previous study of the colon by Malay and his associates, where the long-term (6 months) presence of this inflammatory reaction was particularly impressive. This finding was also observed in stapling of the esophagus where the healing and scarring of the anastomosis was prolonged in its evolution, as compared to the manual sutures, where the healing and scarring became stable in a much shorter time. It is possible that the foci of inflammation surrounding the staples, which remain for a long

time in the tissues, heal by fibrosis and are responsible for the stricture formation. Although metal staples are usually well tolerated by the tissues, the simple prolonged presence of a foreign body with smoldering inflammation may be a deciding factor.

Translated from the French by F.M. Steichen, M.D.

REFERENCES

1. Descottes B: Les procédés de suture automatique sont-ils source de complications réelles? In: Les cancers de l'oesophage en 1984—135 questions. Paris: Maloine, 1985:275–276.
2. Fekete F, Breil Ph: Utilisation des sutures mécaniques dans la chirurgie de l'oesophage (200 anastomoses). Actualités Chirurgicales Masson (Paris) 1:170–173, 1984.
3. Peracchia A, Tremolada C: Anastomose oesophagienne intrathoracique: fistules et sténoses (anastomose manuelle versus anastomose mécanique). Actualités Chirurgicales Masson (Paris) 1:41–50, 1985.
4. Richelme H, Baulieux J: Le traitement des cancers de l'oesophage. Monographie de l'A.F.C. Paris: Masson, 1986:120–121.
5. Wong J, Cheung H, Lui R, et al: Esophagogastric anastomosis performed with a stapler: the occurrence of leakage and stricture. Surgery 101:408–413, 1987.
6. Waxman BP: Large bowel anastomosis II: the circular staplers. Br J Surg 70:64–67, 1983.
7. Steichen FM, Ravitch MM: Stapling in Surgery. Chicago: Year Book, 1984:232–233.
8. Johnston GW: Bleeding oesophageal varices: the management of shunt rejects. Ann R Coll Surg Engl 63:3–8, 1981.
9. Peracchia A, Ancona E, Battaglia G: Dévascularisation oeso-gastrique avec transsection mécanique de l'oesophage par voie abdominale. Encycl Méd Chir (Paris), Techn Chir App Dig 40999, 6:39–40.
10. Buchmann P, Schneider K, Gebbers J: Fibrosis of ex-

perimental colonic anastomosis in dogs after EEA stapling or suturing. Dis Colon Rectum 26:217–220, 1983.

11. Malvy P, Visset J, Lehur PA, et al: Désunion très tardive d'une anastomose colo-rectale mécanique. Rapport d'un cas et revue de la littérature. Approche expérimentale des complications tardives des agrafages circulaires. Chirurgie, 111:650–658, 1985.

12. Swenson O, Merrill K, Peirce C, Rheinlander H: Blood and nerve supply to the esophagus. An experimental study. J Thorac Surg 19:462–479, 1950.

13. Williams DB, Payne WS: Observations on esophageal blood supply. Mayo Clin Proc 57:448–453, 1982.

14. Lehur PA, Robert R, Rogez JM, et al: Vascularisation artérielle de l'oesophage cervical du chien. Arch Biol 97(Suppl):62, 1986.

15. Graffner H, Andersson L, Lowenhielm P, Walther B: The healing process of anastomoses of the colon. A comparative study using single, double layer or stapled anastomosis. Dis Colon Rectum 27:767–771, 1984.

CHAPTER 18

STRICTURE FOLLOWING THE USE OF THE EEA STAPLER

Panagiotis Delikaris, Konstantinos Karamoschos, and Theodoros Diamantis

Since its initial introduction, mechanical stapling, linear as well as circular, has played a progressively more important role in gastro-intestinal surgery. The main reason for the acceptance of staplers is that the mechanical anastomosis is at least as reliable as the manual one. It seems that the use of staplers decreases operating time and results in less trauma to tissues and in an anastomosis with a lower leakage rate.[1] Manufacturers also claim that mechanical anastomoses function earlier than the manually sutured ones.

Anastomotic stricture, on the other hand, seems to be a problem that appears more often with the mechanical than with the manual techniques. We are not aware of comparative studies, but the literature offers previous adequate experience with strictures seen following mechanical colo-rectal anastomoses.[2]

This is a retrospective study of strictures seen following the use of the EEA stapler; the purpose is to correlate the problem with the upper or lower gastro-intestinal tract and the size of the anvil and cartridge.

PATIENTS AND METHODS

Between 1984 and 1987, 71 patients underwent mechanical anastomosis. In 28 patients, the anastomosis was located in the upper gastro-intestinal tract, and in 43 patients it was in the lower gastro-intestinal tract (Table 18-1).

In the upper gastro-intestinal tract, the EEA circular stapler was used for the construction of esophago-jejunal anastomoses in 11 patients; for gastro-duodenal anastomoses of the Billroth-I type in 8 patients; and for esophago-gastrostomy for porto-azygos disconnection because of bleeding esophageal varices in 9 patients (Table 18-2). Esophago-jejunal anastomoses were all carried out following total gastrectomy for gastric cancer. Billroth-I anastomosis was performed following partial gastric resection for benign lesions.

In the lower gastro-intestinal tract, patients could be classified as follows:

Thirty-two resections and colo-rectal anastomoses at different levels of the rectum were performed for colon cancer. Four patients had subtotal colectomy for malignant disease and ileo-rectal anastomosis. Seven patients had colo-rectal anastomosis following segmental colectomy for benign lesions (2 patients with ischemic colitis, 4 patients with diverticular disease, and 1 patient with sigmoid volvulus) (Table 18-2).

Table 18-3 shows the various anvil sizes used in the different types of anastomosis, both in the upper and lower tract.

RESULTS

In the early postoperative period, we experienced stricture of the anastomosis in 12 patients (16%).

Table 18-1. Breakdown by Age and Sex of 71 Patients Undergoing Mechanical Anastomosis in the Gastro-Intestinal Tract with the Circular EEA Stapler

Upper GI Tract (n = 28)
Age: 62.4 (mean), 42–74 (range)
Sex: Male 20, Female 8

Lower GI Tract (n = 43)
Age: 67.2 (mean), 43–78 (range)
Sex: Male 28, Female 15

Table 18-2. Breakdown of Types of Anastomoses

Upper GI Tract (n = 28)
Esophago-jejunal: 11
Porto-azygos disconnection: 9
B1 anastomosis: 8

Lower GI Tract (n = 43)
Malignant (36)
Colo-rectal: 32
Ileo-rectal: 4

Benign (7)
Colo-rectal: 7

Seven patients experienced stricture in the upper gastro-intestinal tract (25%) and five patients had strictures following anastomosis in the lower gastro-intestinal tract (11.6%).

Table 18-3 shows the number of stenoses, or strictures, observed as related to the size of the anvil used and the type of the anastomoses performed. The diagnosis was initially clinical and confirmed with contrast studies and endoscopy.

DISCUSSION

All of our anastomotic strictures were seen in the initial postoperative period. The earliest and main complaint in patients with anastomotic stricture in the upper gastro-intestinal tract was dysphagia to solids soon after oral ingestion of food. Patients experienced frequent and small bowel actions in the lower gastro-intestinal tract. As already mentioned, contrast studies and endoscopy confirmed the diagnosis. It is also interesting to note that the clinical course of our patients was not disturbed by the development of anastomotic strictures. They all responded well and promptly to dilatation, pneumatic in the upper and pneumatic or digital in the lower gastro-intestinal tract. Occasionally, the simple passage of the endoscope was sufficient for treatment, soon after diagnosis had been confirmed.

Anastomotic stricture in the upper gastro-intestinal tract has been seen following surgery for both malignant and benign lesions. In the lower gastrointestinal tract, all anastomotic strictures were experienced following resection for malignant disease.

The size of the anvil used was decided following careful intra-operative estimation of the diameter of the lumen of the gastro-intestinal tract. In analyzing our data, we find a tendency toward stricture in cases where smaller anvils were used. In the upper gastrointestinal tract in 19 patients in whom a 25-mm anvil was used, we found 6 anastomotic strictures (31.5%). When a 28-mm anvil was used (8 cases), we had only 1 stricture (12.5%). In the lower gastro-intestinal tract, in 11 patients in whom a 28-mm EEA stapler had been used, we had 2 anastomotic strictures (18.2%), whereas stricture was seen in only 3 of the 32 cases (10.9%) in which a 31-mm anvil was used.

CONCLUSIONS

We believe that stricture following the use of an EEA stapler should be occasionally expected. The percentage varies, and the problem usually arises in the early postoperative period. Clinically, the problem is minimal in the majority of patients, and symptoms subside promptly with simple dilatation. A word of caution should be raised in the differential diagnosis of stricture in cases in which the previous operation was a resection for cancer.

Table 18-3. Breakdown of Anvil Sizes Used with Circular EEA Stapling Instrument and Number of Stenoses (Parentheses)

Size	Upper GI Tract (n = 28)			Lower GI Tract (n = 43)		
	Esophago-Jejunal	Porto-Azygos	B1 Anastomosis	Colo-Rectal*	Ileo-Rectal*	Colo-Rectal**
25 mm	9 (2)	8 (2)	2 (2)	–	–	–
28 mm	2 (1)	1	5	8 (2)	2	1
31 mm	–	–	1	24 (3)	2	6
Totals	11 (3)	9 (2)	8 (2)	32 (5)	4	7

* For malignant disease
** For benign lesions

CHAPTER 19

STRICTURES AFTER STAPLED ANASTOMOSIS IN COLO-RECTAL SURGERY

J. Cady

The retrospective study of our clinical experience with 705 stapled colo-rectal anastomoses performed from 1977 to 1987, which showed 25 anastomotic strictures (3.5%), led us to review the causes, short and long-term clinical importance, and treatment of these strictures. The histologic examination of four completely resected strictures gave a better understanding of their true morphologic nature.

Of the various techniques used for reconstruction after colo-rectal resection, that of triangulation with partial inversion and partial eversion, used in 21 patients, was not responsible for any strictures. The use of the GIA-TA instruments in the functional end-to-end or Bayonet anastomosis in 293 patients was followed by 3 strictures (1%). The circular anastomosing instrument (original EEA, disposable EEA, CEEA) was applied in 391 patients, with an incidence of 22 strictures (5.6%).

During this same period, 13 strictures were observed that had no relation to the anastomotic technique. Postoperative peri-anastomotic tumor recurrence was seen in 10 of these, radiation fibrosis in 1, and ischemia with retraction of the proximal colon from the anal canal in 2.

CLINICAL EXPERIENCE

Strictures with the GIA-TA Anastomosing Technique

Three cases were observed in female patients, who were 55, 72, and 83 years old. One patient suffered from an elongated sigmoid colon with repeated epi-sodes of volvulus, another from cancer of the right colon, and the third from a diverticular sigmoid abscess mimicking a tumor. Symptoms of anastomotic obstruction in the first 2 patients required re-operation because of the intra-peritoneal location of the two anastomoses, but the stricture in the third patient was asymptomatic and was found only at follow-up examination 1 month postoperatively. Because of its low location, it was dilated manually without any long-term problems. (Table 19-1)

Strictures with the Circular Anastomosing Instrument

A total of 22 strictures were observed in 391 colo-rectal anastomoses in 6 men and 16 women, 23 to 82 years old (average 65 years). The operative indications were cancer in 14 patients, sigmoid diverticulitis and abscess in 5 patients, and miscellaneous rare conditions in the remaining 3 patients. In 3 patients with acute inflammatory disease and peritonitis, the overall condition of the patients and the local findings had been judged satisfactory to permit colectomy and primary anastomosis. (Table 19-2)

These strictures were found at the recto-sigmoid level in 1 patient, high in the rectal stump in 2 patients, in the middle of the rectal ampulla in 8 patients, and at the level of the low rectum or anal canal in 2 patients. The original anastomosis had been end-to-end in 15 patients and side-to-end through an abdominal approach in 7 cases. There were 9 protective transverse colostomies in the overall group of 22 strictures. (Table 19-3)

Table 19-1. Strictures with the GIA-TA Anastomotic Technique in Colo-Rectal Surgery

Ileo-colic anastomoses	1/146 Cases
Ileo-rectal anastomoses	0/28 Cases
Colo-colic anastomoses	0/5 Cases
Colo-rectal anastomoses	2/114 Cases
Total	3/290 Cases (1%)

CLINICAL PRESENTATION

With the exception of one stricture, all others were discovered in the first 3 postoperative months. They were characterized by minimal symptoms or no symptoms at all. Most often, some troubles of transit across the anastomosis or incomplete rectal emptying had been noticed. Strictures that could be palpated by rectal examination appeared like a thin diaphragm with a central opening that did not accept the tip of the index finger; they were found to be uniformly brittle and easy to break up by finger pressure alone.

Radiologic examination of the abdomen showed an intact circle of staples, normal in diameter. Barium enema confirmed the stenotic diaphragm. Endoscopic examination demonstrated a mature scar of the inverted circular edge of the anastomosis, allowing only for a small narrow opening surrounded by inflammatory reaction. However, all of these complementary examinations are not indispensible for the diagnosis of strictures that can be reached by digital examination.

In only one patient, who was lost to followup until the sixteenth postoperative month, did we observe a clinical presentation of distal colon obstruction, due to a thick diaphragm with a pinpoint opening. This patient appeared to have suffered a total loss of anastomotic patency.

TREATMENT

Dilatation

In 20 of 22 patients suffering from stricture following the use of the circular anastomosing instrument, operative correction was unnecessary. The anastomotic lumen stayed patent after one or two digital

Table 19-2. Strictures in Circular Stapled Anastomoses in Colo-Rectal Surgery

Ileo-colic anastomoses	0/17 Cases
Ileo-rectal anastomoses	0/14 Cases
Colo-colic anastomoses	0/1 Case
Colo-rectal anastomoses	22/359 Cases (6%)
Total	22/391 Cases (5.6%)

dilations or after dilatation in the operating room at the time of colostomy closure.

Resection of the Stricture

This resection was achieved through the anus with the use of the disposable curved EEA instrument in one patient. Following partial dilatation of the stricture with a Kelly clamp, the stapling instrument was advanced through the anal canal with the anvil separated from the cartridge. With some circular movement and moderate pressure, the anvil was passed beyond the stenotic diaphragm, the instrument was closed and activated, and the stenotic area was resected. When there is a proximal colostomy, these maneuvers can be accomplished under colonoscopic vision.[1] (*Note:* with the new premium CEEA instrument, a similar procedure can be performed by placing the cartridge and instrument from below upward and advancing the trocar through the stenotic area. Through a laparotomy and colotomy proximal to the stricture, the anvil with its central rod is placed into the hollow rod of the cartridge, after the trocar has been removed. The instrument is then closed and anastomosis is performed. Although this technique requires a laparotomy and a proximal colotomy, it avoids the need for dilatation with a clamp and the relatively "blind" technique described above.)

Laparotomy is also required if the stricture is placed high in the pelvis and cannot be approached through the anal canal without serious risk to the patient. This approach was necessary in our second case, in which the technique previously described, with separate introduction of the stapler with the cartridge and central rod from below and the attachment of the anvil through a proximal colotomy from above, was used.[2] With both of these techniques, dissection of the anastomotic area is avoided.

Strictures After Anastomosis with the GIA-TA Instruments

Only three such strictures (1%) were observed in 293 operations. In one patient, digital dilatation eliminated the problem; in 2 patients, re-operation was required. The first such patient was a 72-year-old woman who presented with small bowel obstruction 7 months after a right hemi-colectomy. At re-operation, the anastomosis had the shape of a "Bishop's miter," probably because of excessive resection of the common GIA introduction site peripheral to the original application of the TA instrument. A repeat functional GIA-TA anastomosis was followed by an uneventful postoperative course and an excellent result 5 years later.

In the second patient, a 55-year-old woman with

repeated episodes of volvulus due to an elongated sigmoid loop, a sequential anastomosis-resection (anastomose-résection intégrée) with the GIA-TA instruments was followed 5 months postoperatively by a large bowel obstruction. The resulting stricture was resected with an end-to-end EEA circular anastomosis; the patient has been well since.

Since the incidence of strictures in the functional or Bayonet GIA-TA anastomosis is only 1%, the study of strictures occurring with stapling instruments is mostly based on the 22 strictures observed after the use of the circular EEA instrument.

HISTOLOGIC ASPECTS

Examination of one of the three strictures observed after the GIA-TA type of anastomosis showed a small opening through this anastomosis due to scar formation of the inverted edges of the GIA staple lines. Histologically, in addition to inflammatory reaction and fibrosis, there was a deviation of the muscle of the bowel with duplication of the thickness of this layer at the level of the inverting GIA lines. This double muscular thickness created a true diaphragm.

Histologic examination of the two resected circular anastomoses showed a normal mucosa with a fibrous submucosa that was, however, nearly normal in thickness. Again, the level of the muscular layer was the site of the pathologic lesion.

This lesion is characterized by muscular hyperplasia that is often associated with moderate fibrosis, but above all, the direction of the muscular fibers is often deviated. In the areas of this directional change, the muscular layer adheres to the regenerated mucosa and its fibers are more or less perpendicular to the mucosa.

In some of the histologic sections, this change in muscular orientation appears as a V-shaped partial duplication.

In one of the two cases, there was a frank generalized inflammatory reaction, and the submucosa was more or less studded with muscle fibers that contained much granulation tissue. This histologic appearance is associated with a total lack of muscularis mucosae, signifying a loss of this tissue layer in the mucosa-covered scar.

The pathologic lesions were interpreted as showing a mechanically created detour in the direction of the muscular layer, with partial or complete duplication at the level of the inverted bowel walls, resulting in a true diaphragm. The potential for stricture formation is probably increased by the presence of inflammatory reaction and fibrosis.

PATHOGENESIS OF STRICTURE FORMATION

Since anastomotic strictures appear to occur more frequently with the use of the circular stapling instrument (22 of 391, or 5.6%) than with other anastomotic stapling techniques in the colo-rectal area (3 of 314, or 1%), the factors associated with circular-stricture formation will be examined and compared to the overall series of colo-rectal stapled anastomoses. The results of the study will be compared by chi^2 analysis.

Factors that do not influence stricture formation are

1. *Patients' sex and age.* The predominance of strictures in 16 of our female patients is proportionate to the greater number of female patients in the group with circular anastomosis (227 of 391 patients). The average age of the patients is the same for males and females.
2. *Pathologic etiology.* In 209 patients with colo-rectal cancer, 14 strictures (6.6%) occurred, as compared to 5 strictures (5%) in 98 patients with sigmoid diverticulitis. In 34 "ideal" emergency operations with colectomy and primary anastomosis in the presence of peritonitis, there were 3 strictures (9%).
3. *Caliber and type of circular anastomosing instrument.* Cartridge sizes of either 28 or 31 mm, as well as the original metal EEA instrument and its successors (the disposable straight and curved instruments), are not predisposing factors in producing strictures. In 44 earlier cases, in which the original metal instrument had been used, 4 strictures were observed.
4. *Anastomotic leak and fistula.* Although 3 strictures were observed in 28 patients with anastomotic leaks (10%), that difference was not statistically significant.

Factors that influence the development of a stricture, which are essentially technical in nature, are

Table 19-3. Results in Stapled Circular Colo-Rectal Anastomoses

Type of Anastomosis	Patients	Leakage	Stricture	Death
Intra-peritoneal	173	1 (0.5%)	1 (0.5%)	5 (2.8%)
Extra-peritoneal	134	11 (8%)	18 (13%)	8 (6%)
Colo-anal	52	18 (35%)	3 (6%)	1 (2%)

1. *Type of anastomosis.* No strictures were observed after anastomosis of the small bowel to the colon (17 patients) or to the rectum (14 patients). All the strictures were found in the group of colo-rectal anastomoses.
2. *Location of the anastomosis.* In 173 anastomoses at the level of the rectosigmoid junction, only 1 stricture was observed. The upper and middle levels of the rectal ampulla were the sites of 18 strictures in 134 patients (14%). The low rectum and the anal canal developed 3 strictures in 52 anastomoses (6%) ($p < 0.05$).
3. *Technical modalities.* With the end-to-end anastomosis (339 cases), only 15 strictures (4%) were observed. With the trans-abdominal side-to-end anastomosis (20 cases), a total of 7 strictures (35%) were found ($p < 0.01$). Proximal diverting colostomy (43 cases) was followed by nine strictures (21%) ($p < 0.01$).

DISCUSSION

The technical method of anastomosis is not the only factor responsible for strictures that complicate the joining of the large bowel ends or of the colon to the rectum. Strictures may be due to unhealthy tissues or to tissues with a diminished blood supply, such as those seen after radiation treatments. In addition, the creation of an anastomosis under tension and the resulting ischemia may produce a retraction of the proximal colon segment and create a stricture. Finally, extensive leaks due to a variety of causes may lead to an inflammatory stricture.

Of the remaining strictures due to the anastomotic technique proper, those found after circular anastomosis are particular in their development and pathologic features. Their incidence equals that of all other technical modes and suture-type materials. Their features are not comparable to those of any of the strictures that happen because of the usual predisposing factors.

These circular strictures have been defined as membranous in character.[2] However, this definition does not correspond to the fact that more than an epithelial mucosal membrane is involved. The scar is hypertrophic and involves the entire wall of the inverted bowel ends. The involvement of the muscular coat in this scar appears to be predominant on histologic examination, with an abnormal configuration of the muscular architecture and a fibrosis that manifests itself with different degrees of intensity.[3]

The diaphragm that narrows the anastomotic lumen develops from the periphery to the center without modifying the alignment of the staples. As time passes, this diaphragm becomes thicker, an evolution

favored by a proximal colostomy diverting the fecal stream from the anastomosis. This type of stricture appears to be inherent in stapled anastomoses with inversion, and is not found with everting triangulating anastomoses. It is, also exceptional to find a stricture after functional end-to-end GIA-TA anastomosis, except for the occasional occurrence in an oval-shaped configuration, where the TA closure of the inverting GIA lines encroaches too much on these lines and keeps them in contact. We have encountered diaphragmatic narrowing of the circular anastomotic lumen, as others have,[4] after EEA anastomosis between the esophagus and the stomach, the colon and the stomach, and the stomach and the duodenum. However, in the lower intestinal tract, these strictures have been described foremost for circular colo-rectal anastomoses.[5–10]

A certain number of hypotheses are not verified by the histologic findings; for example, ischemia[11] and necrosis do not explain a hypertrophic cicatrix with excellent vascularity. Similarly, the inflammation following an anastomotic leak or the one that is the primary indication for resection, in a sigmoid diverticulitis, is not responsible for stricture formation at a statistically significant level. Factors such as patient's sex and age, underlying pathology, instrument size,[12] type of instrument,[13] including the Russian instruments,[14] are not responsible for stricture formation.

The development of these diaphragms appears to be specifically related to the circumferential scar formation of an inverting circular anastomosis. The frequency of this development is probably greater than we have observed, since the initial frailness of the diaphragm may bring about its spontaneous disappearance by the passage of stools. This is why the incidence of strictures is higher in those cases where the anastomosis was protected by a proximal colostomy.[4]

If, however, these strictures are not diagnosed early, and do not disappear spontaneously, they become thicker, although a somewhat altered bowel transit is still possible.

Ultimately, a true obstruction makes itself felt to the patient and to the surgeon. In their early stages, obstructions are simply cured by digital or instrumental dilation, but the later stage of progressive fibrosis and narrowing can only be treated by surgical resection. Fortunately, the need for this was rare in our experience (0.5%), as it was in a review of the literature on this subject.[5]

CONCLUSIONS

Strictures with stapling instruments are specifically related to the inverting nature of the technique employed, especially if the circular anastomosing instrument is used. The incidence of strictures is higher if the anastomosis has been protected by a proximal colostomy. Strictures usually occur within the first 3 months and, if recognized at that early stage, are easily treated by finger or instrumental dilatation.

Re-operation is indicated only if the stricture has evolved into a thick and fibrous diaphragm. In theory, this complication could be avoided by using an everting circular anastomosis. Strictures are a disadvantage of inverting stapling techniques, and have to be compared to the advantages these instruments provide.

Translated from the French by F.M. Steichen, M.D.

REFERENCES

1. Le Treut YP, Castro R, Bouloudnion G, Boutboul R, Bricot R: Résection trans-anale à la pince EEA d'une sténose anastomotique colo-rectale. J Chir (Paris) 119:75–78, 1982.
2. Brain J, Lorber M, Fiddian-Green RG: Rectal membrane: an unusual complication following use of the circular stapling instrument for colorectal anastomosis. Surgery 89:271–273, 1981.
3. Buchmann P, Schneider K, Gebbers J-O: Fibrosis of experimental colonic anastomosis in dogs after EEA stapling or suturing. Dis Colon Rectum 26:217–220, 1983.
4. Graffner H, Fredlung P, Olsson S-A, Oscarson J, Petersson B-G: Protective colostomy in low anterior resection of the rectum using the EEA stapling instrument: a randomized study. Dis Colon Rectum 26:87–90, 1983.
5. Beart RW Jr, Kelly KA: Randomized prospective evaluation of the EEA stapler for colorectal anastomoses. Am J Surg 141:143–147, 1981.
6. Berard PH, Papillon M, Jacquemard R, Labrosse H, Bigay D, Guillemin G: Les anastomoses digestives à la EEA, à propos de 104 cas. Ann Chir 35:403–408, 1981.
7. Berard PH, Papillon M, Jacquemard R, Labrosse H, Bigay D, Guillemin G: L'anastomose colo-rectale basse à la pince EEA dans la chirurgie du cancer du rectum. J Chir (Paris) 118:115–119, 1981.
8. Fekete F, Gayet B, Place S, Bornet P: 380 anastomoses oesophagiennes mécaniques. Techniques et résultats. Ann Chir 40:641–647, 1986.
9. Vignal J, Beaune B, Gruner L, Payan F, Champetier TH: Résultats de 199 viscéro-synthèses en chirurgie colo-rectale. Lyon Chir 83:171–174, 1987.
10. Waxman BP: Large bowel anastomoses. II. The circular staplers. Br J Surg 70:64–67, 1983.
11. Trollope ML, Cohen RG, Lee RH, Cannon WB, Marzoni FA, Cressman RD: A 7-year experience with low anterior sigmoid resections using the EEA stapler. Am J Surg 152:11–15, 1986.
12. Turbelin JM, Arnaud JP, Welter R, Adloff M: Etude comparative des surfaces anastomotiques obtenues par utilisation des sutures mécaniques en chirurgie digestive. J Chir (Paris) 117:541–546, 1980.
13. Blamey SL, Lee PWR: A comparison of circular stapling devices in colo-rectal anastomoses. Br J Surg 69:19–22, 1982.
14. Goligher JC, Lee PWR, Macfie J, Simpkins KC, Lintott DJ: Experience with the Russian model 249 suture gun for anastomosis of the rectum. Surg Gynecol Obstet 148:517–524, 1979.

ADDITIONAL READING

Antonsen HK, Kronborg O: Early complications after low anterior resection for rectal cancer using the EEA TM stapling device: a prospective trial. Dis Colon Rectum 30:579–583, 1987.

Cady J: Les résections-anastomoses colo-rectales mécaniques, à froid et en urgence (comparaison des différentes techniques à propos de 385 cas). Lyon Chir 83:161–165, 1987.

Heald RJ, Leicester RJ: The low stapled anastomosis. Dis Colon Rectum 24:437–444, 1981.

Smith LE: Anastomosis with EEA stapler after anterior colonic resection. Dis Colon Rectum 24:236–246, 1981.

CHAPTER 20

PATTERNS OF LETHAL STAPLE-LINE BREAKDOWN

Hans Rinecker

Comprehensive study of broadly based clinical reports shows that roughly half of the postoperative mortality of gastro-intestinal operations is caused by technical failures of gastro-intestinal sutures. With this in mind, all suture-related fatal outcomes of 1550 consecutive gastro-intestinal operations performed in our institution with staples were analyzed. Because no related deaths were caused by either staple-line bleeding or stenosis, the study concentrated solely on leaks. The analysis was limited to fatal outcomes only because non-fatal temporary leaks are difficult to assess in some anatomic locations.

Gastro-intestinal stapling was used as a standard method without manual over-sewing. Only esophago-jejunostomies with the EEA stapler were routinely covered by manual sutures, because of the tendency of the circular instrument to cause breaks in the outer muscular esophageal ring, which is unprotected by serosa. Total gastrectomies were accomplished using the Longmire procedure; for partial gastrectomies, a Billroth-I reconstruction was preferred. The gastro-duodenostomies were performed with a conical end-to-end TA-stapled triangulation, as described by us some years ago.[1] For all small bowel entero-enterostomies, the functional end-to-end anastomosis was used.[2] Colonic resections were highly standardized. In almost all cases, either a right or left hemi-colectomy was employed. For right hemicolectomies, end-to-side anastomoses were performed with the EEA stapler.

In left hemi-colectomies, continuity was established by trans-anal EEA-stapled anastomoses placed extra-peritoneally. The distal rectal stump was usually closed temporarily with a TA application, followed more recently by double-stapling TA-EEA anastomosis. Within the 1550 cases, 3837 single-stapling applications were made. Nineteen fatal outcomes were demonstrated as being staple-line-related. This equals an overall mortality risk of 1.2% per case, or a fatal risk of 0.5% per single stapler application.

The first question in a detailed analysis is to ask if higher risks of fatal staple-line breakdowns are organ-related. Table 20-1 shows the specific risk per gastro-intestinal organ stapled. Anastomoses between different organs, such as in esophago-jejunostomies or ileo-colostomies, show up twice in this summary, namely in each line of the single organ taking part in the anastomosis. The stapling risk is seemingly somewhat higher at the esophagus. But here only a single patient had been lost, who had undergone operation without manual over-sewing of the esophago-jejunostomy. Since coverage of the staple line has become obligatory at this anastomotic site, no other leak has been observed. Most lethal suture breakdowns with participation of the large bowel occurred before the development of routine preoperative orthograde lavage. Certainly, no single anastomotic site, no single part of the gastro-intestinal tract stands out as carrying an especially high risk for stapler operations.

The second question is the risk distribution related to the different types of stapling instruments employed (Table 20-2). GIA anastomoses can be considered very safe. The performance of the EEA instrument seems to be minimally less reliable. Again, fatal

Table 20-1. Location-Related Risk of Lethal Staple-Line Breakdown

Location	No. of Patients	No. of Breakdowns	Percentage
Esophagus	52	1	2.0
Stomach	910	9	1.0
Duodenum	797	7	0.9
Small intestine	732	8	1.1
Large bowel	350	6	1.7

outcomes after anastomoses performed with more than one type of instrument are counted and recorded for each type participating in the anastomosis.

In the pioneer days of stapling in surgery, the big question concerned the safety of everted mucosa-to-mucosa sutures. These contradicted the then-current dogma of the necessity for serosa-to-serosa approximation (Table 20-3). When trans-anal EEA anastomoses for low anterior resections are routinely done through distal stump closures with the TA instrument, pure serosa-to-serosa apposition does not occur regularly. Nevertheless, the resulting unconventional mucosa-to-mucosa approximation is certainly no less safe than the serosa-to-serosa anastomoses had been, nor is it any less safe than the bulk of anastomoses with mixed inverted and everted staple lines. This is a clinical verification of the surgical principle that holds that the intestinal walls to be sutured should have unimpaired blood supply, be tension-free, and be joined by an air-tight closure, reducing the method of approximation to the level of expertise and preference held by the individual surgeon.

Another question relates to stapler reliability under the condition of local peritonitis. This is difficult to analyze. Peritonitis is often associated with tissue edema, which limits the application of stapling instruments with fixed suture gap geometry. Therefore, patients with marked peritonitis have operations where manual sutures are preferred. To get an idea about staple performance in peritonitis, however, all Hartmann resections were analyzed. After colon resection for perforated diverticulitis and construction of a proximal end colostomy, the distal rectal stump was routinely closed with a TA stapler within the

Table 20-2. Stapler-Type-Related Risk of Lethal Staple-Line Breakdown

Type	No. of Patients	Breakdowns	Percentage
GIA	1315	7	0.5
TA	2367	20	0.8
EEA	149	2	1.3

Table 20-3. Anastomotic-Mode-Related Risk of Lethal Staple-Line Breakdown

Mode	No. of Patients	Breakdowns	Percentage
Mucosa-to-mucosa	969	5	0.5
Mixed	983	13	1.3
Serosa-to-serosa	63	1	1.6

pelvic peritoneum. In spite of manifest fecal contamination of the peritoneum, 66 operations performed that way did not lead to a single rectal stump leak. In the 1550 cases, 61 staple closures or anastomoses were marked by the operating surgeon as especially risky because of local peritonitis. In none of these cases did a fatal anastomotic leak occur. Contrary to traditional belief, local peritonitis probably is not a very bad risk for staple lines.

Stapling techniques still belong to an expanding surgical technology. Hospitals are facing the transition to stapling or are within the training period. In our institution, 13 of the lethal suture disruptions occurred within the first 500 cases, only 4 fatal outcomes occurred within the second 500, and only 2 patients lost their lives because of staple-line complications within the third 500 consecutive operations. This equals a staple-related mortality of 2.6% at first, then 0.8%, and finally 0.4%. So stapling became an extremely reliable method after the first 500 operations had been performed.

Beyond the impressive reliability of improvements related to the accumulation of case numbers, and the slightly higher risk with the EEA instrument, staple-line leaks occur very much at random, in our experience. Nevertheless, a closer look at the clinical course of the 19 patients with fatal suture breakdowns reveals some risk patterns (Table 20-4). All of them carried severe systemic risks. Ten of these 19 patients showed respiratory failures. Arterial partial oxygen pressures of less than 55 mm mercury were registered either pre-operatively or postoperatively as baseline values (e.g., during failed weaning attempts). All of these oxygen values were found before the onset of clinical manifestation of the suture disruptions. Most of these cases involved operations under emergency conditions. Nine of these patients who died postoperatively in the hospital showed severe metabolic disorders. These disorders were manifested either by uncontrolled malignant growth with multiple liver metastases or peritoneal carcinomatosis, or by gross liver failure. Statistical comparison of the partial oxygen pressures and the total protein levels of non-survivors with matched survivor pairs treated by the same operations shows a high significance for both hypoxia and hypo-proteinemia. A third

Table 20-4. Factors for Staple-Line Breakdown

	Respirator Failure or P_aO_2 <55 mm Hg	Malignant Growth, Liver Failure, or Total Protein <50 g/l	Pancreatitis, Enteritis, or Obstruction
Total gastrectomy + colon resection	●	●	
Gastrotomy		●	
Gastro-enterostomy		●	
B-II	●		
B-II	●		
B-I	●	●	●
B-I		●	
B-I	●		
B-I			●
B-II → B-I	●		
Duodenal stump	●		
Duodenal stump	●	●	
Duodenotomy			●
Small intestine resection			●
R colon resection		●	
R colon resection		●	●
Subtotal colon resection		●	●
L colon resection	●	●	
L colon resection	●		●
n = 19	10*	9*	7

* t-Test p < 0.005

group of 6 patients carried mixed risk factors like postoperative necrotizing pancreatitis, severe enteritis, or bowel distention by unrelated postoperative obstruction.

In reviewing the improvement with progressive experience of the staple-related mortality rate (2.6% to a 0.4%), these complications seem to indicate that the initial higher number of fatal outcomes in these successive series of 500 patients each resulted less often from technical incompetence of surgeons inexperienced with stapling than from extended operative indications using complicated stapling procedures on high-risk patients. Certainly, the ease and quickness of stapling operations can make an eager surgeon succumb to the desire to attempt extensive reconstructive procedures in bad-risk cases. Although the indications for the use of staplers has lately been streamlined, this reduction of stapling was not done in favor of manual suturing. Instead, procedures like endoscopic treatment of bleeding gastric ulcers, esophageal varices, and temporary Hartmann colostomies were used in such high-risk patients.

The postoperative staple leaks manifested themselves quite late in the clinical courses (Fig. 20-1). The literature maintains a mean postoperative interval of 3 to 4 days for the first symptoms of a developing suture leak after manual suturing. The diagram for staple failures, however, shows mostly a considerably delayed staple-line breakdown. It is unknown if the very late staple-line disruptions with mucosa-to-mucosa apposition are an expression of the severely disturbed metabolism of this group of non-survivors.

As our last 1000 consecutive patients who underwent operations show, it is possible to perform, with the aid of staplers, reconstructive gastro-intestinal surgery with a suture-related mortality risk of less than 1%. To secure this success, the remaining risk factors, as they emerge out of the experience of this series, should be studied more closely: namely, postoperative respiratory and metabolic failures.

SUMMARY

The probability of lethal suture breakdown is the decisive factor in judging the capability of gastro-

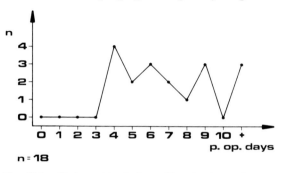

Fig. 20-1. Postoperative leak manifestation interval.

intestinal suturing methods: 1550 stapler operations were retrospectively analyzed for recurring patterns of staple-related disruptions. Nineteen suture breakdowns resulted in fatal outcomes. Anatomic location within the intestinal tract, the type of device used, mucosa-to-mucosa vs. serosa-to-serosa suture, and the presence of local peritonitis do not correlate strongly with breakdown probability. Team experience seems to be of less importance in relation to the choice of a given reconstructive operative technique than in the selection of a risk-adequate treatment-method selection. Respiratory insufficiency or systemic metabolic failure caused by malignancy, sepsis, and liver malfunction emerge as high-risk factors for stapler-related, late breakdowns. These occur with a mean postoperative interval of 8 days.

REFERENCES

1. Rinecker H: Improved stapler-gastroduodenostomy for Billroth I gastric resection. In: Klammernahttechnik in Thorax und Abdomen: Ulrich B, Winter UJ. Stuttgart: Verlag, 1986.
2. Steichen FM: The use of staplers in anatomical side-to-side and functional end-to-end enteroanastomoses. Surgery 64:948, 1968.

Part VI

Stapling in Pulmonary Surgery

CHAPTER 21

STAPLING IN PULMONARY LOBECTOMY AND PNEUMONECTOMY

Th. Junginger

The technical result of pulmonary resection depends in large part on the quality and reliability of the bronchial closure. Both operative methods and suture material are of great importance in achieving a safe bronchial closure. The mechanical bronchial closure using staples has been slowly accepted; in 1972, Boyd and Spencer[1] concluded that stapling techniques in pulmonary surgery were only of limited value. Some 10 years later Lawrence and his associates were able to demonstrate from a poll taken of thoracic surgeons in the United States that half of them used stapling techniques in the closure of bronchi.[2]

A review of the results of experimental and clinical studies will help in establishing the place of stapling techniques in pulmonary lobectomy and pneumonectomy.

EXPERIMENTAL STUDIES

As shown previously by Schmidt, Heuer, and Smith,[3,4,5] the type of suture material used makes no difference in the healing of the bronchus or in the incidence of broncho-pleural fistulae. Rienhoff and his associates demonstrated in 1942 that the use of a minimal but safe amount of suture material, and the coverage of the bronchial stump with a pleural flap, were important factors in the stump's healing.[6] Factors that favored a bronchial leak were infection,[7] diminished blood supply due to extensive dissection around the bronchial stump, failure to close the stump flush with the parent bronchus or trachea,[8,9,10] and finally malignant infiltration at the line of resection.[11]

Scott and his associates demonstrated in an experimental study the importance of the inflammatory reaction after closure of a bronchial stump.[12] By comparing various suture materials after pneumonectomy, they found that the inflammatory reaction to stainless steel staples was less than with any of the other closure materials. Conversely, the wound strength of the stapled bronchial stumps was significantly higher than that with closures of silk or nylon. The authors concluded that bronchial closure with stapling instruments improves healing and reduces the risk of a bronchial leak.

CLINICAL RESULTS

The incidence of broncho-pleural fistulae following stapled closure of the bronchus varies significantly with individual published series. These differences are due to a number of factors that may vary from one study to the other, such as the underlying pulmonary disease, the duration of postoperative observation, the definition of a broncho-pleural fistula, and finally the retrospective character of most clinical series. Comparison between the various studies is therefore limited. Only Gamondes and his associates have examined in a prospective fashion their results of bronchial closures with manual and mechanical techniques following right pneumonectomy.[13]

With the use of the Russian UKB-25 (single staple row parallel to the bronchial axis) and UKL-40 or UKL-60 (double staple row at right angle to the bronchial axis) in bronchial closures after pneumonectomy, the reported frequency of broncho-pleural fistula has varied from 0 to 17% with an average of 5.8% (Table 21-1). The use of the linear TA instruments in bronchial closures for pneumonectomy (Table 21-2)

Table 21-1. Staple Closure of the Bronchus: Pneumonectomy with Russian UKB and UKL Instruments

Author	Year	Instrument	n	BPF	Followup
Ravitch, M.M.[21]	1964	UKB-25	25	0	?
Smith, D.E.[5]	1963	UKB-25	17	3 (17.7%)	9–18 months
Amasov, N.M.[22]	1961	UKL-60	178	8 (4.5%)	2–24 months
Betts, R.H.[20]	1965	UKL-40	40	2 (5%)	?
Dart, C.H.[16]	1970	UKL-40	104	8 (7.7%)	>14 days
			364	21 (5.8%)	

BPF = Broncho-pleural fistula

has led to an incidence of bronchial insufficiency that varies from 0 to 15.3%. The average incidence is 5.15%, which corresponds to the earlier findings with the Russian instruments.

The risk of a bronchial leak after lobectomy is clearly diminished. With the use of the Russian instruments such leaks occur in 0 to 3.8% of all patients; with the TA instruments, the rate is 0 to 4.4%, with average values that are not essentially different between the two types of instruments (Table 21-3). Several authors have attempted to compare the results of mechanical bronchial closures with those of manual closures. Only Gamondes and his associates have answered this query in conducting a prospective study in right-sided pneumonectomies.[13] The rate of right main bronchial insufficiency was 6.5% (2 of 31 patients) with the use of stapling instruments and 3% (1 of 33 patients) with manual techniques. Because of the relatively small number of patients involved in the entire study, these differences were not statistically significant.

In all remaining retrospective studies, no significant difference could be found in the incidence of bronchial insufficiency or broncho-pleural fistulae between manual and mechanical bronchial closures,

with the exception of the historically consecutive comparison of Forrester-Wood, in which the bronchial insufficiency was found to be significantly less with the use of stapling instruments (Table 21-4).[14] The question of how much other factors, such as improved preoperative and postoperative patient care, have influenced these results remains unanswered, especially since closure with manual sutures in parallel time periods has also been associated with an improved outcome.

The comparison of bronchial insufficiency after lobectomy does not show a significant difference between manual and mechanical sutures (Table 21-5). Petterfy observed a diminished frequency of bronchial insufficiency in stapled closures as compared to manual techniques in a substantial series of patients who underwent various, unspecified types of pulmonary resections (Table 21-5).[15]

PERSONAL EXPERIENCE AND RESULTS

Between 1975 and 1987, 233 pulmonary resections were undertaken, first at the Department of Surgery of the University of Köln and then in the Department of General and Abdominal Surgery of the University of Mainz.

Table 21-2. Staple Closure of the Bronchus: Pneumonectomy with the Linear TA Instrument

Author	Year	Instrument	n	BPF	Followup
Dart, C.H.[16]	1970	TA	13	0	>14days
Rutten, A.P.M.[23]	1982	TA	30	0	30 days
Forrester-Wood, C.P.[14]	1980	TA	225	6 (2.7%)	>3 months
Konrad, R.M.[18]	1973	TA	32	1 (3.1%)	?
Irlich, G.[24]	1986	TA	128	4 (3.1%)	?
Hood, M.R.[17]	1973	TA	60	2 (3.3%)	>30 days
Hakim, M.[25]	1985	TA	71	3 (4.2%)	?
Lawrence, G.H.[2]	1982	TA	37	2 (5.4%)	?
Gamondes, J.P.[13]	1983	TA	31	2 (6.5%)	>3 months
Maaßen, W.[19]	1985	TA	89	6 (6.7%)	?
Bazelly, B.[26]	1981	TA	145	12 (8.2%)	>3 months
Hakim, M.[25]	1985	TAPr	59	9 (15.3%)	?
Totals			920	47 (5.1%)	

BPF = Broncho-pleural fistula

Table 21-3. Staple Closure of the Bronchus: Lobectomy

Author	Year	Instrument	n	BPF	Followup
Smith, D.E.[5]	1963	UKB-25	84	1 (1.2%)	9–18 months
Ravitch, M.M.[21]	1964	UKB-25	80	3 (3.8%)	?
Betts, R.H.[20]	1965	UKL-40	45	0	?
Dart, C.H.[16]	1970	UKL-40, TA	167	3 (1.8%)	>14 days
Amasov, N.M.[22]	1961	UKL-60	152	4 (2.6%)	2 months–2 years
Totals			528	11 (2.1%)	
Hood, M.R.[17]	1973	TA	136	0	>30 days
Rutten, A.P.M.[23]	1982	TA	65	0	30 days
Irlich, G.[24]	1986	TA	399	6 (1.5%)	?
Lawrence, G.H.[2]	1982	?	117	4 (3.4%)	?
Konrad, R.M.[18]	1973	TA	23	1 (4.4%)	?
Totals			740	11 (1.5%)	

BPF = Broncho-pleural fistula

Until 1980, bronchial closures were essentially accomplished with manual techniques using interrupted sutures of resorbable material. Since 1980, stapling instruments have been employed with increasing frequency. In comparing the two patient groups, we have found that there is no difference in the disease conditions that lead to operation, except for an increase in resections for metastatic disease in the stapled group (Table 21-6). In the stapled group of patients, we have also found a regression of the number of pneumonectomies in favor of lobectomy, and more peripheral resections (Table 21-7).

A comparison of postoperative complications demonstrates a reduction of broncho-pleural fistulae from 7.1% with manual sutures to 2% with stapled closures (Table 21-8). During this same time period, our postoperative mortality rate was 9.4% in the patient group with manual sutures, as compared to 2.7% in the stapled closure group. During the years of 1980 to 1987, we observed only 1 death due to bronchopleural fistula in an overall group of 148 patients.

From these results we conclude that the mechanical closure of the bronchus is reliable, and have therefore extended its use to the closure of a broncho-

pleural fistula in a 68-year-old patient who had undergone left lower lobectomy 3 years earlier (Fig. 21-1). This patient was hospitalized because of recurrent episodes of fever with left-sided pneumonia; in the course of examination, he was found to have a communication between a broncho-pleural fistula and the stomach (which had herniated into the left chest) (Fig. 21-2). At re-operation it was possible to liberate the lower-lobe bronchial stump close to the level of its take-off beyond the left upper-lobe bronchus and resect the excess stump after closure flush with the left upper-lobe bronchus, without compromise of its lumen. The fistula into the fundus of the stomach was closed manually. The patient has been symptom-free since then (Fig. 21-3).

EVALUATION OF STAPLED BRONCHIAL CLOSURES

From all available evidence it can be concluded that stapling instruments provide surgeons with reliable bronchial closures after lobectomy and pneumonectomy. The comparison with manual sutures does not demonstrate a clear advantage of one technique

Table 21-4. Bronchial Stump Closure: Comparison of Suture and Staple Techniques (Pneumonectomy)

Author	Year	Suture		Stapler			
		n	BPF	n	Instrument	BPF	p
Smith, D.E.[5]	1963	13	2 (15.4%)	17	UKB-25	3 (17.7%)	ns
Forrester-Wood, C.P.[14]	1980	225	25 (11.1%)	225	TA	6 (2.7%)	<0.001
Bazelly, B.[26]	1981	161	7 (4.3%)	145	TA	12 (8.3%)	ns
Rutten, A.P.M.[23]	1982	11	0	30	TA	0	ns
Lawrence, G.H.[2]	1982	45	3 (6.7%)	37	?	2 (5.4%)	ns
Gamondes, J.P.[13]	1983	33	1 (3%)	31	TA	2 (6.5%)	ns

BPF = Broncho-pleural fistula

Table 21-5. Bronchial Stump Closure: Comparison of Suture and Staple Techniques (Lobectomy and Pulmonary Resection)

Author		Suture		Stapler		
		n	BPF	n	Instrument	BPF
Lobectomy						
Rutten, A.P.M.[23]	1982	31	1 (3.2%)	65	TA	0
Lawrence, G.H.[2]	1982	179	1 (0.6%)	117	?	4 (3.4%)
Pulmonary resection						
Peterffy, A.[15]	1979	153	5 (3.3%)	147	TA	2 (1.4%)

BPF = Broncho-pleural fistula

over the other, with the exception of a small comparative prospective study (all other studies are retrospective).[13] One advantage of stapling instruments is their technical simplicity, which has resulted in a diminished incidence of intra-operative difficulties (2.7%) in our experience. Furthermore, closure without opening the bronchus reduces the potential for contamination and can be accomplished rapidly, which has led to a shortening of operating time in various series from 10 to 30 minutes.[16,17,18]

With manual sutures, the placement of individual sutures varies, as does the strength with which these sutures are tied. Staple lines are symmetric and regular, with equal tissue compression.[15] The positioning of a stapling instrument for closure of the left main bronchus below the arch of the aorta can be difficult, especially if a large tumor hinders the introduction of the instrument under the aortic arch. At times we have preferred manual sutures in this situation.[19] Another disadvantage is the inability to inspect the remaining bronchial tree following a classically stapled bronchial closure. If the preoperative endoscopic examination has shown that this intra-operative examination is important to ensure safe resection margins, we have found it useful to open the bronchus distal to the planned level of resection. The bronchial tree can be examined and bronchial closure accomplished at the planned safe level proximal to the bronchotomy. If this precaution is not observed, tumor can conceivably be squeezed into the remaining bronchus proximal to the closure.[20]

The operative steps preparatory to the use of stapling instruments are the same as those observed for manual sutures. In both techniques, extensive dissection with loss of vascular supply and long bronchial stumps should be avoided. The line of resection should be flush with the parent bronchus and accomplish a perfect coaptation of the membranous wall of the bronchus onto the cartilaginous wall without longitudinal twisting. Right and left main bronchi should be closed with the 4.8-mm stapler;[18] the lobar bronchi can be closed with the 3.5-mm staples. The staple instrument is not suited to the closure of the severely inflamed and thickened bronchial walls, since in this case even the 4.8-mm staples may not suffice to hold the abnormally thick bronchial walls.

STAPLED CLOSURES OF THE PULMONARY VESSELS

The fine vascular staples are very useful in the closure of pulmonary vessels. During the course of an extended pneumonectomy, the pulmonary veins can be stapled at their junction with left atrium, especially in a left pneumonectomy. This procedure facilitates and extends the radical nature of an extended pneumonectomy. Similarly, the left pulmonary artery can be closed without any problems flush with its origin from the main pulmonary artery; we have found it easier to achieve the same goal behind the superior vena cava on the right side with the help of a suture ligature. Personally, we prefer the vascular

Table 21-6. Lung Resection: Diagnosis

Diagnosis	Manual sutures 1/75–5/86 n = 85		Stapler 11/80–12/87 n = 148	
	n	Percentage	n	Percentage
Bronchogenic carcinoma	51	60.0	73	49.3
Metastatic tumor	14	16.5	42	28.4
Other tumor	5	5.9	17	11.5
Others	15	17.6	16	10.8

Table 21-7. Lung Resection: Type of Operation

	Manual sutures n = 85		Stapler n = 148	
	n	Percentage	n	Percentage
Pleuropneumonectomy	—	—	3	2.0
Pneumonectomy	19	22.4	18	12.1
Bilobectomy	9	10.6	13	8.8
Lobectomy	36	42.3	76	51.4
Segmentectomy	5	5.9	4	2.7
Wedge resection	5	5.9	32	21.6
Extended resection	7	8.2	2	1.4
Others	4	4.7	—	—

Table 21-8. Lung Resection: Postoperative Complications

	Manual sutures n = 85		Stapler n = 148	
	n	Percentage	n	Percentage
Failed stapling	—	—	4	2.7
Air leakage	—	—	5	3.4
Broncho-pleural fistula	6	7.1	3	2.0
Operative deaths	8	9.4	4	2.7
Broncho-pleural fistula	4	4.7	1	0.7
Pulmonary insufficiency	3	3.5	2	1.4
Postoperative bleeding	—	—	1	0.7
Intestinal bleeding	1	1.2	—	—

closure in various pulmonary resections with ligatures. However, the experience gained with the closure of vessels with staples is very positive (Table 21-9). Death secondary to delayed bleeding has been reported,[19] as has an embolic phenomenon originating at the level of the stapled closure of the left atrium.[17]

CONCLUSIONS

Experimental studies in stapled bronchial closures after lobectomy and pneumonectomy have shown minimal inflammatory reaction and optimal wound strength of bronchi, compared to all other suture materials. In clinical studies, the incidence of broncho-

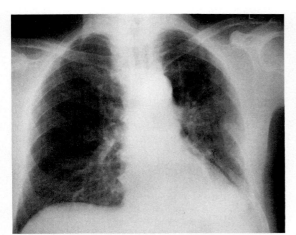

Fig. 21-1. Patient, 68 years old: recurrent septic episodes 3 years following left lower lobe resection.

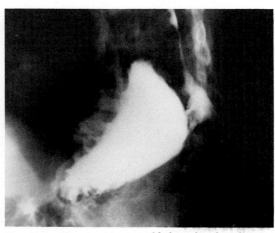

Fig. 21-2. Patient, 68 years old: broncho-pleural-gastric fistula into the fundus of the stomach (herniated into the mediastinum.)

Table 21-9. Lung Resection: Closure of Vascular Structures with Stapler

Author	Year	n	Complications
Betts, R.H.[26]	1965	11	0
Dart, C.H.[16]	1970	35	0
Hood, M.R.[17]	1973	196	1
Rutten, A.P.M.[23]	1982	76	0
Maaßen, W.[19]	1985	40	1

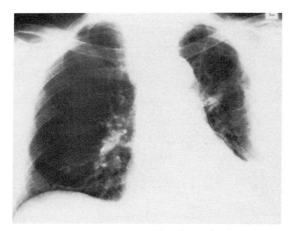

Fig. 21-3. Patient, 68 years old: radiographic examination 6 months after operation for cure of a broncho-pleural-gastric fistula.

pleural fistulae was equal to or less than that of manual sutures. The essential advantages of the stapled bronchial closures are technical simplicity, speed and symmetry of closure, and tissue compression. For these reasons, stapling instruments provide a significant extension in the technical options available to the surgeon intra-operatively.

Translated from the German by F.M. Steichen, M.D.

REFERENCES

1. Boyd AD, Spencer FC: Bronchopleural fistulas—how often should they occur? Ann Thorac Surg 13:195, 1972.
2. Lawrence GH, Ristroph R, Wood JA, Starr A: Methods for avoiding a dire surgical complication: bronchopleural fistula after pulmonary resection. Am J Surg 144:136, 1982.
3. Schmidt Goffi F, Lima Goncalves E: Closure of bronchial stump after pneumonectomy: comparison of some techniques through evaluation of tensile strength of suture. Surgery 42:511, 1957.
4. Heuer GJ, Dunn GR: Experimental pneumonectomy. Bull J Hopkins Hosp 31:30, 1920.
5. Smith DE, Karish AF, Chapman JP, Takaro T: Healing of the bronchial stump after pulmonary resection. Thorac Cardiovasc Surg 46:548, 1963.
6. Rienhoff WF, Gannon J, Sherman I: Closure of the bronchus following total pneumonectomy. Ann Surg 116:481, 1942.
7. Björk VO: Suture material and technique for bronchial closure and bronchial anastomosis. J Thorac Surg 32:22, 1956.
8. Lynn RB: The bronchus stump. J Thorac Surg 36:70, 1958.
9. Stafford EJ: Experimental pneumonectomy with obliteration of the bronchial stump. J Thorac Surg 14:480, 1941.
10. Thomas LC, Behrend A, Mann FC: Experimental pneumonectomy. J Thorac Surg 6:677, 1936.
11. Williams NS, Lewis CT: Bronchopleural fistula. A review of eighty-six cases. Br J Surg 63:520, 1976.
12. Scott RN, Faraci RP, Hough A, Chretien B: Bronchial stump closure techniques following pneumonectomy: a serial comparative study. Ann Surg 184:205, 1976.
13. Gamondès JP, Devolfe Ch, Girard C, Ducerf Ch, Elkirat AM: Sutures mècanique et manuelle des moignons bronchiques dans la pneumonectomie droite: etude comparative chez soixante-quatre opèrès. Ann Chir 37:130, 1983.
14. Forrester-Wood CP: Bronchopleural fistula following pneumonectomy for carcinoma of the bronchus. J Thorac Cardiovasc Surg 80:406, 1980.
15. Peterffy A, Calabrese E: Mechanical and conventional manual sutures of the bronchial stump. Scand J Thorac Cardiovasc Surg 13:87–90, 1979.
16. Dart CH, Scott StM, Takaro T: Six-year clinical experience using automatic stapling devices for lung resections. Ann Thorac Surg 9:535, 1970.
17. Hood MR, Kirksey TD, Calhoon JH, Arnold HS, Tate RS: The use of automatic stapling devices in pulmonary resection. Ann Thorac Surg 16:85, 1973.
18. Konrad RM, Ulrich B, Huth F, Ammedick U, Peters HJ: Die Bronchusstumpfinsuffizienz nach Verwendung des Klammernahtgerätes. Thoraxchirurgie 21:513, 1973.
19. Maaßen W, Stamatis G, Greschuchna D: Klammernahtgeräte in der Chirurgie der Lunge. Chirurg 56:227, 1985.
20. Betts RH, Takaro T: Use of a lung stapler pulmonary resection. Ann Thorac Surg 1:197, 1965.
21. Ravitch MM, Steichen FM, Fishbein RH, Knowles PW, Weil P: Clinical experiences with the soviet mechanical bronchus stapler (UKB-25). J Thorac Cardiovasc Surg 47:446, 1964.
22. Amasov NM, Berezovsky KK: Pulmonary resection with mechanical suture. J Thorac Cardiovasc Surg 41:325, 1961.
23. Rutten APM, Sikkenk PJH: Stapling devices in pulmonary surgery. Neth J Surg 34:5, 1982.
24. Irlich G: Bronchusstumpfinsuffizienz nach Pleuraempyem nach Klammernaht an Bronchus und Lunge in der Thoraxchirurgie In: Klammernahttechnik in Thorax und Abdomen. Ulrich B, Winter UJ: Stuttgart: Verlag, 1986.
25. Hakim M, Milstein BB: Role of automatic staplers in the aetiology of bronchopleural fistula. Thorax 40:27, 1985.
26. Bazelly B, Donzeau-Gouge GP, Daussy M, Vanetti A, Daument Ph: Suture mècanique et manuelle des moignons bronchique dans la pneumonectomie: etude comparative. Presse Med 10:3647, 1981.

CHAPTER 22

STAPLING IN PULMONARY SURGERY

P. Keszler

Surgical staplers have a long tradition of use in Hungary since the development of the first stapling device by Hültl in 1908 and the more popular instrument by Von Petz, former chief surgeon in Gyor-Hungary. This background motivated our interest in the Soviet staplers in 1958—some 30 years ago—after a visit to Amasov's Institute in Kiev.[1,2,3] Since that time, stapling has been an integral part of our operative technique in thoracic surgery.

CLOSURE OF THE BRONCHIAL STUMP BY STAPLING

Our first series, published in 1964, concerned 222 resections performed for tuberculosis, including 26 pneumonectomies. The UKB-25 stapler, inserting a single row of longitudinal staples in the long axis of the bronchus, had been used for closure. This series has been achieved without a single broncho-pleural fistula, evidently reason enough to encourage continued application of the method.[4] Until we became acquainted with the UKL stapler, which inserts two rows of staggered parallel staples at a right angle to the long axis of the bronchus, we believed that the single row of longitudinal staples corresponded best to Sweet's bronchial closing technique. We were concerned that the double staggered row closure might compromise the blood supply of the bronchial stump. After several years of experience with the UKL stapler, we have come to the conclusion that if there is any difference at all in the security of bronchial closure, it is one that favors the UKL instrument, which corresponds to the TA series.[3,5-9]

In two operative series (the first from 1963 to 1967), the operative indications were 3 to 1 for tuberculosis over cancer, whereas in the second study (from 1973 to 1982), this relation reversed to 5 resections for carcinoma for every 1 resection for tuberculosis. The incidence of broncho-pleural fistulae was 5.7% in 173 pneumonectomies of the more recent series vs. 3.2% in the 123 pneumonectomies of the earlier group. It has to be emphasized that the mean age was 12 years older in the recent series (Tables 22-1 and 22-2).

According to the comparative study of Takaro, the incidence of fistulae in 1976 manually sutured mainstem bronchi was 6%, whereas in 647 mechanically closed bronchial stumps, this complication occurred in only 4.3%. This difference, however, is statistically insignificant.[10] The main advantage of the stapling technique is not exclusively related to secure closure of the bronchus, if by comparison modern resorbable atraumatic sutures are used for manual closure and the procedure is carried out by an experienced surgeon.[6-8,11-17]

Advantages of stapling are found in a variety of technical steps:

Symmetry and precision of staples are superior to manual sutures

Stapling is more apt to provide a straight and pouch-less stump

Stapling is a closed procedure eliminating possible aspiration of blood into the remaining bronchial tree, contamination of the pleural cavity, and interference with intra-operative ventilation

Healing is without bronchial stump granuloma

Shortening and simplification of the operative procedure is usually observed.

On the other hand, there are conditions preventing the use of the stapler, such as proximity of a tumor (where open exploration and biopsy of a proposed transection line are unavoidable) or when a sleeve

Table 22-1. Bronchial Closure with UKL-40, 1963–1967—Mean Age: 43 (21–67) Years

		n	Fistula
Resection	Pneumonectomy	123	4 (3.2%)
	Lobectomy	444	1 (0.2%)
	Segmentectomy	83	0
	Total	650	5 (0.7%)
Indication	Carcinoma	130	2 (1.5%)
	Tuberculosis	402	3 (0.7%)
	Other	118	0

resection and bronchoplasty have to be performed. Relative *contraindications* or *technical inconveniences* may also prevail:

Adhesion and penetration of calcified lymph nodes into the bronchial wall make use of the stapler cumbersome, difficult, and even unsafe. The danger of injury to the vessels is considerably increased.

Stapling of the left main stem bronchus meets with difficulties if the tumor originates there. It seems likely that the roticulator can be placed with greater ease into the aortic window, flush with the carina.

Manual closure is preferred by us in left-upper and right-middle lobectomy, because staples may hurt the overlying pulmonary artery. If staple closure is performed, covering of the bronchial stump is essential.

There is no reason to use the stapler on a segmental bronchus, because of the difference between the size of the bronchus and the jaws of the stapler.

General conditions leading to *failure* do not present considerable differences with those observed following manual closure. An early and total reopening of the stump points to technical problems. This dramatic complication occurs in approximately 20% of the reported broncho-pleural fistulae, predominantly in the more-exposed right main-stem bronchus. In our series, the incidence of fistulization was the highest in the second period studied. This is because the total number and proportion of extended resections for bronchial carcinoma was the highest in this period: 27% stage N1 and 12% stage N2 lymph-node involvement. It is evident that blood supply of the bronchial stump suffers damage as lymph nodes are removed from the bronchial stump surroundings, particularly from the carina.

Technical errors such as inadequate use or a discrepancy between staple size and bronchial wall thickness may result in insufficient closure, crushing,

or breaking of the bronchial wall—all ominous complications in aged and emphysematous patients because of poor tissue elasticity.

The surgeon's experience and knowledge of "his" stapler's potential and limits are essential factors in avoiding technical complications. Some authors have reported a higher incidence of bronchial fistulae after pneumonectomy with the hinged-type stapler instead of the proven parallel stapler.[18,19] It is questionable if a real increase in usefulness is gained by frequent modifications of the devices. The correct application of a stapler, regardless of its origin and type, means having knowledge of small, meticulous practical details, which hardly can be described in books or papers, especially since such details belong to the particularities of each instrument. Consequently, if a surgeon becomes fully acquainted with the properties and the use of "his or her own staplers," he or she will probably work with a minimum of technical failures, or at least with fewer failures than if he or she were to repeatedly fall into the temptation to use new and apparently more advantageous instruments without having sufficient time to become familiar with their particularities.

STAPLING OF LUNG PARENCHYMA

Our comments are based on some 4000 staple applications in pulmonary surgery, for which the TA or UKL model is currently used. However, the GIA or UKJ stapler, developed originally for linear anastomosis in gastro-intestinal surgery, is also applied for simultaneous transection and closing of central and peripheral parenchymal cut surfaces.

The basic methods for removing peripheral coin lesions are the tangential and wedge resections that replace the classic segmentectomy. Stapling greatly simplifies the transection of the incomplete fissure in lobectomy.[9,13,14,16,20–25]

Pulmonary tuberculosis is still a health problem in developing countries, where surgical therapy remains an integral component of overall treat-

Table 22-2. Bronchial Closure with UKL-40, 1973–1982—Mean Age: 56 (32–76) Years

		n	Fistula
Resection	Pneumonectomy	173	10 (5.7%)
	Lobectomy	645	7 (1.08%)
	Segmentectomy	237	3 (1.2%)
	Total	1055	20 (1.8%)
Indication	Carcinoma	671	16 (2.3%)
	Tuberculosis	124	2 (1.6%)
	Other	260	2 (0.76%)

ment plans. Therefore, pluri-segmental or trans-segmental resections to remove fibrocavernous or caseous lesions from both the upper and lower lobes have become much easier and safer.[5] These operations, performed under the protection of effective anti-tuberculosis drugs, are successful even in the presence of considerable spreading of disease to the remaining healthier lung tissue, because of the elimination of the traumatizing blunt dissection so characteristic of classic segmentectomy.

Stapling extends the technical limits in the surgical treatment of recurrent spontaneous pneumothorax and bullous emphysema. Of 2000 patients admitted for these conditions, 400 underwent operation, with no postoperative mortality in patients with isolated blebs or bullae. The essential goal in bullous emphysema is the removal of giant or main bullae. With stapling techniques, a maximum of valuable functional parenchyma can be saved and decompressed. The prognosis is determined by the type of bullous disease and the extent of diffuse emphysema in the remaining lung tissue. Because of their deficient elasticity and retractability, emphysematous lung staples, like running sutures, may cause small air leaks. In such cases an uninterrupted suture with 3-0 Dexon or Vicryl is used to cover the staple row; if aerostasis remains unsatisfactory, a thin layer of tissue sealant (Fibrin) is also applied. Very rarely, stapling of fibrotic tissue may result in hematoma formation, producing a temporary opacity on chest x ray and possibly leading to infection if the hematoma is not absorbed.

Stapling is now the most accepted method for the removal of peripheral lesions of unknown origin. Stapling techniques facilitate atypical resections performed as elective procedures in T1, N0 stage carcinoma, an approach that hitherto had been reserved for aged patients with poor general and respiratory conditions. Survival is not inferior to that observed in a comparable group of patients after lobectomy. Indications were therefore extended, and preference is now given to atypical resections in subpleural squamous-cell- or adenocarcinoma in the absence of hilar or mediastinal lymph-node metastases. In 300 patients followed for 5 years or more, the overall survival rate is 36%; the operative mortality rate was 2.4%. Local recurrence was observed in 12% of patients, and more than 30% of the subsequent mortality was from non-carcinomatous causes.

Stapling the most central or even intra-pericardial sections of the great *pulmonary vessels*, possibly the left atrial wall itself, is a considerable contribution to the more radical resection in borderline cases.[23] This method is safer than any other and facilitates within reasonable time limits the accomplishment of operations that might not be possible with conventional techniques. Severe bleeding may result from the retraction of ligated or sutured vessel stumps, a complication avoided by the use of the fine vascular staples placed with the TA-30 or UKS-30.

After discharging the stapler, but before transecting the vessel, insertion of two atraumatic holding sutures into both vessel corners is advisable to hold the stump for inspection. This simple procedure allows control of bleeding in case of a technical failure by applying a Satinsky clamp without delay. In our practice, a single case was experienced in which the staple line failed completely; in 12 cases we were obliged to put one or two additional sutures on bleeding points.

Mechanical sutures are without peer in procedures to remove Pancoast's tumors and tumors of the pleura, chest wall, mediastinum, and diaphragm with extension of or adherence to the lung. Setting the stapler beyond and under the involved part of the lung and proceeding first with stapling and then with transection in healthy parenchyma, the "en bloc" removal of such tumors is considerably facilitated and radically improved.

Additional reasonable and generally accepted fields of applications are resection of solitary or multiple lung metastases and palliative resection of inoperable peripheral tumors when complications like bleeding or abscess formation have to be controlled.

CONCLUSIONS

Pulmonary surgical techniques were the first to benefit from the development of modern stapling devices. Although a lowering in the incidence of broncho-pleural fistulae is observed when the bronchial stump closure is performed with staples, this point remains controversial for some surgeons. It is, however, incontestably true that stapling has brought new concepts and considerable technical facilities to lung resection for tuberculosis, coin lesions of unknown origin, benign tumors, blebs and bullae, and peripheral and metastatic carcinoma. It simplifies and shortens the duration of some embarrassing details of operative technique. Finally, in placing non-reactive staples, tissue reaction and the possibility of infection are decreased.

REFERENCES

1. Amasov NM, Berezovsky KK: Pulmonary resection with mechanical suture. J Thorac Cardiovasc Surg 41:325, 1961.
2. Androsov PI: An instrument for suturing the bronchial stump (UKL-25 and 16). Clin Surg (Tokyo) 17:980, 1962.

3. Petz A: Zur Technik der Magenresektion. Ein neuer Magen-Darmnähapparat. Zentralbl Chir 5:179, 1924.

4. Keszler P, Kozma A: Tapasztalatok UKB-25 szovjet bronchus varrógéppel. Tuberkulózis (Budapest) 1:17, 1964.

5. Goldman A: An evaluation of automatic suture with UKL-60 and UKL-40 devices for pulmonary resection. Dis Chest 46:29, 1964.

6. Guilbert B, Mulsant P, Giffon H, et al: La fermeture des bronches en chirurgie d'exerese pulmonaire. Lyon Chir 75:82, 1979.

7. Pellegrini GF, Mezzetti M, Contessini Avesani E, et al: Clinical experience in the use of automatic stapler for bronchial stump closure. Surgery in Italy 10:215, 1980.

8. Péterffy Á, Calabrese E: Mechanical and conventional manual sutures of the bronchial stump. Scand J Thorac Cardiovasc Surg 13:87, 1979.

9. Ravitch MM, Brown I, et al: Experimental and clinical use of the soviet bronchus stapling instrument. Surgery 46:97, 1959.

10. Takaro T: Use of staplers in pulmonary surgery. Surg Clin North Amer 64:461, 1984.

11. Bazelly B, Donzeau-Gouge GP, Daussy M, Vanetti A, Daumet PH: Suture mechanique et manuelle des moignons bronchiques dans la pneumonectomie. Presse Méd 4:3647, 1981.

12. Gamondes JP, Eloi R, Adeleine P, et al: Étude comparée de la cicatrisation des moignons bronchiques aprés exereses pulmonaire; suture manuelle contre agraffage mechanique. Ann Chir Thorac Cardiovasc 38:188, 1984.

13. Giordani M, Zorzoli A, Sacchi M: Considerazioni su 270 casi di suture mechaniche in chirurgie polmonare. Chir Thorac 4–5:283, 1980.

14. Keszler P: The mechanical suture with UKL-40 and UKL-60 in pulmonary surgery. Dis Chest 56:383, 1969.

15. Keszler P, Romeu FP: Stapling on bronchus, lung parenchyma and lung vessels. In: Delarue et al: International Trends in General Thoracic Surgery, Vol. 4: Esophageal Cancer. St. Louis: Mosby.

16. Ravitch MM, Steichen FM, Fishbein RH, et al: Clinical experiences with the soviet mechanical bronchus stapler UKB-25. J Thorac Cardiovasc Surg 17:454, 1964.

17. Verain Ch, Cayot M, Viard H: Etude comparative des modes de suture automatique et manuelle en chirurgie pulmonaire á propos de 132 resections. Ann Thorac Cardiovasc 33:147, 1979.

18. Hakim M, Milstein BB: Role of automatic staplers in the aethiology of bronchopleural fistula. Thorax 40:27, 1985.

19. Smiell J, Widmann W: Bronchopleural fistulas after pneumonectomy. A problem with surgical stapling. Chest 92:1056, 1987.

20. Betts RH, Takaro T: Use of the lung stapler in pulmonary resection. Ann Thorac Surg 1:197, 1965.

21. Birecka A, Drzewski Z, Goralczyk J, et al: Lungenresektion mit mechanischer Naht. Thoraxchirurgie 12:328, 1964.

22. Dart CH, Scott SM, Takaro T: Six year clinical experience using automatic stapling device for lung resection. Ann Thorac Surg 9:550, 1970.

23. Hood RM, Kirksey TD, Calhoon JH, et al: The use of automatic stapling devices in pulmonary resection. Ann Thorac Surg 16:85, 1973.

24. Hood RM: Stapling techniques involving lung parenchyma. Surg Clin North Amer 64:469, 1984.

25. Mineo TC, De Leo G, Rea S, et al: La nostra esperienza con la suturatrice automatica TA-30 nelle resezioni polmonari. Chir Torac 6:449, 1979.

ADDITIONAL READING

Busalov AA, Mikaeljan AL: Die mechanische Naht des linken Herzohrs. Chirurgija 8, 1955.

Erret LE, Wilson J, Chiu R, Munro DD: Wedge resection as an alternative procedure for peripheral bronchogenic carcinoma in poor risk patients. J Thorac Cardiovasc Surg 90:656, 1985.

Hun N, Deutriax M, Barra JA, et al: Automatic stapling devices (TA and GIA) in lung resection. Poumon Coeur 35:267, 1979.

Steichewn FM, Ravitch MM: Stapling in surgery. Chicago: Year Book, 1984.

CHAPTER 23

STAPLING IN PULMONARY SURGERY: A TEN YEAR EXPERIENCE

A. Van der Tol

In contrast to the experience in other countries, stapling in the Netherlands was more readily adopted by abdominal than thoracic surgeons. However, since 1978 we have been using stapling instruments in all pulmonary operations. In our 10 years of experience, we have found staples extremely useful in sealing pulmonary parenchyma and reducing or even eliminating oozing of blood and leaks of air previously encountered with the traditional techniques of pulmonary parenchymal resections. We have also observed greater ease and safety in bronchial closures with staples, although the clinical impression of their superiority over manual techniques has not been confirmed statistically, in large part because of the absence of meaningful, prospective, comparative studies. Closure of pulmonary vessels with staples is expedient and safe. Our use has only been limited by economical considerations in lobectomies where ligation of segmental branches is equally reliable and fast with manual techniques. However, to consider the cost factor in its right perspective, it is important to account for the total cost of one pulmonary operation, from the day of hospital admission to discharge. This includes costs of hospitalization, radiographic and laboratory examinations, physiotherapy, all professional fees, and amounts to 10,000 guilders in our area ($4,750.00!). With an average use of 2.5 staple cartridges per patient, the cost of stapling is only 3.3% of this total amount, as compared to the cost of physiotherapy, which is approximately 6 to 8%.

CLINICAL EXPERIENCE

Our study is a retrospective one. From 1978 to 1988 we performed operations on 651 patients with the use of staplers. The types of operations are shown in Table 23-1. Of the 214 *pneumonectomies*, 135 were performed on the left side and only 70 on the right side. From an analysis of our patient material, no explanation can be offered for this prevalence of the left side. Three times we observed an empyema without bronchial fistula, and we encountered 5 bronchopleural fistulae, which will be analyzed in detail later on. Re-operation for hemothorax became necessary on 2 occasions for non-staple-related bleeding.

Four patients suffered severe respiratory failure postoperatively. Two patients eventually died. The first, a 59-year-old man with emphysema, had undergone a pneumonectomy for a large-cell carcinoma of the right upper lobe. He was known to have a pre-existing neurologic impairment of muscular function and could not resume breathing on his own postoperatively.

The second patient, a 69-year-old male, developed a rapidly progressing adult respiratory distress syndrome 4 days after right pneumonectomy, which did not respond to intensive treatment. The patient died 4 weeks postoperatively.

A third patient died during operation from a myocardial infarction.

Three times, subcutaneous emphysema developed

Table 23-1. Operations 1978–1988

Operation	n
Pneumonectomy	214
Lobectomy	283
Bi-lobectomy	41
Segmental resection	13
Wedge excision/lung biopsy	37
Excision of bullae and pleurodesis	63
Total	651

that subsided after removal of the chest tube (Table 23-2).

Pulmonary *lobectomy* was performed 324 times, including 41 bi-lobectomies (Table 23-3).

Four patients died: 2 of respiratory failure, 1 of autopsy-proven pulmonary embolism, and the fourth of myocardial infarction (the mortality rate was 1.3%). One broncho-pleural fistula developed, which will be discussed later.

Our clinical experience with various *parenchymal* and tissue-sparing *excisions* for lung biopsy and modified segmentectomy is shown in Tables 23-4 and 23-5. In all 50 cases, only 1 re-operation was necessary. There were no additional serious complications.

Segmental resections and wedge excisions for malignant disease were performed on patients with limited pulmonary function. Sixty-three procedures were accomplished on patients with recurrent or persistent pneumothorax. Resection of bullae and mechanical pleurodesis were achieved in all cases (Table 23-6).

Re-operation was necessary for 2 patients because of bleeding not related to stapling. One patient developed respiratory failure that required several bronchoscopies for removal of retained secretions. One patient needed medical support for cardiac failure. There were no stapler-related complications.

Table 23-2. Pneumonectomy 1978–1988 (n = 214)

Sex distribution	203 M, 11 F
Location	135 L, 70 R
Average age	60.3 yrs; Range: 38–81 yrs
Diagnosis	Non-oat cell carcinoma: 210
	Oat cell carcinoma: 3
	Metastasis: 1
Complications	Empyema: 3
	Broncho-pleural fistula: 5
	Hemothorax: 2
	Respiratory failure: 4*
	Cardiac failure: 4*
	Subcutaneous emphysema: 3

* Mortality rate was 1.4% (3 Patients).

Table 23-3. Lobectomy 1978–1988 (n = 324)

Sex distribution	279 M, 45 F
Location	138 L, 186 R
Age distribution	*Malignant disease:* 62.8 yrs; Range 27–82 yrs
	Benign disease: 49.9 yrs; Range 18–79 yrs
Diagnosis	*Malignant disease:* 296
	Benign disease: 28
Complications	Broncho-pleural fistula: 1
	Hemothorax: 3
	Respiratory failure: 19*
	Cardiac failure: 9**
	Prolonged air leak: 14
	Pulmonary embolism: 1**

* Two patients died in this group; one of cardiac failure, one of pulmonary embolism.
** Mortality rate was 1.3% (4 patients).

STAPLING TECHNIQUES AND RELATED COMPLICATIONS

In all *pneumonectomies*, staples were used to close the main bronchus, the veins, and all but eight arteries.

Intra-operative bronchial air leaks requiring an additional suture appeared twice.

Stapling of arteries was technically impossible in eight cases. Once a Swan-Ganz catheter happened to be caught in the stapled artery. Another time we became aware of having used the wrong cartridge in a venous closure, after the fact; minor bleeding occurred, which stopped spontaneously. These two complications are only remotely related to the use of staplers (Table 23-7).

Table 23-4. Wedge-Excision/Lung Biopsy 1978–1988 (n = 37)

Diagnosis
Benign lesions: 12
Malignant disease: 18
Miscellaneous: 7

Diagnostic Breakdown

Malignant (n = 18)	Benign (n = 12)
Carcinoma: 13	Hamartoma: 4
Hodgkin's disease: 1	Tuberculoma: 4
Metastasis: 3	Non-resolving atelectasis: 1
Carcinoid: 1	Sarcoidosis: 2
	Abscess: 1

Other Relevant Data
Complications: (No staple-related complications)
Hemothorax (intercostal artery): 1
Length of hospitalization (average): 10.4 days
Mortality: (None)

Table 23-5. Segmentectomy 1978–1988 (n = 13)

Diagnosis
  Squamous cell carcinoma: 10
  Benign lesion: 3

No complications

Length of hospitalization (average): 10.1 days

In 324 *lobectomies,* intra-operative bronchial air leaks appeared four times. Twice a tear in the membranous portion of the bronchial stump developed, and this was due to either technical failure or instrument mishandling. Twice we forgot to fire the instrument and achieve bronchial closure (not a strictly staple-related complication). Once we used the wrong cartridge for bronchial closure. Finally, we encountered one bona fide broncho-pleural fistula (Table 23-8).

Stapling of the *parenchyma* was performed 235 times. Parenchymal closures were accomplished in 135 lobectomies, mostly for incomplete fissures (Table 23-9).

Postoperatively, a prolonged air leak resolved with chest-tube drainage only, in 12 patients. The leaks were attributed to alveolar injury. In one case re-operation was indicated, and the leakage appeared to come from a non-stapled area of the parenchyma.

ANALYSIS OF THE INDIVIDUAL ANATOMIC STRUCTURES

Stapled *bronchial closures* were performed 538 times (Table 23-10). A bronchial air leak developed 6 times during operation, requiring an additional suture for complete control. Six broncho-pleural fistulae became apparent postoperatively, 5 after pneumonectomy with an incidence of 2.3% and 1 after lobectomy with an incidence of 0.35%. The diagnosis of broncho-pleural fistula can be difficult to establish, and is most often suspected and confirmed clinically. Radiographic chest examination was a most helpful aid in the detection of fistulae.

A persistent or increasing air bubble in the pleural

Table 23-6. Bulla Excisions for Pleurodesis 1978–1988 (n = 63)

Sex: 50 M, 13 F
Age: 42.9 yrs (average); range 20–81 yrs

Complications
  Hemothorax: 2
  Respiratory failure: 1
  Cardiac failure: 1

No staple-related complications

Table 23-7. Stapling Techniques and Complications: Pneumonectomy 1978–1988 (n = 214)

Number of Staples
Vein: 426*
Artery: 206**

Staple-Related Complications
Bronchial air leak: 2
Swan-Ganz catheter in stapled artery: 1
Arterial stapling technically impossible: 8
Wrong cartridge used on vein (TA-30-35): 1

* Extensive resections with intra-pericardial vein stapling in 22 cases.
** Note that arterial stapling was technically impossible in 8 cases.

space for up to 3 months after operation makes the diagnosis likely. Bronchoscopic diagnosis of a broncho-pleural fistula was possible only once in our experience. In a 73-year-old male we performed a left upper lobectomy for adeno-carcinoma. Persistent and increasing air drainage through the chest tube developed. Bronchoscopy was performed, and a bronchopleural fistula was clearly seen.

Fourteen days after the first operation, the remaining lower lobe was resected and the newly created bronchial stump covered with a pericardial flap. Local antibiotics were administered. There was an uneventful recovery. The patient is in excellent condition 18 months later and free of disease.

The other broncho-pleural fistulae are listed below.

Male, 65, left pneumonectomy for squamous cell carcinoma.
2 months postoperatively: broncho-pleural fistula and recurrent disease
9 months postoperatively: died of metastasis

Table 23-8. Stapling Techniques and Complications: Lobectomy 1978–1988 (n = 324)

Number of Staples
Bronchus: 323*
Vein: 151
Artery: 59
Parenchyma: 135

Staple-Related Complications
Bronchial air leak: 4
Tear in bronchial stump: 2
Broncho-pleural fistula: 1
Forgot to fire the instrument: 2
Wrong cartridge on bronchus: 1

* In 283 lobectomies, there were 275 stapled closures; in 41 bi-lobectomies, there were 48 stapled closures (275 + 48 = 323).

Table 23-9. Stapling Techniques and Complications in the Parenchyma 1978–1988 (n = 248)

Fused fissure (in lobectomies): 135
Bulla resections: 63
Wedge excision/lung biopsy: 37
Segmentectomy: 13

Complications
Prolonged air leak: 13
Staple-related: (none)

Male, 66, left pneumonectomy for squamous cell carcinoma.
2 months postoperatively: broncho-pleural fistula
1 year postoperatively: died of metastasis

Male, 65, left pneumonectomy for squamous cell carcinoma.
3 months postoperatively: broncho-pleural fistula
2 years postoperatively: free of disease

Male, 60, right pneumonectomy for squamous cell carcinoma.
3 months postoperatively: broncho-pleural fistula and empyema
(Patient died 3 weeks after thoracostomy)

Male, 64, right pneumonectomy for squamous cell carcinoma.
2 months postoperatively: broncho-pleural fistula
(Patient died 2 weeks after re-operation)

Stapling of the *vessels* was performed 842 times with no complications whatsoever (Table 23-11).

Stapling of the artery was technically impossible in

Table 23-10. Stapling of the Bronchus: Number of Stapled Closures and Broncho-Pleural Fistulae (BPF)

Procedure	n	BPF
Pneumonectomy	214	5 (2.3%)
Lobectomy	276	1 (0.3%)
Bi-lobectomy	48	
Total	538	6 (1.1%)

Intra-operative bronchial air leaks: 6

Table 23-11. Stapling of the Vessels 1978–1988

Arteries	
Pulmonary:	206
In (bi)lobectomy	59
Veins	
In pneumonectomy:	426
In (bi)lobectomy:	151
Total	842

eight cases: the stapling apparatus appeared to be too short or presented problems with complete encircling of an occasional wide artery. In our opinion, a 90° curved clamp should be developed that accommodates the cartridge of the instrument and thus facilitates encircling of the artery.

In stapling the pulmonary artery, minimal oozing around the staples may occur. This should be treated by tampon compression and will always subside spontaneously. The new cartridge with three staple lines will avoid this always-minimal bleeding.

The advantages of stapling arteries are determined by local conditions. Sometimes suture ligation might be hazardous, because a running suture closure is time-consuming or may even be technically impossible.

CONCLUSIONS

Our series confirms the generally held impression that the incidence of broncho-pleural fistulae is reduced with the use of bronchial staplers and continues to diminish with increasing experience in the use of mechanical sutures. Vascular closures are safe and fast. Economical considerations limit their use for us to pneumonectomies and major vascular trunks in lobectomies. Parenchymal closures with staples have been far superior to any other method in our hands. However, stapling instruments and the techniques required to place mechanical sutures are not foolproof, nor are they totally free of problems and complications: a review of our experience leads to the conclusion that many or most of these can be avoided with increasing experience and exercise of sound surgical judgments.

CHAPTER 24

THE USE OF STAPLING DEVICES IN PULMONARY SURGERY

G. Antypas, A. Hatzinis, and S. Bathrellou

At the Metaxa's Memorial Hospital in a recent 24-month period, 254 patients underwent operations primarily for pulmonary carcinoma (group A): 160 patients had pneumonectomies, 90 had lobectomies. Stapling devices were used exclusively in these procedures for ligation of the pulmonary veins and artery and for closure of the bronchus. The parameters studied were (a) operating time, (b) amount of blood loss and blood replacement, (c) postoperative complications, (d) postoperative length of hospital stay, (e) patient tolerance, and (f) total hospitalization costs. We compared the results with a similar series of patients who underwent operations in the immediate previous period without the use of stapling devices (group B). Operating time for patients of group A was decreased by 50% as compared to group B.

The total blood loss in group A was decreased by one third and the blood replacement by one fourth of the amounts of group B. The postoperative complications in group A were atelectasis in 3 patients (1.2%) and wound infections in 5 patients (2%). No broncho-pleural fistulae were observed in any of these patients.

In group B, the postoperative complications were atelectasis in 11 patients (4.4%), wound infection in 9 patients (3.6%), pulmonary emboli in 3 patients (1.2%), and broncho-pleural fistulae in 8 patients (3.2%). Postoperative hospitalization in group A lasted an average of 13 days, and in group B, 18 days.

The decrease in hospital stay and the significant limitation of postoperative complications appear to offset the higher cost of stapling devices.

DISCUSSION

Closure of the bronchial stump with manual sutures is achieved with a line of individual sutures placed at variable distances from the cut edge of the stump, and tied with different degrees of strength. Therefore, the tissue compression at various points of the stump edges is not uniform. These two parameters influence the healing of the bronchial stump. With staples, the closure and the stump edges are in symmetric alignment and the tissue compression is the same throughout the staple line. Two other factors that influence the healing are the size of the stump and the material used for closure. As long as the stump closure is flush with the parent bronchus or trachea and the material used for closure is nonreactive, the cause for failure to heal is related only to tissue viability.

Pneumonectomy after stapled bronchial closure is possible without the placement of chest drainage tubes, as demonstrated by our comparative study of 65 patients.

CONCLUSIONS

The use of stapling devices in pulmonary cancer surgery has reduced postoperative complications, is well tolerated by patients, limits the need for and volume of blood replacement, and reduces the duration of operation and length of hospital stay, making it more cost-effective.

CHAPTER 25

STAPLING IN PULMONARY PARENCHYMAL RESECTIONS

Nguyen Huu, Y. Raut, J.A. Barra, Ph. Mondine, J. Monod, and Hoan Vu Nguyen

The most spectacular and satisfying use of the TA and GIA instruments has been in their application to parenchymal resections in pulmonary surgery. Stapling of the lung parenchyma is certainly used much more widely than the few published reports would indicate, while a much larger volume of publications is reserved for stapling instruments used on the hilar elements, most significantly the bronchus. In this chapter we will discuss our technique of parenchymal pulmonary stapling and present the results obtained in 1243 patients who underwent operations from 1976 to 1987 with the use of the TA and GIA instruments.

OPERATIVE TECHNIQUE

As a rule, the TA and GIA instruments are applied to the collapsed pulmonary parenchyma (double lumen endo-tracheal Carlens tube). This approach facilitates the operative procedure and makes parenchymal resections much safer, by allowing precise placement of the jaws or arms of the instruments and avoiding lacerations of the expanded lung. Furthermore, the collapsed lung facilitates readjustments in the placement of the instruments while the lesion to be incorporated in the resected specimen is seen and palpated with greater ease.

If, however, a parenchymal resection of any size becomes necessary on the inflated lung, it is important to delineate the margins of resection, if necessary by stay sutures or by temporary compression with a vascular clamp outlining the future lines of staple placement.

If the parenchymal resection is undertaken on the collapsed lung with the TA or GIA instruments, the lesion is held between thumb and index finger and

the instruments are placed at a safe distance, some 2 to 2.5 cm from the periphery of the lesion. In both techniques it is important to choose the size of the staples judiciously. We are also in the habit of touching the resection lines with gauze soaked with beta-dine.

Following either one of these two techniques, the lung is re-inflated to examine hemostasis and aerostasis. From time to time it is necessary to complete the staple line with an interrupted suture to control a localized bleeding point or an air leak. For this purpose we have also used hemostatic clips, careful pinpoint electro-coagulation, and sealing with biologic glues. In general, one or two sutures are necessary at the point of crossing or overlapping of two staple lines. Using these techniques we have achieved parenchymal resections extending from the simple stapling of parenchymal lacerations to trans-segmental resections that straddle several adjacent segments.

COMPLETION OF INTERLOBAR FISSURES WITH THE PARAHILAR TUNNEL TECHNIQUE

The separation of an incomplete fissure can be accomplished as either the first or last step of lobectomy. As the first step, completion of a fissure helps in the mobility of a given lobe to gain better access to the hilar structures. This technique can be used on an inflated or collapsed lung. A tunnel is created lateral (above the vessels from the surgeon's postero-lateral point of view) to the vessels and bronchi; it starts from the middle of the oblique fissure to the mediastinal surface on the left and from the junction of horizontal and oblique fissures to the mediastinal aspect on the right. This dissection is performed sharply to the level of the arteries in the fissures and to the level of the veins on the mediastinal side. Once a safe plane is obtained, blunt dissection by an educated finger tip or "peanut" cotton dissector is easy. A vessel loop is passed through the tunnel to help in guiding the instrument (TA or GIA) into place (Fig. 25-1). If the TA instrument is used, the anvil-carrying arm of the instrument is advanced through the tunnel. With the GIA instrument, the application can be performed safely from the periphery of the fissure into the tunnel (Fig. 25-2).

If the fusion or adherence between two lobes is relatively peripheral, then the stapling instruments can be applied as the final step after all of the hilar vessels and the bronchus of the lobe have been dissected, stapled, and transected.

Stapling instruments are also very useful in the repair of superficial pulmonary lacerations from intraoperative handling or external trauma.

PULMONARY PARENCHYMAL EXCISIONS

The difficulties encountered in these excisions vary according to their extent and anatomic site. For biopsies of peripheral, superficial lesions, we use a dou-

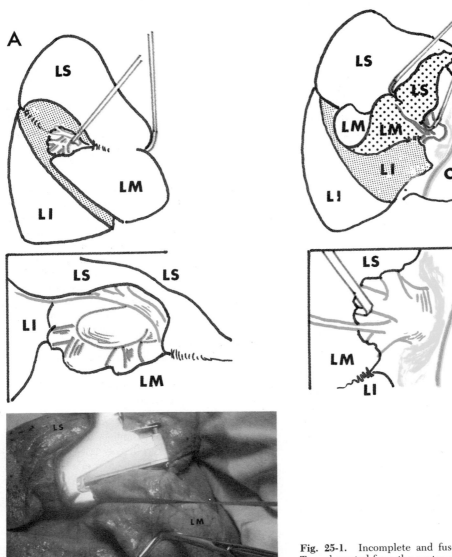

Fig. 25-1. Incomplete and fused interlobar fissure. *A.* Tunnel created from the center of the horizontal fissure to the mediastinal aspect. *B.* Placement of the TA-90 through the tunnel with the anvil guided by the vessel loop.

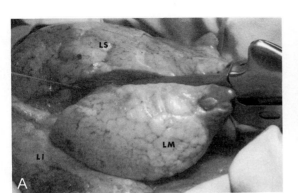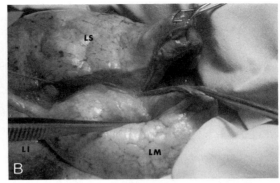

Fig. 25-2. *A.* Incomplete fissure technique using the GIA instrument from the periphery of the horizontal fissure to the parahilar tunnel marked by the vessel loop. *B.* The resulting closures of the upper and middle lobes on both sides of the instrument application are shown.

ble application of either GIA or TA instruments in a tangential or cuneiform (wedge) fashion (Fig. 25-3). The area of resection, including the lesion to be biopsied, is held with a Duval clamp.

ANATOMIC SEGMENTECTOMY

This technique is used in the resection of a single segment, as well as in the excision of several segments such as the apical-posterior segments of the upper lobe, the lateral segment of the middle lobe, the lingula, and the superior segment of the lower lobes. These operations are indicated for more cen-

trally located lesions that do not allow a peripheral biopsy.

The operation starts with the dissection of the vessels and bronchus that supply a given segment (Fig. 25-4). Following transection of the segmental bronchus, the remaining lung is inflated, and the intersegmental plane is opened by following the stem of the spreading intersegmental veins centrally and the demarcation between collapsed and inflated lung peripherally (previously known as the "peeling" procedure). The TA-90 (4.8) is then positioned along this demarcation line, the lung is collapsed, and the instrument is closed by encroaching—if possible—on the segment to be resected to preserve the intersegmental venous arborization.

TRANS-SEGMENTAL RESECTIONS

If the lesion is in the periphery of the lobe, the approach is from the lung margins by using transsegmental planes that involve a portion of several adjacent segments. In these resections, which may involve only one, two or, more exceptionally, even three lobes, the surgeon is not limited by segmental boundaries. There are three types of trans-segmental resections (Fig. 25-5):

1. Peripheral trans-segmental resections are easy to accomplish with the TA-90 instrument; they result in the amputation of a mass of tissue situated at the free periphery of a lobe, such as the apex of the upper lobe or the peripheral half of the lingula or middle lobe.
2. Pyramid-shaped trans-segmental resections are actually extended cuneiform (wedge) resections that require repeated applications of staple instruments. Usually, the GIA stapler is applied twice to delineate the separation of the speci-

Fig. 25-3. Localized superficial resections and stapling of lacerations.

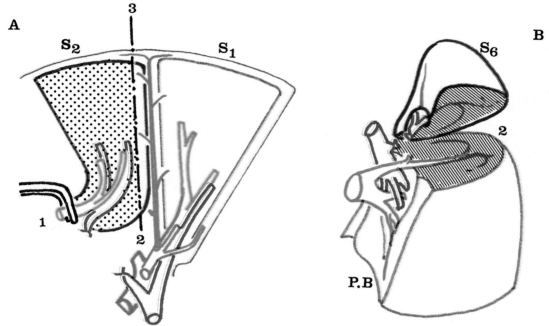

Fig. 25-4. Trans-segmental resections.

men from the remaining healthy lung. The TA-55 or TA-90 instrument is then applied perpendicular to the broncho-vascular pedicle of the segments to connect both GIA staple lines at the base of the resection (Fig. 25-6A).

3. With the lung collapsed, it is possible to do an extended deep resection of a tumor situated on the convex surface of the lung. The resulting change in the configuration of the lung is that of a "well" or "pit." As the lung is re-inflated with

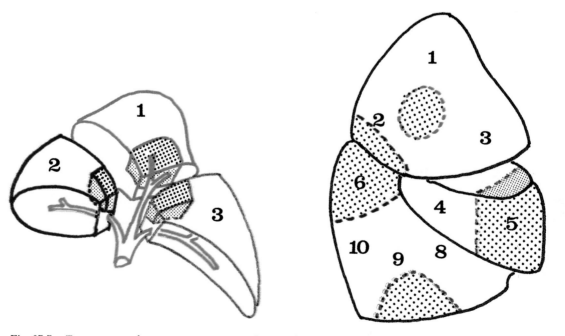

Fig. 25-5. Trans-segmental resections in anatomic planes with stapling of parenchyma.

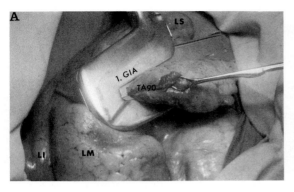
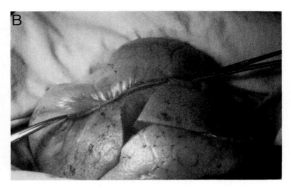

Fig. 25-6. *A.* Application of the TA-90 instrument perpendicular to the hilar segmental elements, after two parallel applications of the GIA instrument have been accomplished. The TA instrument connects both GIA lines. *B.* "Well" or "pit" excision of a lesion of the convex aspect of the upper lobe. Following re-inflation, the staple line placed with a TA-90 instrument is air- and water-tight and the lung does not rupture at the staple line.

a competent staple line, the initial depression tends to be corrected somewhat (Fig. 25-6*B*).

These extended parenchymal resections, usually easy to accomplish, can be made difficult by the changing consistency of the pulmonary parenchyma in patients with diffuse infiltrations and induration, or in patients with thinned-out parenchyma (such as in emphysematous bullous disease). If the parenchymal infiltration has definite limits, a larger excision in healthy parenchyma may be indicated; if this is impossible, a lobectomy may be necessary. If, on the other hand, the parenchyma is thinned out and the instruments are used for the closure and resection of emphysematous bullae, we reinforce the 3.5-mm staple line with a running suture of fine absorbable material or with biologic glue applied along the staple line.

If the blebectomy is performed with the lung collapsed, it is possible to place a TA-90 onto the healthier base of a given bleb or bulla. In this fashion staples are held better, and the bulla can be resected "en bloc" without preliminary opening of the bulla. Fortunately, most spontaneous pneumothoraces are caused by one or several small blebs that can be easily resected distal to the placement of a TA stapler in healthy pulmonary parenchyma.

RESULTS

The intra-operative imperviousness of the staple line is uniformally excellent. Only rarely are additional, limited steps necessary to assure hemostasis or aerostasis here and there. To avoid mechanical problems, it is important to watch the alignment of the cartridge with the penetration of the tissue pin into the corresponding hole in the anvil, especially with the scissor-like closing of premium TA instruments.

In the long-term followup, the staple line continues to be well aligned; in fact, it is difficult to determine the participation of the staples in the occasional postoperative complication. For this reason, we will only consider here those complications that are due to either bleeding or air leaks.

The interstitial hematoma along the staple line is clearly due to this method. As a rule, this opacity, seen on chest radiography, clears spontaneously after a few weeks. We have observed four incidents of important hemorrhage after anatomic excisions in which the staplers had been used on both the parenchyma and the corresponding hilar structures. At reoperation, none of these bleeding sites were found at the level of the vascular stumps or at the lines of parenchymal transection.

On two occasions, prolonged air leaks occurred following the resection of large apical emphysematous bullae that had been responsible for a spontaneous pneumothorax in young patients. These patients required several re-operations and chest-tube drainage lasting well over 1 month.

Since 1976, when we started to use stapling instruments in our department, we have rarely had to establish prolonged chest-tube drainage of persistent pleural spaces due to discrete air leaks. In fact the only postoperative pleural spaces observed were due to a separation of the lung from the apex of the chest wall or the diaphragm. These spaces have routinely disappeared with well directed respiratory physiotherapy, and none of them have required an additional re-operation.

DISCUSSION AND CONCLUSIONS

The double row of staples applied with the TA and GIA instruments is a safe, non-ischemic, flat suture line, especially if it is applied on the collapsed lung parenchyma. The excellent quality of the parenchymal healing has been obvious in our re-operations done for reasons related to the disease and in a series of experimental studies on dogs that were sacrificed either 8 days or 6 months after the operation. The rust-proof steel of the staples is well tolerated and the line of staples in the "well-" or "pit-like" resections disappears in the depths of these resections without any untoward result. The B-closure of these staples preserves the blood supply beyond the line of closure as shown by us on the injection-corrosion studies in dogs. Because of their reliability and safety, staplers facilitate a faster liberation of the lobar fissures and expedite wedge resections for biopsy. They make tissue-sparing resections possible if necessary, either as conventional anatomic segmentectomies or as intersegmental resections. Staplers have totally changed the technique of operations for bullous emphysema and for traumatic laceration of the pulmonary parenchyma. Finally, the possibility of resecting several segments is not limited to a given lobe but can be applied to adjoining segments in different lobes.

Translated from the French by F.M. Steichen, M.D.

BIBLIOGRAPHY

1. Allan A, et al: Recent experience of the treatment of aspergilloma with a surgical stapling device. Thorax 41(6):483–484, 1986.
2. Allen Th: Technic of resection of localized bullous disease of the lung. Ann Surg 37:671–676, 1971.
3. Amasov NM, Berezovsky KK: Pulmonary resection with mechanical suture. J Thorac Cardiovasc Surg 41(3):325–335, 1961.
4. Arcerito S: The automatic stapling devices: a real progres in the resection of pulmonary tissues. Chir Ital 33(1):135–140, 1981.
5. Cook WA, Lee CW, Yon KD, Santos GH: Pulmonary resection autosuture technique. NY State J Med 74:967, 1974.
6. Dart CH Jr, Scott SM, Takaro T: Six year clinical experience using automatic stapling devices for lung resections. Ann Thorac Surg 9(6):535–550, 1970.
7. Hood RM, Kirksey TD, Calhoon JH, Arnold HS, Tate RS: The use of automatic stapling devices in pulmonary resection. Ann Thorac Surg 16:85–98, 1973.
8. Hood MR: Stapling techniques involving lung parenchyma. Surg Clin North Am 64(3):469–480, 1984.
9. Irlich G, et al: Automatic stapling devices in the surgery of the lung and the bronchial tree. Langenbecks Arch, Chir 355:459–463, 1981.
10. Kirksey TD, Arnold HS, Calhoon JH, Hood RM: Techniques of pulmonary resection: tradition and travail. Ann Thorac Surg 9:525, 1970.
11. Lawson WR, Hutchison J, Longland CJ, Haque MA: Mechanical suture methods in thoracic and abdominal surgery. Br J Surg 64:115–119, 1977.
12. Maassen W, et al: Surgical staplers in surgery of the lung. Chirurg 56(4):227–231, 1985.
13. Monod JE: Sutures automatiques et exérèses pulmonaires. These de Doctorat en Medecine. Brest, Mai 1980.
14. Moritz E, et al: Automatic suturing devices in lung surgery. Wien Klin Wochenschr 94(7):189–192, 1982.
15. Nguyen Huu, Raut Y, Monod J, Nguyen Hoan Vu: Bilan de sept années de suture automatique en chirurgie pulmonaire. J Chir (Paris) 122:187–191, 1985.
16. Nguyen Huu, Doutriaux M, Barra JA, Monod JE: Suture automatique et chirurgie pulmonaire. Poumon Coeur 35:267–275, 1979.
17. Ravitch MM: Experience with a second generation of stapling instruments in general and thoracic surgery. Bull Soc Intern Chir 31:502–509, 1972.
18. Reuter MJP: Les sutures mécaniques en chirurgie digestive et pulmonaire. Doctoral Thesis, Strasbourg 1982.
19. Rutten AP: Stapling devices in pulmonary surgery. Neth J Sur 34(5):211–215, 1982.
20. Steichen FM, Ravitch MM: Stapling in Surgery. Chicago: Year Book, 1984.
21. Takaro T: Use of staplers in pulmonary surgery. Surg Clin North Am 64(3):461–468, 1984.
22. Verain Ch, Cayot M, Viard H: Etude comparative des modes de suture automatique et manuelle en chirurgie pulmonaire. A propos de 132 résections. Ann Chir: Chir Thorac Cardiovas 33(3):147–150, 1979.

CHAPTER 26

THE VALUE OF STAPLERS IN OPERATIONS FOR SPONTANEOUS PNEUMOTHORAX

D. Schröder, A. Thiede, O. Meinicke, and H. Hamelmann

The concept of idiopathic, spontaneous pneumothorax applies to those forms that occur primarily in young patients with apparently normal lung tissue and a generally predictable clinical course. A "symptomatic" pneumothorax, on the other hand, is usually associated with bullous emphysema, cystic lesions, or clustered blebs; such lesions are due to the destruction of the pulmonary parenchymal architecture.

Although the idiopathic pneumothorax is thought to be associated with ill-defined constitutional factors, histologic studies show that the idiopathic form does not develop without some morphologic alterations of the lung surface.[1] Hence, the idiopathic pneumothorax enters within the definition of the symptomatic form. The clinical and pathologic manifestations are limited in extent[2,3] and vary to a degree that seems to justify separate descriptions (Table 26-1).

To establish a base for surgical treatment, we define recurrent pneumothorax as a failure of the primary successful treatment, regardless of the post-therapy duration of pulmonary expansion without air leak and notwithstanding the possibility that the pathologic character and morphology of the recurrence may be different from the original or previous lesion.

A gradual therapeutic response to the various clinical and pathologic presentations of pneumothorax has been followed by us since 1978, when we started a prospective clinical series with yearly followup examinations of all patients.[4] The following *therapeutic procedures* were used:

1. Tube thoracostomy with water-sealed drainage for a minimum of 7 days. For complicated pneumothorax, additional chest tubes might be inserted and left in place for more than 10 days.
2. Thoracoscopy with electrocoagulation, fibrin sealing of parenchymal leaks, and tube thoracostomy. Thoracoscopy is useful in young people if prolonged suction fails to expand the lung and small cystic lesions cannot be identified by tomography and CT Scan. It is also useful in patients with a high operative risk for open thoracotomy.
3. Thoracotomy with tangential parenchyma-sparing lung resection, using staplers or manual suture techniques, in association with parietal pleurectomy and fibrin-sealing of parenchymal defects.

From 1978 to the end of 1987, 137 patients (104 men and 33 women) were admitted for 172 treatments. In 85% of these patients, a yearly followup chest x ray was obtained. Patients with more than one episode of pneumothorax (n = 6) are listed only once with their final treatment. Sixty-two patients (45%) were transferred from other hospitals after primary treatment with chest-tube drainage had failed. They are included with the patients whose primary treatment was unsuccessful, and therefore cause a bias towards increased complexity in the composition of the overall group (Tables 26-2, 26-3).

Twenty-eight of 81 patients suffered a recurrence after primary treatment with chest-tube drainage for a minimum of 10 days. The period in which relapse

Table 26-1. Age Distribution in Patients with Pneumothorax

Age Group	Male	Female	Total
10–19	3	4	7
20–29	30	11	41
30–39	16	4	20
40–49	14	2	16
50–59	11	3	14
60–69	10	6	16
70–79	10	2	12
80–89	0	0	0
90–99	0	1	1
Totals	104	33	137

occurred ranged from 15 days to 83 months. In this group, one 71-year-old patient died because open thoracotomy was impossible due to poor pulmonary function. The cause of death was diffuse fibrosis of both lungs, confirmed by the post-mortem examination. In 17 of the 28 cases, the cause of recurrence could be determined and the patients were successfully treated by open thoracotomy. One of these 17 patients, 69 years old, died after thoracotomy because of her underlying disease.

Fifty-six patients underwent open operation after primary treatment by drainage proved unsuccessful, because of early or repeated recurrences. In this group, 3 patients, aged 69, 73, and 78 years respectively, died because of respiratory insufficiency. We performed 67 transaxillary thoracotomies with a 30-day hospital mortality rate of 6%. A lobectomy was done in a single case (honeycombed lung fibrosis). Anatomic segmental resections always proved impossible because the disease extended beyond the segmental margins.

In 35 of 67 open thoracotomies, we used the linear stapling instruments for the tangential resection of blebs (Fig. 26-1). In the average case, the transaxillary approach provides satisfactory access to all lobes for the placement of the stapling devices. In 22 cases, the resection surfaces were sutured by conventional techniques (Fig. 26-2). In the remaining 10 cases,

Table 26-2. Management of Primary Pneumothorax (n = 137)

Primary Treatment	No. of Cases	No. of Recurrences	No. of Deaths
Chest tube	81 (59%)	28 (36%)	1 (1%)
Thoracoscopy	7 (5%)	1 (14%)	0
Thoracotomy	49 (36%)	0	3 (6%)

Table 26-3. Management of Recurrent (Secondary) Pneumothorax (n = 29)

Secondary Treatment	No. of Cases	No. of Recurrences	No. of Deaths
Chest tube	11 (38%)	0	1 (10%)
Thoracoscopy	0	0	0
Thoracotomy	18 (62%)	0	3 (18%)

fibrin adhesives and electrocoagulation only were applied. Of the 67 patients, we performed an apical pleurectomy in 45 instances. There was no recurrence in these 45 patients observed over a 10-year period.

DISCUSSION

Properly employed stapling devices are more convenient than hand sutures and technically superior in the division of incomplete fissures and resection of wedges of pulmonary parenchyma. However, the opportunity to demonstrate the superiority of mechanical stapling over the manual suture techniques by statistical methods may be an impossible task unless huge studies are undertaken. As such prospective series, especially for tangential parenchymal lung resections, are unlikely to occur, our recommendations are limited to the experience gained by this prospective study.

As there is no effective preventive or curative treatment of the primary disease that causes spontaneous pneumothorax, surgical procedures are limited to the management of complications of such disease. Therefore, the objectives of pneumothorax therapy focus on eliminating the peripheral lung lesion and

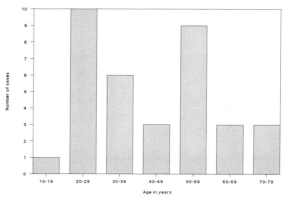

Fig. 26-1. Application of staplers sorted to age distribution.

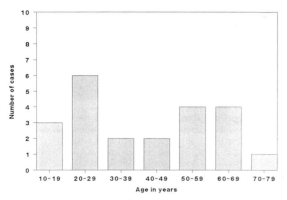

Fig. 26-2. Application of sutures sorted to age distribution.

avoiding functional respiratory damage by extended parenchymal resection.

Because of the structural and functional transformations of the lung tissue in elderly patients with emphysematous lung disease, one has to consider and expect a higher rate of mortality, which was 6% in the group of patients over 65 years old (there was no mortality in the group under 65 years of age). Elderly patients suffer not only from restrictive obstructive lung disease, but also from the resultant cardiorespiratory impairment. These risk factors justify an individual approach to treatment to satisfy each specific clinical presentation and to recommend exploration only after closed tube thoracostomy has failed. Uncomplicated pneumothorax in young individuals is usually due to a rupture of an emphysematous bleb that is mainly in the apical portion of the upper lobe, and usually does not herald the onset or presence of generalized emphysematous disease. Although some of these cases may represent an early stage of emphysema or the rupture of an isolated lung cyst, excision of the subpleural blebs or cysts has proven to be efficient, with low morbidity and recurrence rates.

TECHNICAL CONSIDERATIONS IN THE MANAGEMENT OF PNEUMOTHORAX

The operative management of pneumothorax complicated by localized bullae and representing the focal end stage of diffuse emphysema is much more difficult than the handling of the limited condition in the young individual. This is especially true if the atrophic bullae have a thin outer shell and the tissue is not firm enough to accept a primary airtight and durable suture line by either interrupted or continuous manual suture techniques.

Because of the tissue destruction, loss of parenchymal elasticity, and decrease in lung substance, a conventional manual suture produces additional puncture lesions of the lung surface. These punctate wounds grow into small linear tears from the additional air pressure produced by many fine bronchial communications into the base of the bulla.

The use of staples provided by the TA-55, TA-90, and GIA instruments, while technically more convenient, contributes above all precision, efficiency, and reliability to the tangential pulmonary parenchymal closures in these young and elderly groups of patients.

Since the stapler compresses the spongy lung parenchyma and holds it immobilized while all the staples (mechanical sutures) are placed simultaneously, tissue trauma is alleviated and the aerostatic seal is greatly improved around the fine staples, which are both the needle and the suture material. The pulling of a thread through thin tissue is thus eliminated. If necessary, areas of small air leaks can be "silenced" with the application of fibrin adhesive.

CONCLUSIONS

Following the recurrence of pneumothorax after chest-tube drainage therapy only, we recommend an open surgical approach.[4] Parietal pleurectomy with excision of the responsible parenchymal lesions has proven to be the most effective treatment, with no second recurrences in our 10-year series. Stapling is highly beneficial to patients with bullous emphysema, since a tight closure of the rigid, thin, and atrophic tissue can be provided with more ease only by tissue compression, immobilization, and simultaneous placement of the mechanical suture line.

REFERENCES

1. Masshof W, Höfer W: Zur Pathologie des sogenannten idiopathischen Spontanpneumothorax. Dtsch Med Wochenschr 98:801–805, 1973.

2. Senac JP, Giron J, Aguado JL, et al: L'interet de la tomodensitometrie dans le bilan pre-therapeutique des pneumothorax spontanes idiopathiques de l'adulte. A

[1] Auto Suture Company, division of the United States Surgical Corporation, Norwalk, Conn., USA
* Tissucol[R] IMMUNO GMBH, Heidelberg, West Germany. Beriplast[R] HS BEHRINGWERKE AG, Marburg, Germany.

propos de vingt-cinq cas. Ann Radiol (Paris). 28(8):586–591, 1985.

3. Vincent M, Celard P, Pinet F, Loire R, Brune J, Galy P: La radiologie du pneumothorax spontane du sujet jeune. A propos de deux cents cas. Sem Hop Paris. 60(11):759–765, 1984.

4. Schröder D, Thermann M: Aetiologie und Therapie des Spontan-pneumothorax. Fortschr Med 102:1071–1076, 1984.

5. Pawlowicz A, Droszcz W: Pulmonary function and alpha-1-antitrypsin levels in patients after so-called idiopathic spontaneous pneumothorax. Bull Eur Physiopathol Respir 23(1):1–4, 1987.

ADDITIONAL READING

Burford ThH, Ferguson ThB: Congenital lesions of the lungs and emphysema. In: Sabiston DC Jr, Spencer FC: Gibbon's Surgery of the Chest. Philadelphia: WB Saunders, 1976:611–649.

Giese W: Atemwege und Lungen. In: Doerr W, Giese W, Leder L-D, Remmle W: Organpathologie (Band I). Stuttgart: Thieme, 1974.

Jagdschian V: Der Spontanpneumothorax und seine Behandlung unter Berücksichtigung dystrophischer Lungenveränderungen. Langenbecks Arch Klin Chir 304:437–446, 1963.

CHAPTER 27

TECHNIQUE OF TISSUE SAVING PULMONARY RESECTIONS (USING THE LINEAR GIA STAPLING DEVICES)

John M. Keshishian and Greg Groglio

The use of stapling devices on lung tissue is not a new procedure. This chapter concerns our experience with currently used techniques of pulmonary parenchymal resection, which has been referred to as non-anatomic tissue sparing or (irreverently) "heretical" resection.

At the present time, approximately 80 to 85% of all pulmonary resections in the United States are for bronchogenic carcinoma. A high percentage of these patients are elderly with some elements of chronic obstructive pulmonary disease and cardiac involvement as well.

A reduction in operating time and anesthetic exposure is an important aspect of the total care of this type of patient. These two factors are interdependent. By refining anesthetic techniques, one can reduce operating times; by refining surgical techniques, we can further reduce the total exposure to anesthesia.

We based the development of the following protocol on our experience with linear stapling instruments.

MATERIALS AND METHODS

If it is determined by radiologic studies (such as chest films, tomograms, CAT Scans, MRI, or any combination of these) that a lesion appears to be resectable by saving lung tissue and that such an "economical" resection is reasonable from a therapeutic point of view, the following approach is used:

If pulmonary function tests indicate that the afflicted lung may be collapsed during thoracotomy, a double-lumen endotracheal tube is used to adminis-ter inhalation anesthesia. Following thoracotomy, the lesion is identified, and the feasibility of and rationale for a tissue-saving procedure are established intraoperatively. On request, the anesthesiologist deflates the exposed lung, which is then grasped with Duval clamps and elevated into the field. The area to be resected is delineated by inspection and palpation. Suitably long, straight vascular clamps are then applied to the collapsed lung tissue, outlining the area to be resected. The clamps are closed and opened, then quickly removed. The linear GIA stapling device is now applied to fit into the groove created by the vascular clamp. The instrument halves are matched and locked, the staples are fired, and the knife blade is advanced simultaneously. This maneuver is repeated as many times as is necessary until the specimen has been resected. The lung is gently re-expanded. The stapled edges are examined closely for incomplete hemostasis or aerostasis. Occasionally, cautery or an interrupted mattress suture may be required to secure a bleeding point.

The remaining areas of lung need not be approximated unless there is danger of torsion.

RESULTS

One hundred twenty patients were considered suitable for stapled parenchymal lung resections. In half of the patients, findings proved unsatisfactory for a lung-sparing procedure. Of the 61 patients in whom parenchymal resections could be carried out, there was no morbidity or operative mortality. Chest tube drainage was not required after 48 to 72 hours, and many patients had minimal or no air leakage.

CHAPTER 28

THE USE OF ABSORBABLE HEMOSTATIC CLIPS IN PULMONARY RESECTIONS

Huu Nguyen, Hoan Vu Nguyen, J.A. Barra, Y. Raut, Ph. Mondine, and
S. Castel-Dupont

Of the various synthetic resorbable sutures used with great regularity by surgeons since 1970, two that belong to a second generation—the lactomer and the polydioxanon—have been molded into hemostatic clips (1980).

The main characteristic of these new hemostatic clips that differentiates them from their metallic predecessors is the presence, at their free ends, of a locking system that prevents both spreading of the arms of the clip and sliding of the clip along the long, or transverse, axis of the vessel.

At present two types of resorbable synthetic clips exist:

The polysurgiclips of lactomer (PSC) of the U.S. Surgical Corporation

The Absolok clips made of PDS introduced by the Ethicon Corporation (Fig. 28-1).

The polysurgiclips are provided with a double interlocking system at their open end and with dentate profiles of arms, or jaws, of the clip preventing slippage. These clips are presented in preloaded, sterilized, disposable, automatically activated application instruments. The great advantage of this presentation is the fact that the cleared vessel can first be held by the empty claws of the delivery instrument. Only after a perfect placement has been selected is the polysurgiclip discharged from the instrument and placed onto the vessel with maximum visibility and safety.

The Absolok clips have a longitudinal and transversal interlocking mechanism at their open ends and smooth jaws, or arms. Each clip has two lateral projections to guide them into the placement instrument, which is reusable. The clips are for single use only, and are presented in cartridges of five or ten clips. While these cartridges are economically more advantageous, each clip has to be loaded into the placement instrument individually.

EXPERIMENTAL STUDIES

Following our introduction to these clips in October of 1983, we planned to study their use in anatomic pulmonary resections because they appeared reliable with their interlocking systems at their open ends. Also, the vessels in pulmonary resections are within a low pressure circulation. Our thesis was first tested experimentally on 25 large (40 kg) dogs and 5 rabbits. As shown in Table 28-1, we have placed these clips not only on large pulmonary vessels in the

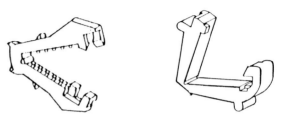

Fig. 28-1. Resorbable synthetic hemostatic clips with interlocking closure. *Left:* Polysurgiclips, a double interlocking system with dentate jaws preventing slippage. *Right:* Absolok clips, a longitudinal and transversal interlocking system with smooth jaws.

Table 28-1. Placement of Hemostatic Clips in Experimental Study Involving 25 Dogs and 5 Rabbits

Site	No.	Diameter
Pulmonary vessels	25	8–9 mm
Carotid arteries	6	6–8 mm
Femoral artery	7	7–8 mm
Splenic artery	3	6 mm

animal, but also on systemic vessels such as the carotid, femoral artery, and splenic artery.

The results of these experimental studies were especially encouraging in as much as the hemostasis obtained with the clips was instantaneous intra-operatively, without any need for complementary manual ligatures. The long-term follow-up of these animals did not show any hematomas, secondary hemorrhage, or death by hemorrhage. At autopsy of animals sacrificed between 1 week and 6 months postoperatively, the clips were found to be reliably closed during the first 3 weeks after operation and to have lost their coloration, but remained perfectly identifiable after 1 to 2 months. Within 6 months the clips had lost their original shape and were recognizable as a small, whitish foreign body, surrounded by a well delineated fibrotic scar, in a clean thorax without any adhesions to speak of.

Histologically, the resorbable clip appears as an amorphous, fragmented foreign body surrounded by a thin shell of fibrosis (Fig. 28-2). Our results confirmed those of Lerwich[1] and Ray et al.[2] who have shown that these new materials are perfectly well tolerated in a living biologic environment.

CLINICAL APPLICATION

Encouraged by these experimental results, we have used the polysurgiclips and the Absolok clips in human pulmonary resections since June of 1984. In Table 28-2, the various operations in which absorbable clips were used are shown, such as lobectomy, bi-lobectomy, segmentectomy, and pleuri-segmentectomy (e.g., excision of lingula, superior segment of the lower lobes, or apical-posterior segments of the upper lobes). We have also observed the clips in 10 pneumonectomies, following an attempt to first limit the operation to a lobectomy. This experience has allowed us to verify the excellent hemostasis obtained with the clips intra-operatively, before moving to pneumonectomy.

SURGICAL TECHNIQUE

Following the complete and satisfactory isolation of the vessel to be ligated, we place two clips at a distance of 10 mm from each other. Transection of the vessel is achieved one-third of the way from the peripheral clip and two-thirds the distance from the central clip to preserve a safe stump centrally of some 5 to 6 mm. If the vessel can only be isolated for a distance of 1 cm, the two clips can be placed so that the transection takes place very close to the peripheral clip. If the isolated vessel measures only 5 to 6 mm, it is safe to place a clip on the central portion of the vessel and to reserve transection for the very last step of the hilar dissection.

We have frequently used the TA-30-V (vascular) on the central portion of the vessel and a clip on the peripheral portion. At times, the better part of valor is to simply use a classic manual ligature or to place the vascular staples centrally and a manual ligature peripherally. However, with the technique as initially described, the intra-operative hemostasis is perfect in all instances. We have never had to use an additional manual ligature, although at times before

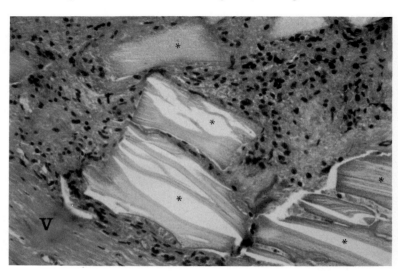

Fig. 28-2. Histologic aspect of resorbable hemostatic clips at 3 months after operation. The clips (asterisks) are fragmented and surrounded by inflammatory reactions; V = vessel wall.

Table 28-2. Operative Procedures

Procedure	No.
Segmentectomy and pleuri-segmentectomy	7
Lobectomy	42
Bi-lobectomy	11
Complementary pneumonectomy (following lobectomy)	10

transecting a vessel, we have placed a second central clip if there were doubts about the safety of the original clip placement. In the immediate postoperative period, we have not observed a hemorrhagic episode that would have forced re-operation or the administration of blood. The quantity and character of the fluid drained from the chest postoperatively resembles that observed after manual ligature of all vessels or after stapling closure of the vessels.

A summary of postoperative complications is presented in Table 28-3.

DISCUSSION

The experimental study and clinical application of hemostatic clips demonstrate the reliability and safety of these new absorbable vascular occlusion devices for pulmonary vessels with a caliber of 8 to 9 mm. However, placement of these clips is subject to certain strict rules.

The first rule is to match the size of the clip to that of the vessel, thus avoiding the danger of a short clip including the vessel wall in the interlocking system. Conversely, the use of an excessively long clip could create a problem with slippage. It is important to clear the vessel over a sufficient length to obtain vessel stumps of at least 5 mm beyond the central clip. The closing of the locking mechanism is important and should be heard and felt by the surgeon.

The use of resorbable clips presents many advantages. Their materials, polydiaxanon and lactomer, are perfectly well tolerated in a living biologic milieu, being comparable to biologic resorbable substances. Their slow, predictable, and total resorption through simple hydrolysis is more than satisfactory to assure permanent hemostasis of the vascular stumps in-

Table 28-3. Postoperative Complications

Hemorrhage requiring re-intervention	0
Clotted hemothorax	0
Prolonged bleeding (requiring transfusion)	0
Broncho-pleural fistula	1
Prolonged air leak (more than 10 days)	2
Interstitial hematoma	1
Atelectasis requiring flexible bronchoscopy	10

volved in the process of natural scarring.[1,2,3] After 67 months, the basic substance disappears completely from the patient.[4]

The clips are inert in magnetic fields and do not cause distraction to the CT scan. This makes followups with scanning and magnetic resonance imaging much easier.[5,6,7]

Compared to traditional manual sutures and ligatures, clips are a simpler, faster, and easier method, especially in areas that are deep and narrowly accessible to the fingertips.

The disadvantages associated with these clips include their volume, which forces the surgeon to take special precautions not to dislodge them by catching them in a compress. Also, these absorbable clips are more expensive than manual ligatures and the classic metallic V-shaped clips. However, these two disadvantages are compensated by the many advantages they have thus far presented in our experience. Up to now, publications have only mentioned their use in the occlusion of lymphatic and small vessels, mostly in large excisions for cancer, with the exception of clips used for the cystic artery,[8] vessels of the greater omentum,[9] vessels of the adrenal glands,[10] and ligature of the internal saphenous vein.[11]

In conclusion, the resorbable clips with interlocking mechanisms at their open ends are a technical advance in pulmonary resections for the ligature of vessels measuring from 9 to 12 mm in diameter. They offer all of the advantages of metallic clips without their disadvantages: speed, simplicity, ease of placement, and biologic compatibility, as well as safety if postoperative irrigation is required. Postoperative radiologic followups are greatly simplified with these clips.

Translated from the French by F.M. Steichen, M.D.

REFERENCES

1. Lerwich E: Studies on the efficacy and safety of Polydioxonone monofilament absorbable suture. Surg Gynecol Obstet 156:51–55, 1983.
2. Ray JA, Doddi B, Regula D: Polydioxanone, a novel monofilament synthetic absorbable suture. Surg Gynecol Obstet 153(4):497–507, 1981.
3. Schaeffer CJ, Colombani PM, Geelrded GW: Absorbable ligating clips. Surg Gynecol Obstet 154(4):513–516, 1982.
4. Champault G, Faure P, Patel JC: Le "résorbable en chirurgie." J Chir (Paris) 123(1):45–51, 1986.
5. Marks WM, Collen PW: Computed tomography in the evaluation of patients with surgical clips. Surg Gynecol Obstet 151(4):557–558, 1980.
6. New PFJ, Rosen BR, Brady TJ, et al: Potential hazards and artefacts of ferromagnetic and non ferromagnetic surgical and dental materials and devices in nuclear

magnetic resonance imaging. Radiology 147(1):139–148, 1983.

7. Weese JL, Rosenthal MS, Gould H: Avoidance of artifacts on computerized tomograms by selection of appropriate surgical clips. Am J Surg 147:684–687, 1984.

8. Allan A, Cooper MJ, Leaper DJ: A new absorbable ligating clip for use in cholecystectomy. J R Coll Surg Edinb 29(1):53–54, 1984.

9. Clarke-Pearson DL, Creasman WT: A clinical evaluation of absorbable polydioxanone ligating clips in abdominal and pelvic operations. Surg Gynecol Obstet 161(3):250–252, 1985.

10. Geelhoed GW: Hemostatic clips. Contemp Surg 23(10): 75–79, 1983.

11. Harjola PT, Ala-Kulja K, Heikkinen L: Polydioxanone in cardiovascular surgery. Thorac Cardiovasc Surg 32(2):100–101, 1984.

ADDITIONAL READING

Castel-Dupont S: Clips synthétiques résorbables et exérèses pulmonaires réglées. These de Doctorat en Medecine, Brest 1987.

Documentations ETHNOR-ETHICON.

Documentations Auto-Suture France.

Michel F: Biological tolerance to PDS absorbable clips: a comparison with metallic ligating clips: Eur Surg Res 18(2):122–128, 1986.

Nguyen Huu, Nguyen HV, Raut Y, Briere J: Clips synthétiques résorbables et exérèses pulmonaires. J Chir (Paris) 1985 122(6-7):415–419, 1985.

Nguyen Huu, Nguyen HV, Barra JA, Raut Y, Castel-Dupont S: Clips synthétiques résorbables et exérèses pulmonaires. Notre expérience clinique. J Chir (Paris) 1987 124(2):113–118, 1987.

Ponsot Y, Michel F: Etude expérimentale d'un clip hémostatique résorbable. J Chir (Paris) 1984 121(1):33–37, 1984.

Part VII

Stapling in Esophageal Surgery

CHAPTER 29

STAPLING IN ESOPHAGEAL RESECTIONS

Hiroshi Akiyama and Masahiko Tsurumaru

In esophageal surgery, the technique of anastomosis is the most important step in the reconstructive phase. In our earlier experience, esophago-jejunostomy was accomplished with manual sutures. More recently, with the development of stapling devices, mechanical gastro-intestinal anastomoses have gained wide acceptance. In fact, considerable advantages, such as procedural uniformity and shortened operative time, are well recognized.[1-4] In our clinic, comparative studies revealed essentially similar results for both mechanical and manual anastomoses in the incidence of anastomotic leakage and postoperative stricture. Therefore, shortening of operative time assumed an important role in favoring the mechanically stapled over the manually sutured anastomosis.

MATERIALS AND METHODS

At the Department of Surgery of Toranomon Hospital, 652 instrumental anastomoses in upper gastro-intestinal operations were performed during the period between 1980 and 1987.

Among these 652 instrumental anastomoses, 631 (97.5%) were esophageal anastomoses after resection for adenocarcinoma of the lower esophagus and proximal stomach, all performed with the EEA instrument (US Surgical Corporation). The most frequently used loading unit was the EEA-28 (Table 29-1).

OPERATIVE TECHNIQUE

The circular anastomosing stapler is most commonly used in mediastinal and abdominal esophago-jejunostomy. It is also used in the neck for the anastomosis between a free jejunal graft and the transected end of the proximal thoracic esophagus. Anastomosis to the cervical esophagus or pharynx, however, can be more easily accomplished by manual suturing.

The end-to-side esophago-jejunostomy is preferred over the end-to-end method, because of technical simplicity and the ease with which the EEA can be positioned by inserting the cartridge carried by the instrument into the lumen of the transected end of the jejunum. A similarly constructed manual anastomosis would provide the same advantage as with the EEA, of creating an anastomotic lumen that is the size of the esophageal opening. Since the site of anastomosis is located on the anti-mesenteric wall of the jejunum, its blood supply is not compromised by the anastomosing procedure.

ANATOMIC CHARACTERISTICS OF THE ORGANS TO BE ANASTOMOSED

Esophagus

Unlike other parts of the alimentary tract, the esophageal wall is only covered by a very thin adventitial layer and no serosa. Careful operative handling of the esophagus is mandatory to avoid adventitial damage. Special care should be taken if the vagus nerves are to be transected to mobilize the abdominal esophagus. Since both vagal nerve trunks are embedded within the muscle layer deep to the adventia, transection of the vagus nerves will inevitably injure the adventitial and muscle layers at the site of transection. Therefore, foresight dictates that the level of vagal nerve transection should be distal to the one planned for anastomosis. The objective is to spare the anastomotic site the disadvantage of a damaged adventitial layer.

The muscle layer of the esophagus is thicker, compared to other levels of the alimentary tract. There-

Table 29-1. Instrumental (EEA) Esophageal Anatomoses: Types of Operations

Reconstruction after lower esophagectomy and total gastrectomy: 600
Reconstruction after lower esophagectomy and cardiectomy: 36
Bypass: 7
Free jejunal transfer: 9
Total: 652

fore, in fashioning the purse-string suture at the transected end of the esophagus with the special purse-string instrument (PSI), inadvertent inclusion of the opposite esophageal wall with through-and-through needle passage may occur.

At other times, the thick muscle excludes the mucosal layer from the course of the needle and therefore from participation in the purse-string and subsequent circular anastomosis. The act of inserting a long straight needle through the purse-string instrument, while working in a crowded sub-diaphragmatic area, is often technically impossible and always tedious. Finally, the longitudinal esophageal muscle fibers, composing the only layer of the esophageal wall other than mucosa-submucosa, are predisposed to tearing as the circular in-and-out purse-string suture, placed at a right angle to the longitudinal muscle bundles, is tightened. Thus we prefer an over-and-over whip stitch of the esophageal cut end that includes the thick muscle wall and the mucosa, often retracted to a higher level.

Jejunum

The jejunal wall is relatively thin, with prominent mucosal folds. Occasionally, the mucosal folds offer a certain degree of resistance not only to insertion but also to extraction of the EEA instrument. A torn jejunum may result from excessive force applied to maneuver the instrument in and out of such a delicate situation. Therefore, the size of the jejunal lumen is an important factor to consider while determining the size of the cartridge used. In fact, the size of the cartridge is occasionally decided by the caliber of the jejunal lumen, rather than by that of the esophagus.

STEPS IN ANASTOMOSIS

Jejunal Preparation

An intestinal loop of adequate length with sufficient blood supply to avoid tension should be chosen. The jejunal loop is elevated, usually to the level of the inferior pulmonary vein, through the retrocolic route. Adequacy of the esophageal hiatus for the passage of the jejunum should be assured simultaneously. If the hiatal opening is too tight, additional incisions are made to widen it. Another point to emphasize is that the mesenteric axis of the elevated intestine should not be twisted, which would compromise its vascular supply.

Purse-String Suturing of the Transected Esophagus

For the placement of the purse-string at the transected end of the esophagus, a purely manual technique is preferred over the one that makes use of the purse-string instrument for reasons previously described.

Akiyama's esophageal clamp (Fig. 29-1) is applied approximately 1.5 cm proximal to the transected end of the esophagus. A running purse-string suture, over and around the transected edge, is commenced with the needle directed from the lumen outward as shown in Figure 29-2. In this manner the mucosal layer is certain to be included with each passage of the needle. The ideal suture material used for the purse-string should be smooth to handle, strong to hold, and secure to tie: a 1-0 silk suture with an atraumatic needle is often used. A meticulous suturing technique demands that each stitch be placed on a seam line approximately 3 mm from the cut edge.

In between each penetration of the stretched-out wall, an interval of 4 to 5 mm is recommended. A faulty technique, such as an insufficient number of stitches, will result in failure of the purse-string effect around the central shaft of the EEA instrument, especially by missing parts of the retracting mucosa. Too many stitches will make it difficult to tie the knot. The distance between the cut line and the seam line should vary in proportion to the size of the loading

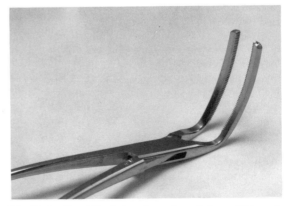

Fig. 29-1. Specially designed esophageal clamp (Akiyama) holds the esophagus securely without traumatizing mucosa.

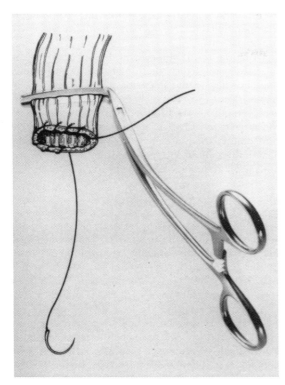

Fig. 29-2. Running suture around the transected edge of the esophagus with application of Akiyama's esophageal clamp.

unit used: within a reasonable range this distance can be more generous for the EEA-31 than for the EEA-25. Otherwise, excessive tissue will separate the circular suture from the central rod as the purse-string effect around the rod is produced.

Insertion of the Instrument into the Jejunum

The size of the cartridge-anvil normally used by us is 28 mm in diameter. To choose the most appropriate anvil for smooth insertion of the EEA instrument, several factors should be taken into consideration, including diameter, spasticity or elasticity, and strength of the mucosae of the jejunal and esophageal walls.

The bare central rod of the EEA instrument, followed by the cartridge, is inserted into the open jejunum. At some 8–10 cm from the open jejunal end, the tip of the central rod is advanced through an antimesenteric stab wound and capped with the anvil.

Insertion of the Anvil into the Esophagus

The esophageal wall is held with three or four triangular atraumatic lung clamps. Smooth insertion of

the anvil into the esophageal lumen is essential. Gentle stretching of the esophageal wall with centrifugal traction on the lung clamps will guarantee the widest possible lumen for easy insertion, as shown in Figure 29-3. After the esophageal lumen is fully stretched, Akiyama's esophageal clamp, which was proximally applied, is removed to provide unimpeded insertion of the anvil.

With a large esophageal lumen, no difficulty should be expected with the instrument insertion. However, when the esophageal lumen is small and the wall fragile, particular maneuvers are required to achieve an atraumatic insertion. The lateral cross-sectional area of the anvil is smaller than the transverse or horizontal one. With the central rod positioned at a right angle to the axis of the esophageal lumen, the anvil can be inserted into the lumen with its smallest possible lateral cross-sectional area, as shown in Figure 29-4. In fact, the central rod can only be advanced obliquely in relation to the axis of the esophageal lumen because of space limitations imposed by the anatomy of the operative field. With half of the peripheral rim of the anvil initially inserted into the esophageal lumen, the central portion of the anvil is moved into position while the anterior esophageal wall is stretched out by the hooking effect of the anterior peripheral rim inserted first. The remaining posterior half of the peripheral rim is then slipped into the lumen with a downward tilt of the center rod. Gentle traction on the atraumatic clamps stretching the esophageal wall helps to smooth the insertion of the instrument. With the new CEEA instruments, which permit separation of the anvil and central rod from the hollow shaft of the cartridge, this maneuver is greatly simplified.

The purse-string is then tightened around the center rod. After all indicated precautions have been taken, the anvil is closed against the cartridge and the stapling mechanism is activated (Table 29-2).

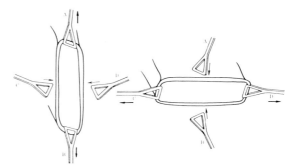

Fig. 29-3. Stretching the esophageal lumen with soft triangular clamps.

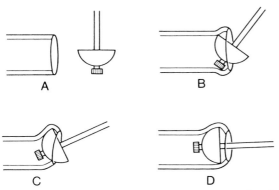

Fig. 29-4. *A–D.* Principles of atraumatic insertion of anvil.

Withdrawal of Instrument

A sterile towel is placed right below the instrument to surround the contaminated cartridge and anvil after its withdrawal. For the withdrawal of the instrument, the same principles are observed as for its insertion. Verification of anastomosis is made (Table 29-2).

Closure of the Jejunal Limb

In end-to-side esophago-jejunostomy, the closure of the jejunal limb will create a pouch that should not be too long or too short. Closure of the jejunal limb too close to the esophago-jejunal anastomosis will result in anastomotic constriction.

In Wong's report, anastomotic stricture after EEA- or ILS-stapled anastomosis was noted more frequently (EEA 20%, ILS 10%) than in manually performed anastomosis (8.7%).[5] Therefore, the over-

Table 29-2. Complications of 636 Instrumental Esophago-Jejunostomies

Intra-Operative Complications
Laceration of esophageal mucosa: 14 (2.2%)
Bleeding from the anastomotic sites: 7 (1.1%)
Total: 21 (3.3%)
Postoperative Complications
Leakage of anastomosis: 15 (2.4%)*
Stricture of anastomosis: 14 (2.2%)
No Operative Mortality

* Fourteen of the 15 leaks were minor, and were demonstrated as a small "speck" radiographically.

whelming advantage of stapling is the shortening of the operative time. No operative mortality was noted in 636 patients.

While the result of mechanical esophageal anastomosis was satisfactory, the use of an intestinal stapler does not negate the need for sound surgical techniques. Mastery of the technique of manual suturing is a prerequisite. To use the instruments effectively, the surgeon must possess mature judgment and technical ability based on sound surgical principles in the anatomic approach to adequate exposure of the operative field, atraumatic handling of organs, and respect for tissue integrity.

CONCLUSIONS

Among 636 mechanical esophageal anastomoses using the EEA stapler, leaks occurred in 15 cases (2.4%). Of these, 14 were small leaks visualized only radiographically. As a late complication, anastomotic stricture was seen in 14 cases (2.2%) (Table 29-2). For all cases with stricture, balloon dilatation only was successful. There was no operative mortality. Mechanical anastomosis was useful, particularly in esophageal anastomosis through a left thoracoabdominal or abdominal approach. However, for special anastomoses such as the pharynx or cervical esophagus, manual suture still plays an important role. It should be kept in mind that even in stapled anastomoses, the importance of basic surgical techniques cannot be overemphasized.

REFERENCES

1. Akiyama H, Tsurumaru M, Watanabe G, Ono Y, Udagawa H, Suzuki M: Development of surgery for carcinoma of the esophagus. Amer J Surg 147:9–16, 1984.
2. Ravitch MM: The use of stapling instruments in surgery of the gastrointestinal tract, with a note on a new instrument for end-to-end low rectal and esophagojejunal anastomoses. Aust N Z J Surg 48:444–447, 1978.
3. Ravitch MM, Steichen FM: A stapling instrument for end-to-end inverting anastomoses in the gastrointestinal tract. Ann Surg 189:373–381, 1979.
4. Steichen FM, Ravitch MM: Mechanical sutures in esophageal surgery. Ann Surg 191:373–381, 1980.
5. Wong J, Cheung H, Lui R, Fon Yw, Smith A, Siu KF: Esophagogastric anastomosis performed with a stapler. The occurrence of leakage and stricture. Surgery 101: 408–416, 1987.

CHAPTER 30

STAPLED ANASTOMOSES IN ESOPHAGEAL RESECTIONS

Xiao-Mai Huang

Carcinoma of the esophagus and cardia is much more prevalent in China than in most other countries. Its age-adjusted death rate is 31.6/100,000 in males and 15.9/100,000 in females. In frequency it ranks next to stomach cancer and occurs in 26.5% of male and 19.7% of female patients who compose the malignant tumor registry. In Linxian County, the well known highest risk area in China, the age-adjusted mortality rate reaches 161/100,000 in males and 103/100,000 in females.[1] Therefore, esophageal cancer is a common disease in most hospitals in China, especially in the five northern provinces. For instance, in our hospital of 1200 beds, including 40 beds for thoracic surgery, we perform 350 major general thoracic operations yearly, of which about 40% are for esophageal resection.

The figures in Table 30-1 give the results of surgical treatment of esophageal cancer in China.

INTRATHORACIC GASTRO-ESOPHAGEAL ANASTOMOTIC LEAKS

This is a serious complication after esophageal resection and reconstruction of continuity. About 30 to 50% of the patients with anastomotic leaks died of grave infections.[2] Table 30-2 shows the incidence of anastomotic leaks from some reports in recent years.

Although in China the incidence of anastomotic failure has dropped to between 2 and 3%, in comparison to 10 years ago, when it was above 5%, anastomotic failure still remains a problem.

MEASURES TAKEN TO REDUCE OR ELIMINATE THE OCCURRENCE OF ANASTOMOTIC LEAK AND FISTULA[3]

Esophageal Flap Formation with Intussusception into the Lumen of the Stomach

After resection of the tumor, a 2-cm longitudinal full-thickness incision is placed along both sides of the esophageal stump ("Fishmouth"). The two flaps obtained by this maneuver are then inserted into the stomach lumen through an opening on the anterior gastric wall. A double layer of interrupted sutures from the intact muscular esophageal wall proximal to the flaps to the seromuscular tunic of the stomach is placed, without suturing of the mucosal layers.

Tunnel-Shaped Gastro-Esophageal Anastomosis

Incisions are made—the proximal one through the sero-muscular layer of the gastric fundus, the distal

Table 30-1. Results of Surgical Treatment of Esophageal Cancer in China

Author	No. of Resections	Operative Mortality	5-Year Survival	10-Year Survival
G.J. Huang (Beijing)[7]	1373	4.1%	29.6%	22.5%
S.L. Fang (Linxian)[2]	5507	2.8%	36.8%	17.2%
X.M. Huang (Beijing)[8]	936	2.3%	26.7%	19.4%

Table 30-2. Incidence of Anastomotic Leaks from Recent Reports

Authors	No. of Resections	Incidence of Leaks	
		Manual	Mechanical
Bardini R., et al. (Italy)[9]	258		4.2%
Blum M., et al. (FRG)[10]	135	11.1%	12.3%
Peracchia A., et al. (Italy)[11]	467		10.4%
Fang, S.L., et al. (China)[2]	5507		3.8%
Du X.Q., et al. (China)[12]	150	3.2%	2.7%

one through the entire gastric wall thickness—to form a muscular tunnel of 3 cm in length and 3.5 to 4.0 cm in width. The open end of the esophagus is passed through the tunnel and anastomosed to the incised gastric mucosa at the lower end of the tunnel. The anastomosis is then covered with the seromuscular tunnel wall.[4]

Wrapping of the Pedicled Omentum Around the Anastomosis[5]

The above-described methods had the benefit of embedding anastomotic lines and reducing the incidence of anastomotic leaks. But they are time-consuming and do not entirely eliminate leaks and fistula formation.

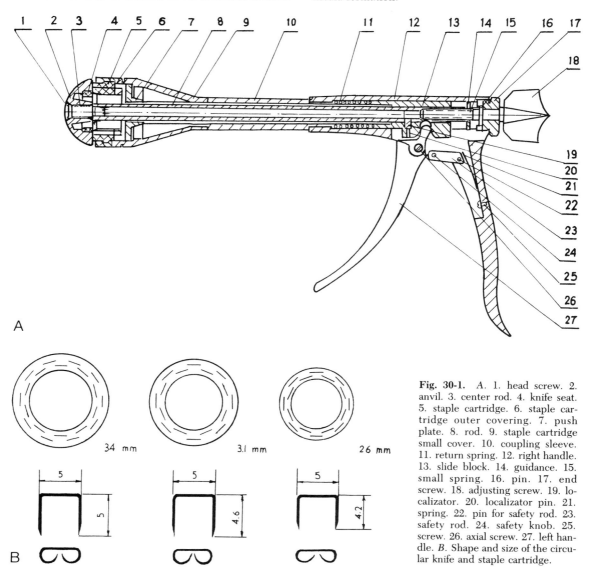

Fig. 30-1. *A.* 1. head screw. 2. anvil. 3. center rod. 4. knife seat. 5. staple cartridge. 6. staple cartridge outer covering. 7. push plate. 8. rod. 9. staple cartridge small cover. 10. coupling sleeve. 11. return spring. 12. right handle. 13. slide block. 14. guidance. 15. small spring. 16. pin. 17. end screw. 18. adjusting screw. 19. localizator. 20. localizator pin. 21. spring. 22. pin for safety rod. 23. safety rod. 24. safety knob. 25. screw. 26. axial screw. 27. left handle. *B.* Shape and size of the circular knife and staple cartridge.

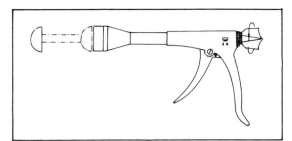

Fig. 30-2. Close the instrument's safety rod to separate it from the center rod by turning the adjusting screw counterclockwise. Withdraw the center rod and the anvil. (The center rod and the anvil are integral.)

Mechanical Suturing with Stapling Devices

Based on our experience, we think this is the logical solution to eradicate anastomotic leaks.

DEVELOPMENT OF MECHANICAL SUTURES IN CHINA

Mechanical suturing in esophageal surgery was started in 1972 by Dr. L.F. Shao with an instrument of his own design, but it was then used only in two or three hospitals. Since 1978, the Shanghai Medical Instrument Corporation has produced a tube-shaped digestive tract stapling instrument (Fig. 30-1). Thereafter, application of mechanical suturing was widely adopted in most large hospitals in China. Now, the accumulated number of cases might be over 3000 for gastro-esophageal anastomosis alone.

Our tube-shaped stapling instrument utilizes a double staggered row of tantalum staples to accomplish the anastomosis. Extra tissue is cut off by a circular knife on the inside of the staple lines as the circular anastomosis is created. Security of the anastomosis and hemostatic effect are thus ensured. Stapling and cutting are accomplished simultaneously (Figs. 30-2 through 30-10).

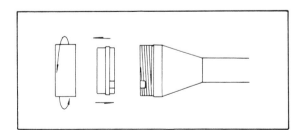

Fig. 30-3. The plastic staple cartridge with pusher, staples, and circular knife inside is fitted on the staple cartridge sleeve by removing the metal covering of the instrument. The convex block in the plastic cartridge must be correctly inserted into the gap of the cartridge sleeve, then the metal covering fastened.

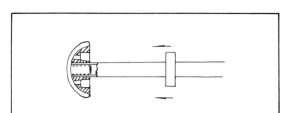

Fig. 30-4. The plastic knife seat is placed into the anvil.

PERSONAL EXPERIENCE AND RESULTS

We published our results with 575 cases of gastro-esophageal anastomosis with the circular stapling instrument, since 1980, in the Chinese Journal of Surgery (August 1987). The incidence of anastomotic leaks was 1.3% (8/575). Before 1980, we used manual suturing in 355 esophageal resections: the incidence of anastomotic leaks was 5.6% (20/355).[6] The difference is statistically significant. The incidence of anastomotic stricture was 1.9%. From July 1985 to April 1988, we have performed 313 consecutive operations with intrathoracic anastomoses using the stapling instrument. There were no anastomotic leaks.

The factors that may cause a leak are:

1. Error in anastomotic technique
2. Insufficient blood supply or undue tension at the anastomotic site
3. Infection

If one can strictly adhere to the basic principles of surgical technique and is equipped with experience in esophageal surgery, all three of these factors could be avoided, especially the second and third factors.

In manual anastomotic technique, individual technical competence is important, and there is an occasional fault as part of the learning curve. An anastomosis may appear perfect, but actually one suture may be too tight or too loose, which finally leads to a leak. With the mechanically stapled anastomosis, the

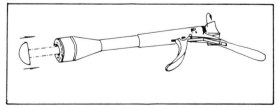

Fig. 30-5. The center rod is inserted into the center hole of the instrument body. Align markings on the center rod with the direction of the handle first. When it contacts with the screw hole on the center rod, the adjusting screw must be turned clockwise to allow the anvil to come close to the staple cartridge.

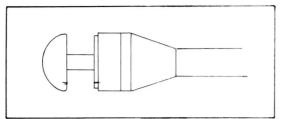

Fig. 30-6. *Caution:* Before using, examine the anvil to make sure it is in line with the markings on the plastic cartridge. Do not use the stapling instrument if there is non-alignment or displacement. Otherwise, the instrument is ready for use.

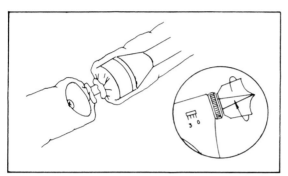

Fig. 30-7. Introduce the instrument into the intestine or tissue to be stapled, then open the tissue gap by turning the adjusting screw counter-clockwise until adequate space is available to place both ends of the tissue structures to be anastomosed between cartridge and anvil. The tissue should be securely tied to the exposed portion of the center rod with a purse-string suture.

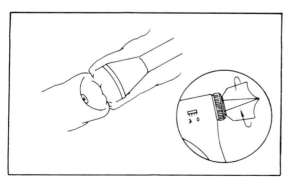

Fig. 30-8. To staple tissue, close the instrument gap by turning the adjusting screw clockwise. Be sure not to exert excessive pressure to prevent injury to the tissue. The tissue thickness, when pressed, is indicated by the graduation of stem. *Caution:* If the center rod is detached from the adjusting screw, clamp the step on the center rod with forceps and realign the center rod with the adjusting screw (see Fig. 30-6).

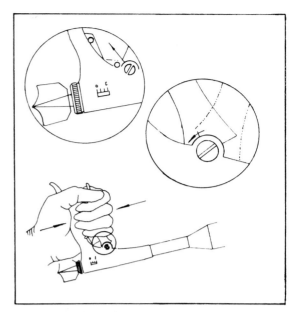

Fig. 30-9. Release the safety from the locked position. Squeeze the left handle firmly, all the way, so that the left handle corner contacts the right handle body. The anastomosis is complete.

importance of individual technical expertise is reduced, and the learning curve is much flatter. The reliability and safety of the stapled anastomosis generally surpasses that obtained with manual suturing.

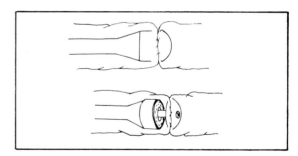

Fig. 30-10. Separate the anvil from the instrument body by turning the adjusting screw counter-clockwise. Incline the front of the instrument body to both sides in turn, so that the anvil is withdrawn from the part to be anastomosed. Then remove the instrument gently and slowly. *Note:* After withdrawing the instrument, the center rod is taken off by turning the adjusting screw counter-clockwise; meanwhile, remove the knife seat within the anvil with excised tissue. Remove the metal covering by turning counter-clockwise. In removing the plastic staple cartridge, pay attention to the following: 1. Be sure that the excised tissue is round and complete. In case of irregularities or incompleteness, sew a few stitches at the corresponding part. 2. When inspecting, do not touch the blade of the circular knife to avoid cutting your finger.

We observed eight leaks in our previous 575 cases of stapled anastomosis, but not a single leak has occurred in our last 313 consecutive cases. Our only explanation for these results is the now routinely added step after mechanical suturing of telescoping the esophagus into the gastric wall 1 to 2 cm above the anastomotic line. This additional step reduces the tension on the anastomotic line, protects it from direct exposure to the thoracic cavity (prevents possible contamination), and promotes adhesion and healing.

REFERENCES

1. Huang GJ: Epidemiology of esophageal cancer in China. Abstract of International Esophageal Week, Munich, Sep. 14–19, 1986:17.
2. Fang SL, et al: Results of surgical treatment in 6123 cases of carcinoma of esophagus and gastric cardia. Chinese Journal of Surgery 25:452, 1987.
3. Zhong BL, et al: Esophageal flaps formation with intussusception into the stomach after esophageal resection. Abstracts of the 5th Conference on Thoracic and Cardiovascular Surgery of Chinese P.L.A., Wuhan, Oct. 1987.
4. Zhang J, et al: The rational use of tunnel-shaped gastroesophageal anastomosis. Abstracts of the 5th Conference on Thoracic and Cardiovascular Surgery of Chinese P.L.A., Wuhan, Oct. 1987.
5. Zhi LC, et al: Application of the pedicled omentum suturing around the gastric esophageal anastomosis. Abstracts of the 5th Conference on Thoracic and Cardiovascular Surgery of Chinese P.L.A., Wuhan, Oct. 1987.
6. Kang LY, et al: Experience in application of the circular stapler device. Chinese Journal of Surgery 25:456, 1987.
7. Huang GJ, et al: Late results of surgical treatment for carcinoma of the esophagus. Chinese Journal of Surgery 25:449, 1987.
8. Huang XM: Experience in surgical treatment of 1139 cases of carcinoma of esophagus and cardia. Abstracts of 2nd German-Chinese Medical Conference, Munich, Sep. 19–22, 1987.
9. Bardini R, et al: Mechanical sutures in esophageal surgery. Personal experience. Abstract of International Esophageal Week, Munich, Sep. 14–19, 1986:80.
10. Blum M, et al: The influence of stapled anastomosis compared to hand made anastomosis on complication rate and mortality after resection of esophagus carcinoma. Abstract of International Esophageal Week, Munich, Sep. 14–19, 1987:81.
11. Peracchia A, et al: Esophago-visceral anastomotic leaks: prevention, diagnosis, treatment. Abstract of International Esophageal Week, Munich, Sep. 14–19, 1986:82.
12. Du XQ, et al: Clinical experience in 150 cases using the tube shaped anastomotic staples. Abstract of International Esophageal Week, Munich, Sep. 15–19, 1986:81.

CHAPTER 31

LONG GASTROPLASTIES WITH THE GIA STAPLER IN ESOPHAGEAL SURGERY

J.M. Collard, J.B. Otte, M. Reynaert, P.J. Kestens

From January 1979 until April 1988, 113 patients required a long gastroplasty for replacement of the esophagus or as a by-pass procedure. The underlying illness was esophageal carcinoma in 99 patients (80 squamous cell carcinomas, 18 adenocarcinomas, 1 sarcoma), pharyngo-laryngeal squamous cell carcinoma in 9, caustic esophagitis in 4, and an instrumental perforation in 1 patient.

METHOD

Esophagectomy and Bypass Techniques

Esophagectomy was subtotal in 94 patients and total in 9 patients; a bypass procedure was performed in 10 patients. Esophagectomy was carried out by a right thoracotomy via the fifth intercostal space, midline laparotomy, and left cervicotomy at the anterior border of the sternomastoid muscle in 83 cases; by left thoraco-phreno-laparotomy with incision of the diaphragm and left cervicotomy in 5 cases; by median sternotomy, midline laparotomy, and left cervicotomy in 1 patient;[1] and by blunt dissection without thoracotomy in another 14 patients. The 10 by-pass operations were performed through midline laparotomy and left cervicotomy.

Intrathoracic cancers were removed by a right thoracic approach and "en bloc" resection according to Skinner,[2] consisting of a wide dissection of the posterior mediastinum with excision of all the fatty and fibrous tissues surrounding the trachea, the main bronchi, the pericardium, the right pulmonary vein, and the thoracic aorta.

When a significant respiratory insufficiency was present, a trans-hiatal dissection without thoracot-omy was chosen.[3,4,5] This approach is also used when total esophagectomy is associated with a pharyngo-laryngectomy.[6,7] In benign diseases, as in caustic burns or instrumental perforations, the left thoracic approach is preferred.

Gastroplasty

A variety of techniques were used to achieve gastroplasty, but some modifications taking into account the specific anatomy of Caucasian people have been introduced (Fig. 31-1). The technique of Akiyama[8] was used 100 times: the greater omentum is separated from the gastro-colic ligament, the short gastric vessels and the left gastric artery are divided, and the posterior wall of the antrum and the first portion of the duodenum are elevated from the pancreas as far as the gastro-duodenal artery. When it is necessary to pull the gastroplasty up to the pharynx, it is helpful to perform an extended Kocher maneuver. This permits a better mobilization of the stomach if it is associated with division of the right gastric vessels and incision of the mesenteric root to the origin of the superior mesenteric artery. As a consequence, it is possible to advance the duodenal arch and the pancreas up to the diaphragmatic crus. The dissection of the lesser omentum, close to the lesser curvature as in a highly selective vagotomy, elongates the lesser curvature. The stomach is incised and simultaneously closed with the GIA stapler near and parallel to the lesser curvature, starting from a level some 3 to 4 cm above the pyloric ring. The stomach is further lengthened by straightening the upper part of the greater curvature, thus taking advantage of its elasticity. The gastric staple line is covered by seromuscular inter-

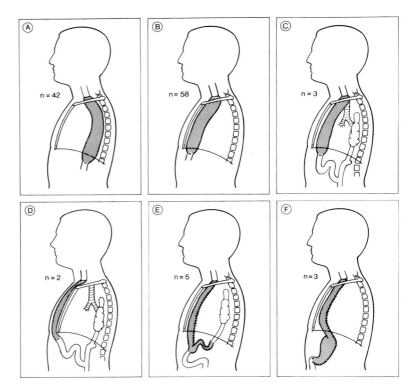

Fig. 31-1. *A.* Isoperistaltic gastroplasty in the posterior mediastinum. *B.* Isoperistaltic gastroplasty in the substernal space. *C.* Kirschner's procedure with the gastric tube in the substernal space. *D.* Kirschner's procedure with the gastric tube in the presternal space. *E.* Postlethwait's procedure. *F.* Reversed tube of Gavriliu.

rupted stitches. A pyloromyotomy is preferable to a pyloroplasty, which shortens the pyloric area. To guide the gastric tube into the neck, we use a Mousseau-Barbin tube and insert the stomach into a plastic bag lubricated with sterile oil. This protects the omental fringes along the greater curvature from being caught in the mediastinal structures during the ascent. The cervical anastomosis, initially made in one layer with interrupted sutures, is now performed in one layer by means of a continuous suture, taking the full thickness of the esophageal wall and the extramucosal layers of the gastric wall. To prevent mediastinitis from a cervical fistula, it is wise to attach the apex of the gastroplasty tube to the posterior aspect of the sternal notch so that the anastomosis will stay in the neck during the postoperative period. Furthermore, it is helpful to bring the omental fringes along the upper part of the greater curvature into the neck with the stomach to establish a barrier between the cervical area and the chest. A feeding jejunostomy is always performed before closure of the abdomen.

The technique of esophageal substitution by Kirschner[9] was used five times, mainly for tracheoesophageal fistulae. This procedure consists of drainage of the esophagus by a Roux-en-Y jejunal loop and bypass of the tumor with the stomach through the presternal or the substernal space. The bypass gastroplasty is accomplished using Akiyama's technique.

When there is a broncho-esophageal fistula, a jejunostomy is performed in the jejunal loop, draining the esophagus, which allows the air insufflated by assisted ventilation to leave the digestive tract during the postoperative period.

A reverse gastric tube of Gavriliu[10] was performed three times. This technique requires the division of the stomach along the greater curvature by the GIA stapler from the prepyloric area up to the left side of the cardia to perform a reversed tube vascularized by the left gastro-epiploic vessels. Removal of the spleen is not always necessary; if it is not done, the spleen has to be mobilized and placed upside down.

In five cases, the esophageal tumor was by-passed by placing an isoperistaltic tube with gastric continuity according to Postlethwait.[11] In this technique, the creation of the gastric tube along the greater curvature is started immediately above the pyloric ring. A short incision in the anterior and posterior prepyloric walls is necessary to introduce the GIA stapler. Vagotomy and pyloroplasty are the rule.

The substitute gastroplasty was placed in the posterior mediastinum in 42 cases, in the substernal space in 69 cases, and in the presternal space in two.

RESULTS

The patients were divided into two groups: group I, made up of 33 patients who underwent treatment at the beginning of our experience (1979 until

1983); and group II, made up of 80 patients who underwent operations between 1984 and 1988. The operative mortality rate was reduced from 24% (8/33) in group I to 2.5% (2/80) in group II (p < 0.001). The causes of death in group I were pneumonia in 5 cases, mediastinitis in 2, and a cardiac arrest in 1. In group II, 1 patient died from renal failure following the preoperative administration of cisplatinum, and another died from respiratory failure. A cervical fistula (Tables 31-1, 31-2) occurred in 42% (14/33) of the patients in group I, and in only 6% (5/80) in group II (p < 0.001). There were 16 fistulae in 64 patients in whom interrupted sutures were used, and only 3 in 49 patients in whom the anastomosis was performed by a continuous suture (p < 0.01). The fistulae healed spontaneously in 17 patients and were responsible for a fatal mediastinitis in 1 patient and required resection-anastomosis in another patient. Disruption of the gastric suture line occurred only once and required a drainage operation. Stricture of the cervical anastomosis occurred in 12 cases in group I (36%) and in 12 cases of group II (15%) (p < 0.005); 18 of these occurred after interrupted sutures (28%) and 6 occurred after continuous suture (12%) (p < 0.05). The narrowing usually occurs 4 to 6 weeks after the operation and requires bougienage, which is successful after 1 or 2 sessions.

DISCUSSION

Choice of the Stomach

After subtotal esophagectomy for cancer or benign disease, digestive continuity can be restored by various types of substitute organs. The long coloplasty, the technique of choice in the past,[12] was still popular recently with some teams.[13–15] Sixty years ago, Kirschner described a procedure using the stomach to take the place of the esophagus after subtotal esophagectomy.[8] The stomach was forgotten as an esophageal substitute during several decades until Gavriliu,[10] Akiyama,[8] Gignoux,[16] and Postlethwait[11] restored this organ to surgical favor. The main inconveniences of the coloplasty (compared to the gastroplasty) are the necessity for three anastomoses instead of only one, the potential for contamination by colon contents, the variability of the colonic vascular anatomy, the possibility of kinking of the colon tube,

Table 31-1. Cervical Anastomosis: Occurrence of Fistulae and Stenoses

Complication	Group I	Group II	
Fistula	14/33	5/80	(p < 0.001)
Stenosis	12/33	12/80	(p < 0.005)

Table 31-2. Occurrence of Fistulae and Stenoses by Suture Technique

Complication	Interrupted Suture	Continuous Suture	
Fistula	16/64	3/49	(p < 0.01)
Stenosis	18/64	6/49	(p < 0.05)

and a generally higher postoperative mortality rate. A coloplasty should be used today only if the stomach is not available—in case of caustic gastritis, for example—and when the stomach is too short to reach the mouth after pharyngo-laryngectomy.[7] In Caucasian people, the use of a jejunal loop as described for Asian people is often impossible.

Gastroplasty Techniques

Akiyama, in Japan, has described the technique to reach the neck easily using the stomach after subtotal and total esophagectomy.[8,17] With Goldsmith as his coworker,[18] Akiyama has shown the anatomic differences between Japanese and American individuals: in Japanese people, the length of the lesser curvature, pyloric mobility, and length of the greater curvature are greater than in American people. The only disadvantage in Japanese people is the greater distance between the costal angle and cardia, so that it is more difficult to reach the neck with a plasty placed in the substernal space. In 1983, Maillard and Hay[19] estimated the gain one can expect from various maneuvers: 0 to 10 cm with the Kocher maneuver, 0 to 3 cm by mesocolon and mesenteric elongation procedures, 4 to 11 cm with gastric tubulization, and 4 to 8 cm by using the posterior mediastinal route. In 1985, Koskas[20] compared various types of gastroplasty: the reversed tube appears to be longer than the isoperistaltic tube, the latter being longer than the entire stomach.

In our experience, reaching the base of the neck after subtotal esophagectomy is usually no problem. Some difficulties can appear when the gastric tube has to be brought up to the base of the tongue and the posterior wall of the oro-pharynx after pharyngolaryngectomy with esophagectomy.[7,21,22] The techniques described by Maillard and Koskas can be helpful.

The posterior mediastinal route is the shortest and avoids, at the apex of the gastroplasty, a bayonet effect encountered when the substernal route is used. This route should now only be employed in cases of palliative resection or bypass procedures. The presternal space is reserved for rare situations, such as a non-resectable tumor of the cervico-thoracic junction, or as a salvage route. The gastric tube should be as large as possible: Thomas and Le Quesne in Great Britain[23] and Koskas and Gayet in France[20] have studied both the anatomy of the submucosal vessels originating, and particularly the anastomoses between the vessels depending, on the left gastric artery, and the anatomy of the submucosal vessels depending on the right and left gastro-epiploic arteries. When the left gastric and the left gastro-epiploic arteries are divided, the fundus is supplied by the right gastro-epiploic artery, mainly through the submucosal network of the lesser curvature and to a lesser extent through the submucosal vessels, which depend on the left gastro-epiploic artery.

A pyloromyotomy or pyloroplasty has been the rule in this series: its usefulness is controversial,[21,24] but in the gastric longitudinal division, vagotomy-pyloroplasty prevents peptic perforation of the right side of the stomach, according to Postlethwait.[25] Lastly, the use of the GIA stapler shapes the stretched stomach much better than does the manual section of this wall. The disruption of the suture line occurs very rarely: there was but one case at the beginning of our experience.

Cervical Anastomosis

The usual complications at this level are postoperative leakage and stricture. In our series, they were frequent at the beginning, but they have been reduced to acceptable rates through improvement of the surgical experience, and perhaps through the use of a continuous suture instead of interrupted stitches. Unlike intrathoracic leaks, cervical fistulae heal spontaneously within a few days or weeks in the majority of cases. Sometimes they need resection followed by a new anastomosis. To prevent such accidents, one has to construct a healthy, long gastroplasty without any tension. In the postoperative period, it is helpful to assure continuous emptying by a nasogastric tube: in case of dilatation of the transposed organ, the increase of the intraparietal tension can compress the submucosal vessels and compromise the blood flow to the apex. The vascularization of the top of the plasty can be recorded by a Doppler[26] or laser-Doppler probe[27] to be sure that the anastomosis will be performed in an area with adequate blood supply.

The use of mechanical staplers is controversial.[3,28,29] Strictures occur 4 to 6 weeks postoperatively. They are more frequent after cervical than after intrathoracic anastomosis,[30] and mechanical sutures seem to increase their incidence.[29,31] Strictures usually respond to one or two dilatations, but some patients have to be submitted to several dilatations during the first year.

Postoperative Mortality

A few years ago, esophageal surgery was known to be hazardous, and the postoperative mortality rate was high. Today, although this rate is still about 15% in two recent collective series,[28,32] a very low mortality rate has been published by some experienced teams.[17,33] In this series, the postoperative mortality rate has been reduced to 2.5% for the last 80 patients through improvement of the perioperative management, better knowledge of surgical techniques, and increasing experience.

CONCLUSIONS

The stomach is the first-choice organ for esophageal substitution today. It can reach the neck easily, and even reaches the base of the tongue when special steps are employed. The GIA stapler affords technical ease and safety. In experienced hands, subtotal and total esophagectomy have a low mortality rate and allow the patient to eat a normal diet. Cervical leakage and strictures, the most common postoperative complications, are usually benign and become less frequent as the surgeon gains experience.

SUMMARY

From January 1979 to April 1988, 113 long gastroplasties have been performed with the GIA stapler, 103 times after esophagectomy and 10 times as a bypass procedure. The indication was esophageal carcinoma in 99 patients, pharyngo-laryngeal carcinoma in 9, caustic esophagitis in 4, and instrumental perforation in 1. The gastroplasty was made according to Akiyama in 100 operations, to Gavriliu in 3, to Kirschner in 5, and to Postlethwait in 5. The gastroplasty was placed in the substernal space in 69 cases, in the posterior mediastinum in 42, and in the presternal space in 2. The cervical anastomosis was initially performed by interrupted sutures in one layer (64 cases). The operative mortality rate fell from 24% among the first 33 patients (group I) to 2.5% among the 80 more-recent patients (group II) ($p < 0.001$). There were 14 cervical fistulae in group I (42%) and 5 (6.7%) in group II ($p < 0.001$); there were 16 leaks among 64 interrupted sutures and 3 among 49 continuous sutures ($p < 0.01$). A cervical stricture occurred in 12 cases of group I (36%) and in 12 cases of group II (15%) ($p < 0.005$), in 18 cases after interrupted sutures (28%), and in 6 cases after a continuous suture (12%) ($p < 0.05$). A localized disruption of the gastric suture required a drainage operation in 1 patient in group I.

REFERENCES

1. Ong G, Lam K, Lam P, Wong J: Resection for carcinoma of the superior mediastinal segment of the esophagus. World J Surg 2:497–504, 1978.
2. Skinner D: En bloc resection for neoplasms of the esophagus and cardia. J Thorac Cardiovasc Surg 85:59–71, 1983.
3. Liebermann-Meffert D, Luescher U, Neff U, Ruedi T, Allgower M: Esophagectomy without thoracotomy: is there a risk of intramediastinal bleeding? Ann Surg 206:184–192, 1987.
4. Orringer M, Orringer J: Esophagectomy without thoracotomy: a dangerous operation? J Thorac Cardiovasc Surg 85:72–80, 1983.
5. Wong J: Transhiatal esophagectomy for carcinoma of the thoracic esophagus. Br J Surg 73:89–90, 1986.
6. Akiyama H, Hiyama M, Miyazono H: Total esophageal reconstruction after extraction of the esophagus. Ann Surg 182:547–552, 1975.
7. Collard JM, Otte JB, Hamoir M, et al. Experience with 38 esopharyngolaryngectomies for esophagyngolaryngeal cancer. Communication, 10th World Congress of the CICD, Copenhagen, 1988.
8. Akiyama H, Miyazono H, Tsurumaru M, Hashimoto C, Kawamura T: Use of the stomach as an esophageal substitute. Ann Surg 188:606–610, 1978.
9. Kirschner M: Ein neues verfahren der oesophagoplastik. Arch Klin Chir 114:606, 1920.
10. Gavriliu D: Les cancers de l'oesophage en 1984: 135 questions. Paris: Maloine Editions, 1984:150–151.
11. Postlethwait R: Technique for isoperistaltic gastric tube for esophageal by-pass. Ann Surg 189:673–676, 1979.
12. Belsey R: Reconstruction of the esophagus with left colon. J Thorac Cardiovasc Surg 49:33–53, 1965.
13. Otte JB, Lerut T, Collard JM, Brecx JF, Gruwez J, Kestens PJ: Les plasties coliques de l'oesophage. Acta Chir Belg 82:389–396, 1982.
14. Peracchia A, Tremolada C, Buin F, Ancona E: Le traitement chirurgical de l'oesophage thoracique. Acta Chir Belg 82:355–358, 1982.
15. Postlethwait R: Colonic interposition for esophageal substitution. Surg Gynecol Obstet 156:377–383, 1983.
16. Gignoux M, Segol Ph, Ollivier JM, Bricard H: L'oesophagoplastie cervicale dans le traitement du cancer de l'oesophage. Lyon Chir 74:262–264, 1978.
17. Akiyama H, Tsurumaru M, Kawamura T, Ono Y: Principles of surgical treatment for carcinoma of the esophagus. Ann Surg 194:438–446, 1981.
18. Goldsmith H, Akiyama H: A comparative study of Japanese and American gastric dimensions. Ann Surg 190:690–693, 1979.
19. Maillard JN, Hay JM: Etude anatomique des gastroplasties. Communication. Journées Chirurgicales de Colombes, Paris, 1983.
20. Koskas F, Gayet B: Etude anatomo-technique avec injection vasculaire des oesophagoplasties gastriques rétrosternales chez le cadavre. Actualités Digestives 2:67–68, 1985.
21. Lam K, Choi T, Wei W, Lau W, Wong J: Present status of pharyngogastric anastomosis following pharyngolaryngo-esophagectomy. Br J Surg 74:122–125, 1987.
22. Peracchia A, Ancona E, Tremolada C, Buin F, Ruol A, Narne S: Comparison between different techniques for the reconstruction of the cervical esophagus resected for cancer. In: Demeester T, Skinner D, eds: Esophageal Disorders, Pathology, and Therapy. New York: Raven, 1985:405–408.
23. Thomas D, Langford R, Russel R, Le Quesne L: The anatomical basis for gastric mobilization in total esophagectomy. Br J Surg 66:230–233, 1979.
24. Huang G, Zhang DE, Zhang DA: A comparative study of resection of carcinoma of the esophagus with and without pyloroplasty. In: Demeester T, Skinner D, eds: Esophageal disorders: pathophysiology and therapy. New York: Raven Press, 1985:383–388.
25. Salizzoni M, Hay JM, Lacaine F, Boudinet A, Pagano G, Maillard JN: Esofagoplastica palliativa per il cancro dell'esofago. Minerva Chir 38:257–262, 1983.
26. Hay JM: Quels sont les problèmes posés par le remplacement de l'oesophage? In: Les cancers de l'oesophage en 1984. 135 questions. Paris: Maloine Editions, 1984:158–159.
27. Kudo T, Abo S, Itabashi T: Prognosis of esophageal substitute in tissue viability and anastomotic leakage. In: Siewert J, Hölscher A, eds: Diseases of the Esophagus. Berlin: Springer-Verlag, 1988:522–525.
28. Giuli R: Enquête du groupe oeso. In: Les cancers de l'oesophage en 1984: 135 questions. Paris: Maloine Editions, 1984:401–424.
29. Peracchia A, Tremolada C: Anastomose intrathoracique, fistules et sténoses, anastomose manuelle versus anastomose mecanique. Actualités chirurgicales. 86ème Congrès Français de Chirurgie. I, 41, 1985.
30. Segol P, Gignoux M, Marchand P, Couque M, Bricard H: Oesophagectomie pour cancer de l'oesophage. Etude comparative de l'oesophagectomie subtotale et de l'oesophagectomie partielle. Communication, "The Belsey 75th Birthday celebration meeting," Louvain, 1985.
31. Wong J: Les risque postopératoires immédiats. In: Les cancers de l'oesophage en 1984: 135 questions. Paris: Maloine Editions, 1984:227.
32. Richelme H, Baulieux J: Le traitement du cancer de l'oesophage. Rapport du 88ème Congrès Français de Chirurgie, Masson Editeur, 1986.
33. Huang G, Wu Y: Carcinoma of the esophagus and gastric cardia. Springer-Verlag (New York), 1984.

ADDITIONAL READING

Akiyama H, Hiyama M: A simple esophageal by-pass operation by high gastric division. Surgery. 75:674–681, 1974.
Collard JM, Otte JB, Fiasse R, et al: Bilan préopératoire et traitement chirurgical du cancer épidermoïde de l'oesophage. Acta Gastroenterol Belg 49:588–601, 1986.

CHAPTER 32

ANASTOMOSIS OF THE CERVICAL ESOPHAGUS TO A GREATER CURVATURE ISOPERISTALTIC TUBE OR COLON SEGMENT WITH STAPLING INSTRUMENTS

N. Kockel and B. Ulrich

After subtotal esophagectomy, cervical anastomosis is preferred to intrathoracic anastomosis because of a reduction in complications and better longitudinal control of submucosal tumor extension or emboli. Nevertheless, fistulae occur frequently after cervical esophago-gastrostomy—in about 30% of these anastomoses.[1,2,3] Although most fistulae heal within 20 days, the hospital stay is increased on an average of 10 days. To achieve a safer, more reliable anastomosis, we have used stapling instruments since 1987. An extremely long gastric tube is essential.

TECHNIQUE

This tube can be created along the greater gastric curvature in an isoperistaltic fashion with the use of the Aeskulap-Ulrich staplers, a set of three instruments (short linear, long linear, and curved) that are a modification of the Yamagishi devices. Following retrosternal pull-through, some 6 to 10 cm of redundant tube length are available in the neck for end-to-side esophago-gastrostomy (Figs. 32-1, 32-2, 32-3). Through the open end of the redundant gastric tube, the circular stapler with a 21-mm cartridge and without the anvil is placed into the tube lumen (Figs. 32-4, 32-5). The center rod is made to exit through a stab wound in the over-sewn staple line, some 6 to 8 cm beyond the open end of the stomach tube (Fig. 32-5). After attaching the anvil and advancing it into

the open lumen of the esophageal stump, the esophageal purse-string is tied (Figs. 32-6, 32-7). The circular instrument is closed and fired; end-to-side esophago-gastrostomy is then accomplished (Fig. 32-8). The excess gastric tube is closed with the TA-55 (Fig. 32-9). The integrity of the stapled anastomosis is tested by instillation of about 100 ml of methylene blue through a nasogastric tube (Fig. 32-10).

PATIENTS AND METHODS

During the period of January 1987 to March 1988, we performed 11 stapled anastomoses in the neck after resection of the thoraco-abdominal esophagus. The mean age of our patients was 62.5 ($\pm$8.8) years. There were 10 men and 1 woman. The tumor was localized 3 times in the upper, 3 times in the middle, and 5 times in the lower third. Histologically, there were 7 squamous cell carcinomas and 4 adenocarcinomas (Barrett's type). The tumor size was staged according to UICC classification: T1 in 2, T2 in 4, T3 in 3, and T4 in 2 cases. The resection was thought to be curative in 8 patients and palliative in the 3 T3 patients. A trans-hiatal technique was possible 8 times; on 3 occasions a right thoracotomy was necessary. For reconstruction, the stomach was used in 10 patients and the colon in 1 patient who had undergone gastric resection for ulcer previously. The retrosternal passage of the substitute organ was used 7

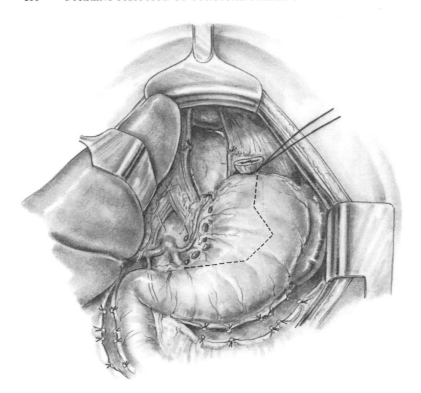

Fig. 32-1. Outline of the isoperistaltic greater curvature gastric tube, based on the right gastroepiploic artery and right and left gastro-epiploic arcades.

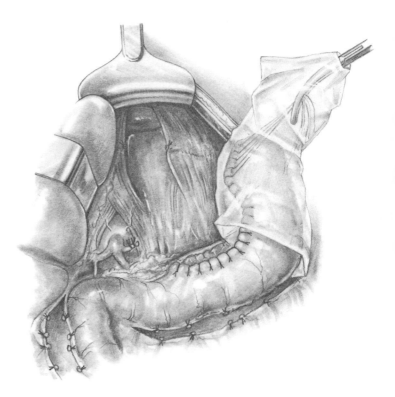

Fig. 32-2. The lesser curvature of the stomach has been resected with the esophagus and all pertinent lymph nodes. The staple line of the gastric tube is reinforced with manual sutures; a Kocher maneuver is performed and the tube is wrapped in a plastic pouch to facilitate pull-through into the neck.

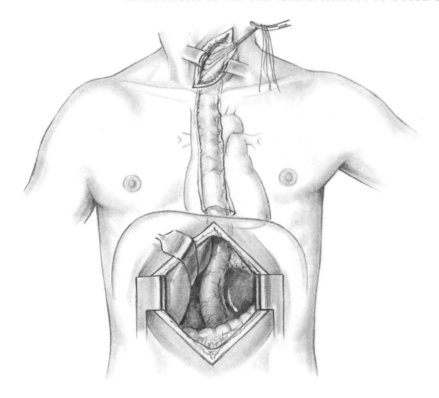

Fig. 32-3. Following retrosternal or posterior mediastinal advancement into the neck, the redundant portion of proximal gastric tube is pulled out through the cervical incision.

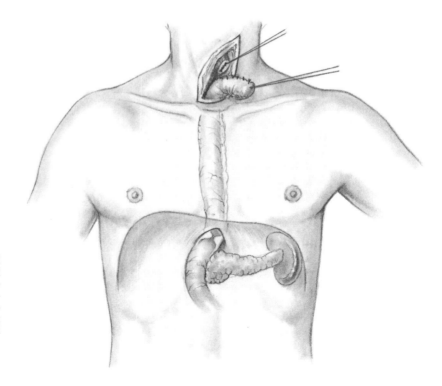

Fig. 32-4. Anastomosis will take place between the cervical esophagus and the medial, stapled-sutured aspect of the gastric tube in an end-to-side fashion. A purse-string has been placed around the esophageal stump.

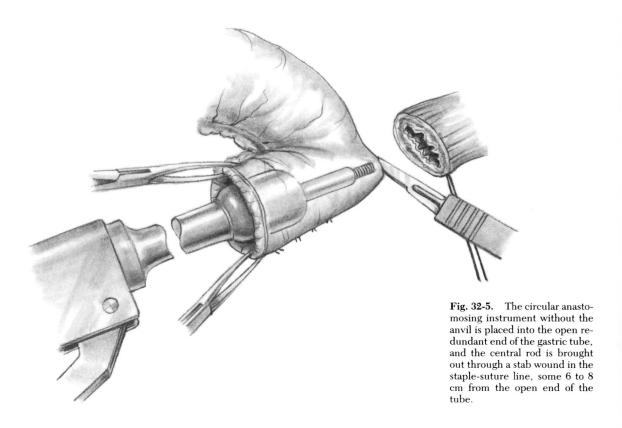

Fig. 32-5. The circular anastomosing instrument without the anvil is placed into the open redundant end of the gastric tube, and the central rod is brought out through a stab wound in the staple-suture line, some 6 to 8 cm from the open end of the tube.

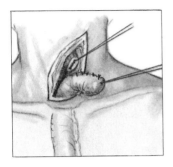

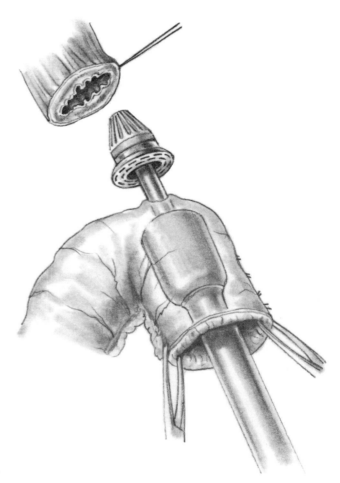

Fig. 32-6. The anvil is attached to the central rod.

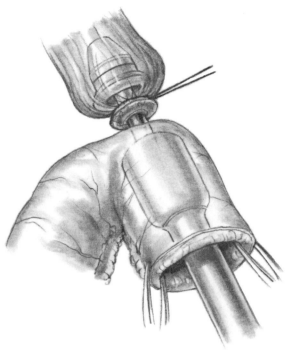

Fig. 32-7. The anvil is advanced into the lumen of the cervical esophagus and the purse-string is tied around the central rod.

times and the mediastinal route on 4 occasions. In 10 cases the ILS-21 was used, and in 1 patient the 25-mm ILS was used. The leakage rates of stapled and hand-sewn anastomoses of our historically consecutive experience were compared and tested by the four-field test.

RESULTS

There was 1 postoperative death within 30 days because of renal and pulmonary failure. There were no postoperative fistulae (Table 32-1), and a significantly lower leakage rate (p < 0.05) was observed than with hand-sewn anastomoses performed before 1987. In the early postoperative period, 2 patients died from their tumors. The other 8 patients lived longer than 8 months. Four of these patients developed a stricture of the esophago-gastric anastomosis, which was caused by local tumor recurrence in 3. Only 2 months after operation, the fourth patient developed a complete fibrous stricture resisting bouginage and laser treatment. This patient had to undergo re-operation with a new hand-sewn anastomosis. Our stricture rate related to technique is therefore 12.5%.

DISCUSSION

Including our own, 55 cervical stapled anastomoses are mentioned in the literature (Table 32-2). The overall leakage rate is 1.8% with EEA, ILS, and SPTU instruments, as used by various authors. Wong also mentions the stapler size used (ILS-25).[4] There are differences in the technical approach. West[5] and Sugimachi[6] introduce the stapler through an incision into the antrum from the abdomen, whereas Wong[4] and Imamura[7] place the stapler through an incision into the highest point of the gastric tube, as we do.

Insertion of the stapler through a gastrotomy in the antrum is possible only if the gastric tube is transposed antesternally and a long incision from the cervical region down to the abdomen is made (Sugimachi).[6] An alternate approach is described by West and colleagues in one case:[5] Before retrosternal interposition of the stomach, they resected the clavicular head. From our experience, this technique is only possible in patients with a wide epigastric angle and short thorax.

We noticed one anastomotic stricture; Wong and Imamura did not observe any. Since West and Sugimachi do not mention this possible complication, we calculated a stricture rate of 3.8% in 28 patients. The reason for a lower stricture rate in stapled cervical, as compared to thoracic, anastomoses is not apparent. In a review of the literature, Wong calculated a stricture rate of 14.5%, the same rate as in his own series of 141 patients. He noticed a correlation between stricture rate and stapler size. Within 13.5 months after operation, Wong noticed no stricture with the ILS 33-mm instrument, while the rate was 25.9% with the EEA 25-mm or ILS 25-mm. Since only small cartridges can be applied in the neck, the low stricture rate is surprising. Could the degree of reflux play a role? Reflux in itself does not seem to be the only responsible factor, since strictures are normally definitively remedied with one or two dilations.[4]

Another reason for the development of a stricture may be found in the lack of mucosa-to-mucosa apposition. In this case, healing is by second intention with granulation tissue and delayed epithelialization. Furthermore, the circumferentially placed non-absorbable staples restrict the capacity of the lumen to dilatate. Thus, smaller-sized staplers carry a higher incidence of stricture.

CONCLUSIONS

Staples can be used for cervical esophageal anastomoses with a low leakage rate. The low rate of strictures, so far observed in a small series of patients, has to be confirmed by further clinical experience.

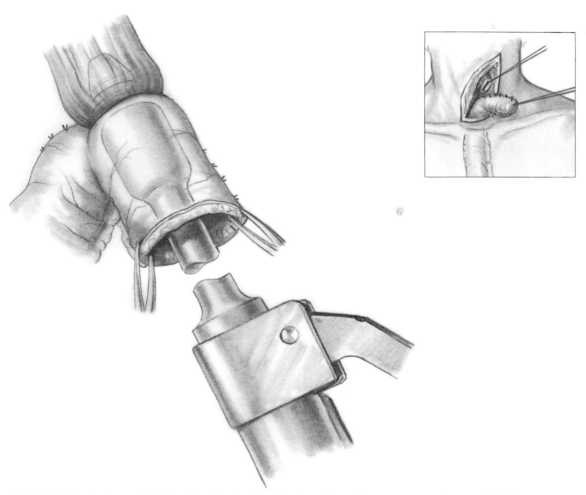

Fig. 32-8. The circular stapler is closed and activated, and end-to-side esophago-gastrostomy is accomplished.

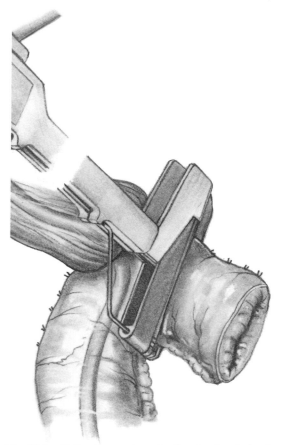

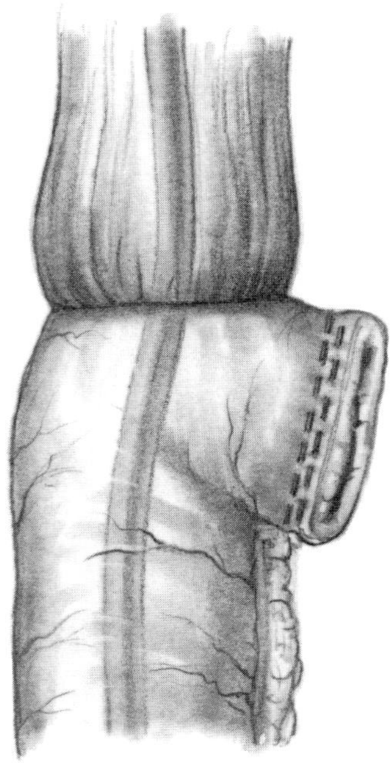

Fig. 32-10. The integrity of the stapled anastomosis is examined with 100 ml of methylene blue injected through a nasogastric tube.

Fig. 32-9. Following anastomosis, the circular stapler is disengaged and the excess gastric remnant is closed near the anastomosis with a linear stapler and removed.

Table 32-1. Esophageal Resections with Cervical Anastomoses: Manual vs. Stapling Techniques

Location	Substitute	n	Hand-sewn	Leaks	Stapler	Leaks
Surgical Clinic University Dusseldorf* (12/80–7/84)	Stomach	88	88	26	–	–
	Colon	9	9	–	–	–
Juliusspital Wurzburg** (8/84–9/86)	Stomach	5	5	1	–	–
Surgical Clinic** Dusseldorf-Gerresheim (1/87–3/88)	Stomach	11	1	0	10	0
	Colon	1	–	–	1	0
	Jejunum	1	1	1	–	–
Totals		116	104	31 (29.8%)	11	0

* Director: Prof. Dr. K. Kremer
** Director: Prof. Dr. B. Ulrich

Table 32-2. Occurrence of Leaks and Structures with Stapled Anastomoses

Author	Year	Stapler	n	Leaks	Stricture
West et al.[5]	1981	EEA	1	0	?
Sugimachi et al.[6]	1981	EEA	11	0	?
		SPTU	17	1	?
Imamura et al.[7]	1987	EEA	10	0	0
Wong et al.[4]	1987	ILS-25	5	0	0
Ulrich et al.[8,9]	1988	ILS-21	10	0	1
		ILS-25	1	0	0
Totals			55	1 (1.8%)	1 (of 26: 3.8%)

REFERENCES

1. Siewert JR, Roder JD: Chirurgische Therapie des Plat-ten-epithelcarcinoms des Ösophagus—Erweiterte Radikalität. Langenbecks Arch Chir 372:129–139, 1987.
2. Ulrich B, Kasperk R, Grabitz K, Kremer K: Die Oe-sophagus-resektion ohne Thorakotomie beim Carci-nom—Erfahrungsbericht über 100 Fälle. Chirurg 56:251–260, 1985.
3. Ulrich B, Grabitz K, Kockel N: Ergebnisse der Magen-hochzugs-operationen ohne Thorakotomie bei der Be-handlung des fortgeschrittenen Ösophaguskarzinoms. Zentralbl Chir 109:1033–1043, 1984.
4. Wong J, Cheung H, Lui R, Fan YW, Smith A, Siu KF: Esophago-gastric anastomosis performed with a stapler: the occurrence of leakage and stricture. Surgery 101: 408–415, 1987.
5. West PN, Marbarger JP, Martz MN, Roper LC: Esoph-ago-gastrostomy with EEA stapler. Ann Surg 193:76–81, 1981.
6. Sugimachi K, Ikeda M, Ueo H, Kai H, Okudaira Y, Inokuchi K: Clinical efficacy of the stapled anastomosis in esophageal reconstruction. Ann Thorac Surg 33:374–378, 1982.
7. Imamura M, Ohishi K, Tobe T: Retrosternal esophago-gastrostomy with the EEA stapler. Surg Gynecol Ob-stet 164:368–371, 1987.
8. Ulrich B, Kockel N: Collare Stapler-Anastomosen nach Ösophagusresektion: Vortrag. 105. Kongress der Deut-schen Gesellschaft für Chirurgie, München, Apr. 8, 1988.
9. Ulrich B, Kockel N: Zur Operationstechnik der Magen-schlauchbildung beim Ösophagusersatz. In: Chirur-gische Gastroenterologie mit interdisziplinären Ges-prächen Nr.2 S.43–46. Hameln: TNM-Verlag, 1986.

CHAPTER 33

TOTAL OR PARTIAL ESOPHAGEAL REPLACEMENT OR BYPASS FOR BENIGN CONDITIONS OF THE ESOPHAGUS

Bryce Gayet

The approach to a benign lesion of the esophagus depends on the general condition of the patient, the diagnosis (perforation, peptic esophagitis, acute or chronic chemical burn, achalasia, papillomatosis, persistent epithelial dysplasia), the intensity of the clinical presentation, the histologic biopsy findings, and the surgeon's attitude toward these various factors. In many instances there is no clear-cut answer to the varied presentations of these benign lesions. In reviewing 61 patients who have recently had esophageal substitute procedures for benign conditions, we will attempt to define the indications and the technical modalities of these therapeutic approaches.

METHODS

Between 1979 and 1987, 61 esophageal substitute operations were performed in 59 patients (2 patients had two operations), using gastroplasty in 14 procedures (Figs. 33-1, 33-2, 33-3) and coloplasty in 47 procedures (Fig. 33-4). The indications were lye burn (36), peptic esophagitis (10) non-dilatable stricture in 7, deep ulcer in 2, and severe dysplasia in 1, traumatic injuries (7: 5 were instrumental perforations), benign tumor (3), benign stricture (2), megaesophagus (1), papillomatosis (1), and severe dysplasia (1). The breakdown between the two types of substitution used for each one of these indications is shown in Table 33-1. There were 43 esophageal replacements extending into the neck with anastomosis at that level, and 18 shorter substitution segments

connected to the esophagus in the chest. Except for 5 patients who underwent operations for lye stricture, all patients had an esophagectomy (92%).

The preoperative preparation of patients consisted of a general assessment; examination of the respiratory function, including upper gastro-intestinal endoscopy; contrast study of the esophagus and stomach; tomodensitometry; and, more recently, echoendoscopy. There were no preoperative examinations that related specifically to the substitute organ used; however, barium enema and colonoscopy were added if a patient had had symptoms of colon disease. In addition to a low-residue diet, all patients were prepared with a regimen of mechanical cleansing of the large bowel and intestinal antibiotics that were in general use at a given period of the study for bowel preparation and general prophylaxis. The pulmonary status was especially addressed with preoperative physiotherapy and broad-spectrum antibiotics for 1 week.

The gastric substitutes used for replacement were all large isoperistaltic tubes created by resecting the lesser curvature with the GIA stapler applied some five to seven times, except for one antiperistaltic, reverse greater curvature gastric tube of Gavriliu. Coloplasty was achieved with the transverse colon based on the superior branch of the left colic artery in 44 of 47 operations. Vascular competence was examined intra-operatively by temporary atraumatic clamping of the vessels to be ultimately sacrificed, after the colon had been mobilized. If the superior branches of

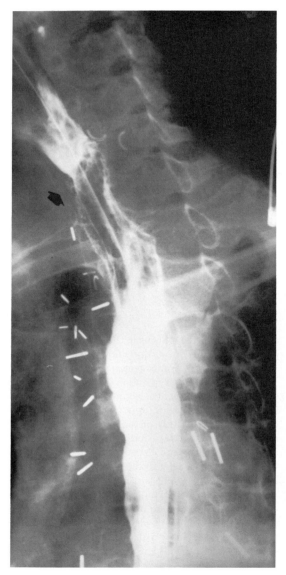

Fig. 33-1. Cervical esophago-gastrostomy with long gastroplasty.

the left-colic vessels appeared to be precarious, the transverse colon was used in an antiperistaltic fashion on two occasions. One patient had two coloplasties, in which the ileum and right colon were used the second time around.

The substitute organs reaching into the neck were elevated 39 times through a retrosternal route, 3 times through the posterior mediastinum, and once through a presternal tunnel. The anastomosis to the esophagus was accomplished with staplers on 40 occasions and manually in the remaining 21 operations. The specific techniques were side-to-end anastomosis

to the pharynx on three occasions, end-to-side 53 times, and end-to-end anastomosis to the esophagus 5 times. For colo-gastric anastomosis, the site was on the posterior aspect of the stomach; an anti-reflux gastric valve was created, as was a pyloroplasty, whenever a patient had undergone vagectomy together with the esophageal resection. On 9 occasions, a total gastrectomy had to be added to the esophagectomy. The colo-jejunostomy was end-to-side, using the Roux-en-Y principle for the jejunal loop.

RESULTS

None of the patients who received a coloplasty died. Only 1 death occurred after esophago-gastrectomy with esophago-gastric anastomosis in the chest in a patient with cirrhosis who underwent operation

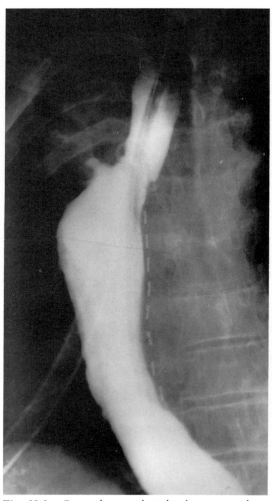

Fig. 33-2. Gastroplasty with right thoracic esophago-gastrostomy.

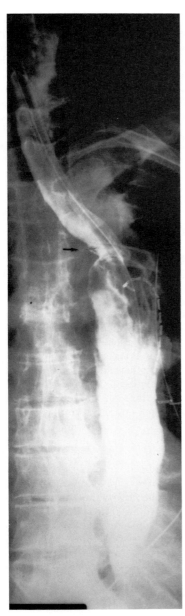

Fig. 33-3. Gastroplasty with left thoracic esophago-gastrostomy.

urgently after esophageal perforation (Table 33-2). In 1 patient with coloplasty, massive necrosis occurred, requiring a second operation for excision of the necrotic colon segment and creation of a new substitute organ using the stomach.

Five anastomotic fistulae (11.6%) were observed in the neck, draining through the drainage site, and were treated non-operatively. With these cervical leaks, the anastomosis had been performed twice

with the ILS, once with the EEA, and twice by manual technique. The operation had been performed three times for lye burn, once for perforation following irradiation of the esophagus, and once for esophageal trauma. We did not observe anastomotic leakage in the chest. However, following a Belsey-type operation, a localized necrosis of the colon cul-de-sac necessitated re-intervention and resection of the blind end with the TA stapler. Routine radiologic contrast study on the seventh postoperative day showed an asymptomatic blind fistula in 1 patient after retrosternal coloplasty with manual anastomosis, for endoscopic perforation of the esophagus. This was initially treated by exclusion of the anastomosis proximally and distally.

Early postoperative complications were 5 recurrent nerve paralyses (3 after esophagectomy for acute caustic burns), 3 pulmonary infiltrates that receded with treatment, and 1 subphrenic abscess. There has been no leakage from the pyloroplasties or from the colo-colic or colo-gastric anastomoses.

In the long-term followup, 14 patients (11 of them with chemical burns) required dilatation for anastomotic strictures (23%). In fact, 1 of these strictures was due to almost complete sclerosis and fibrosis of an entire coloplasty; this patient received a second coloplasty.

Twelve of the 14 strictures and 5 of the 7 suture leaks occurred in patients with retrosternal placements of the substitute organs. Dumping syndrome in 4 patients and persistent diarrhea in 5 were addressed with the prescription of specific diets for these conditions. Finally, some 60% of all patients complained of episodes of reflux, of which 6 were disabling. Two of these were from bile reflux following a jejuno-colic anastomosis; 1 patient developed repeated episodes of pulmonary aspiration. To improve this condition, 3 patients underwent reoperation. In 2 patients, a total duodenal diversion was performed, and in 1 a Roux-en-Y colo-jejunal anastomosis was done to overcome this handicap. In summary, of 59 patients with benign lesions of the esophagus, 35 (59%) have had a simple uncomplicated postoperative course; 73% of all patients had no functional impairments at the conclusion of the study.

DISCUSSION

Indications for Esophageal Replacement or Reconstruction

The indication to create a substitute esophagus in benign conditions depends entirely on the nature of the benign lesion. Following chemical or caustic (lye, acid) burns, the decision is an easy one after either emergency esophagectomy for extensive necrosis or

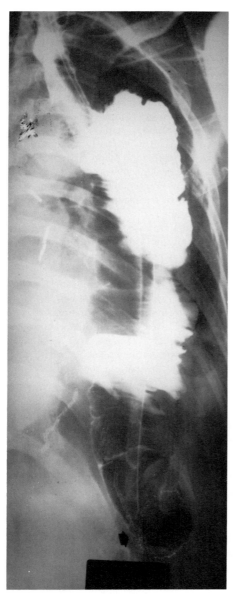

Fig. 33-4. Esophago-coloplasty.

extensive and necessitates total esophagectomy with anastomosis in the neck to the substitute organ.

Even advanced cases of peptic reflux esophagitis rarely require excision and replacement of the lower esophagus. Rather, the complications of esophagitis (such as non-dilatable or recurrent strictures in spite of a well functioning anti-reflux procedure, penetrating ulcers with hemorrhage, and the rare instance of histologic evidence of a premalignant or early malignant lesion) are the reasons to excise and replace the lower esophagus. Of 115 patients seen during the same period of this study with advanced peptic esophagitis, only 10 patients required resection. To use a gastric tube in these cases may invite further postoperative reflux, which is especially debilitating in this general context. For this reason we prefer the left colon interposition described by Belsey.[2]

In the early part of this study, 5 of 47 patients with esophageal perforation were treated by emergency resection, substitution, and primary anastomosis. The high mortality rate of this approach, together with our increasing confidence in the primary suture of the perforation—with or without proximal and distal esophageal exclusion—have made us abandon it for benign perforations. Primary suture of the perforation is further enhanced by the fact that the esophagus can be excluded temporarily by the use of absorbable staples through the entire thickness of the gastro-esophageal junction and cervical, lateral pharyngostomy or esophagostomy, while the repair of the perforation is drained with a chest tube. Following healing of the perforation and removal of the chest tube, the lateral pharyngostomy can be discontinued or repaired. The gastro-esophageal junction reopens spontaneously within 10 to 14 days; in this fashion, the need for a second reconstructive procedure of the esophagus, so often required after "classic" exclusions,[3,4] has become unnecessary.

Indications for Esophageal Resection

The need for one-stage esophageal resection and substitution is less clearly established. Esophagectomy can be justified by the type of the lesion, be it esophageal necrosis or suspicion of malignancy, or it can become necessary for technical reasons, such as in esophago-gastrectomy and anastomosis to the esophagus in the chest. In patients in whom substitution of the entire esophagus is indicated with anastomosis in the neck, it is possible to achieve retrosternal bypass and leave the excluded esophagus in place.

Benign lesions that are predisposed to cancer or premalignant are a special problem. Resection may be technically difficult and even dangerous in pa-

perforation, or because of long-term late extensive stricture that resists all efforts at dilatation. In these cases the stomach is a poor choice, since the burn may have severely damaged the submucosa and muscular layers that carry the blood supply, even though this damage may be grossly inconspicuous. Except for caustic burns that are localized to the cervical esophagus or pharynx (which if absolutely indicated can be treated by free jejunal transplants[1] with microvascular anastomosis), the majority of all chemical burns is

Table 33-1. Diagnoses and Types of Operations

Diagnosis	Coloplasty		Gastroplasty	
	Cervical	Thoracic	Cervical	Thoracic
Lye burn	34	1	1	0
Peptic esophagitis	0	6	0	4
Trauma	4	0	1	2*
Papillomatosis	0	0	1	0
Mega-esophagus	0	0	0	1
Severe displasia	0	1	0	0
Benign tumor	1	0	0	2
Benign stricture	0	0	1	1
Totals	39	8	4	10

* One patient died because of cirrhosis after esophago-gastrectomy with intrathoracic anastomosis for perforation of the esophagus.

tients with conditions such as caustic burns, but it would be difficult to follow such patients with direct examinations, since the esophagus is excluded. Indirect means of diagnosis, such as CT scanning and magnetic resonance imaging, could only help if the tumor has reached a certain volume.[5,6] In this case esophagectomy is justified, especially in the young patient and if done by an experienced surgical team.

Choice of Substitute Organ

A variety of substitute organs are available to the surgeon:

1. The entire stomach, the stomach without the lesser curvature shaped into a wide isoperistaltic tube, and the reverse gastric tube
2. The right, transverse, or left colon
3. A jejunal Roux-en-Y loop with supplemental vascularization in the neck, if necessary
4. A free jejunal transplant with microvascular anastomoses in the neck in patients who require a simultaneous laryngeal reconstruction for benign lesions of the cervical esophagus and the pharynx[7–10]

The postoperative nutritional status is comparable in patients who have received an isoperistaltic gastric substitute or a coloplasty.[11,12] Similarly, the postoperative results of functional scintigraphy, manometric measurements, and pH determination show insignificant differences for the various procedures; pyloroplasty, however, is not useful in gastroplasties without vagectomy, and the colon and ileum tolerate acid secretion and protect the esophagus from acid regurgitation.[13–16]

In our series, the stomach has been used more frequently for shorter replacements with anastomosis in the chest. The colon was reserved for the longer replacements or bypasses with anastomosis in the neck. The colon was also prescribed by gastric involvement with lye or by previous gastric operation. More recently, our clinical results with regard to nutrition, regurgitation, and dumping have led us to prefer the coloplasty if this choice is possible. Based on both preoperative vascular contrast studies show-

Table 33-2. Complications

Procedure	n	Fistulae	Stenoses	Deaths
Coloplasty				
Cervical	39	4*	11	0
Thoracic	8	1**	1	0
Gastroplasty				
Cervical	4	2	1	0
Thoracic	10	0	1	1
Totals	61	7 (11%)	14 (23%)	1 (1.6%)

* One anastomotic fistula was diagnosed by radiologic contrast study.
** Due to localized necrosis of the colic cul-de-sac after end-to-side esophago-colostomy.

ing more reliable vascular arcades on the left and our preference to preserve the ileocecal valve, we have used the transverse colon, as described, in 46 of 47 patients with only one case of immediate postoperative necrosis of the colon transplant.

Details of Operative Technique

Some of the operative maneuvers and steps that complete any operation for esophageal substitution influence the quality of short- and long-range results. However, the contribution by some other operative steps to the quality of life is debatable, steps such as pyloroplasty, cervical or thoracic level of anastomosis, peristaltic direction, and anatomic location of the substitute organ (intrapleural, posterior mediastinum, retrosternal, or even presternal). Our experience has led us to the following conclusions:

1. Pyloroplasty or pyloromyotomy after each esophago-coloplasty is desirable, since we had to perform re-operations to improve gastric emptying in patients with reflux into the coloplasty segment from pylorospasm. This finding was not limited to patients in whom a gastric substitute had been used.
2. We prefer an intrathoracic anastomosis if the location of the lesion makes this possible, since the functional results are superior to those of cervical anastomosis and the dissection avoids the danger of a recurrent nerve paralysis.
3. We prefer isoperistaltic direction of the colon segment, since in some patients peristaltic contractions in the colon segment contribute to active regurgitation.[15]
4. We prefer the posterior mediastinal route, if possible. This is the shortest distance to the esophagus in the chest and in the neck. Furthermore, postoperative dilatations are much easier to accomplish with the substitute organ in this position. We have not performed any esophageal replacement that leaves the substitute organ in the pleural space.

The dissection of the mid-colic vessels is important in the preparation of the transverse colon. These vessels may arise from a short common trunk with the right colic vessels; more often they originate directly from the superior mesenteric vessels and bifurcate more or less early, to establish a bridge between right and left marginal colic arcades. Both vessels are tied close to their origin from the superior mesenteric artery and vein. The superior branch or branches of the left colic artery arise from the inferior mesenteric artery. This ensures a sufficient length of colon to reach any level in the chest or neck. At times it is necessary

to interrupt one or two sigmoid vessels to allow greater mobility of the superior branches of the left colic artery. Our smaller incidence of vascular complications (4.2%) is due to the care taken never to use a segment of colon in which the marginal arteries do not continue to pulsate after the artery that will ultimately be sacrificed has been clamped temporarily. Furthermore, we attach great importance to the careful preservation of the venous drainage. In the only case of necrosis due to vascular impairment, the arteries of the transverse colon segment continued to pulsate at the time of re-operation while the venous drainage was totally deficient. Incision of the white line of Toldt on the right and left side and elevation of the right and left colon ensure a safe colo-colic anastomosis.

Stapling Instruments

The use of circular mechanical suture instruments has not totally eliminated anastomotic leaks and fistulae in the neck but has greatly facilitated cologastric anastomosis. The frequency of postoperative anastomotic strictures does not appear to increase with the use of staplers, in our experience. This incidence was high in those patients who underwent operations for caustic burns (30.5%, or 11 of 36 patients), as compared to 12% (3 of 25 patients) in all other diseases, with 2 of 3 occurring after anastomotic leaks and fistulae.

CONCLUSIONS

The long-range followup has shown in our patients that the colon does not always tolerate acid or biliary reflux, the first leading to ulcerations and the second to pain.[2,18] Because of this experience, we think it is important to associate vagotomy, gastric drainage, and gastroplication around the colon. If the anastomosis is between the colon and the jejunum because of previous or concomitant total gastrectomy, the reconstruction for the jejunum should be in the Roux-en-Y fashion. In three patients in whom this was not done, re-operation became necessary because of crippling reflux. The functional results and the modest incidence of peri-operative complications have increased our enthusiasm for esophago-coloplasty in patients with benign conditions of the esophagus and excellent prospects of long-term survival; hence, the quality of life should be at the same optimal level.

Translated from the French by F.M. Steichen, M.D.

REFERENCES

1. Katsaros J, Banis JC, Acland RD, Tan E: Monitoring free vascularized jejunum grafts. Br J Plast Surg 38: 220–222, 1985.

2. Belsey R, Clagett OT: Reconstruction of the esophagus with left colon. J Thorac Cardiovasc Surg 49:33–55, 1965.

3. Gosset D, Sarfati E, Celerier M: Les perforations de l'oesophage thoracique. A propos de 14 cas opérés. J Chir (Paris) 123:607–610, 1986.

4. Vidrequin A, Mangin P, Beck M, Bresler L, Boissel P, Grosdidier J: Exclusion oesophagienne par agrafes résorbables. Lyon Chir 84:167–168, 1988.

5. Hopkins RA, Postlethwait RW: Caustic burns and carcinoma of the esophagus. Am J Surg 194:146–148, 1981.

6. Appelquist P, Salmo M: Lye corrosion carcinoma of the esophagus. A review of 63 cases. Cancer 45:2655–2658, 1980.

7. Akiyama H, Miyazono H, Tsurumaru M, Hashimoto C, Kawamura T: Use of the stomach as an esophageal substitute. Ann Surg 188:606–610, 1978.

8. Postlethwait RW: Surgery of the esophagus. New York: Appleton-Century-Crofts, 1979.

9. Androsov PI: Blood supply to mobilized intestine used for an artificial esophagus. Arch Surg 73:917, 1956.

10. Roka R, Niederle B, Piza H, Ehrenberger K, Grasl M: Reconstruction of the pharynx and the cervical esophagus with free transplanted jejunum. In: Siewert JR, Hölscher AH, eds: Diseases of the Esophagus. Berlin: Springer-Verlag, 1988.

11. Hanna EA, Harrison AW, Derrick J: Long-term results of visceral esophageal substitutes. Ann Thorac Surg 3:111–118, 1967,

12. Ando N, Ikehata Y, Ohmori T, Abe O: Prospective studies on postoperative nutritional status in patients with esophageal carcinoma as evaluated from various substitutes for reconstruction: gastric tube versus colon interposition. In Siewert JR, Hölscher AH, eds: Diseases of the Esophagus. Berlin: Springer-Verlag, 1988.

13. Okada M, Nishimura O, Sakurai T, Tsuchihashi S, Juhri M: Gastric functions in patients with intrathoracic stomach after esophageal surgery. Ann Surg 204:114–121, 1986.

14. Hölscher AH, Voit H, Siewert JR, Buttermann G: Function of the intrathoracic stomach. In: Siewert JR, Hölscher AH, eds: Diseases of the Esophagus. Berlin: Springer-Verlag, 1988.

15. Little AG, Scott WJ, Ferguson MK, et al: Functional evaluation of organ interposition for esophageal replacement. In: Siewert JR, Hölscher AH, eds: Diseases of the Esophagus. Berlin: Springer-Verlag, 1988.

16. Moreno E, Calleja IJ, Landa JI, Jover JM, Gonzalez I, Gomez M: Functional study of ileocolic interposition after esophagectomy and total esophagogastrectomy. In: Siewert JR, Hölscher AH, eds: Diseases of the Esophagus. Berlin: Springer-Verlag, 1988.

17. Ventemiglia R, Khalil KG, Frazier OH, et al: The role of preoperative mesenteric arteriography in colon interposition. J Thorac Cardiovasc Surg 74:98–108, 1977.

18. Fékété F, Hugentobler JP, Breil P: Ulcères anastomotiques des oesophagoplasties coliques. Ann Chir 36: 334–339, 1982.

CHAPTER 34

EARLY TRANS-HIATAL ESOPHAGECTOMY IN SEVERE CAUSTIC BURNS OF THE UPPER DIGESTIVE TRACT

M. Celerier

Of 679 patients admitted for oral ingestion of caustic material, 50 underwent emergency esophago-gastrectomy because of organ necrosis. In our earlier experience, we used thoracotomy for esophagectomy in 13 patients, of whom 10 died (mortality rate of 76%). Since 1979, we have been performing trans-hiatal esophagectomy and abdominal gastrectomy as indicated without opening the chest. The mortality rate in 37 patients was 35%, with 11 of 13 deaths due to tracheo-bronchial necrosis.

PATIENTS AND METHODS

From January 1970 to October 1987, 679 adults were admitted to our department for oral ingestion of caustic material, most often in an attempt to commit suicide (622/679). Eighty-seven patients had severe burns of the upper digestive tract justifying emergency operation. Fifteen patients did not undergo operations because their lesions were too severe following a late diagnosis. Fifty patients underwent esophago-gastrectomy, 13 from 1970 to 1979 through open thoracotomy for the esophagectomy and 37 since 1979 through a trans-hiatal approach without thoracotomy. The responsible agents are summarized in Table 34-1. The approximate quantities of the ingested agents varied from 30 to 400 ml for lyes and from 100 to 300 ml for acids.

All patients underwent esophageal examination with a fiberoptic endoscope as soon as they were admitted, without concern for the time elapsed from ingestion to hospital admission. The lesions were classified into three stages and a diagram showing the depth and the extent of the burns was established. In the 37 patients who underwent transhiatal esophagectomy, this survey revealed a second-degree burn (deep ulceration) in 2 patients, a combination of second- and third-degree burns (deep necrotic lesion) in 15 patients, and a third-degree burn (no remaining viable mucosa, deep necrosis, or deep ulcers) in 20 patients.

Examination with a fiberoptic bronchoscope either before or immediately after the esophageal procedure was performed in the 31 last patients who underwent an emergency operation. The findings were normal in 9 patients, showed tracheal erythema in 13 patients, and diffuse or partial necrosis of the back wall of the trachea and left main-stem bronchus in 9 patients.

Time elapsing from ingestion to operation is summarized in Table 34-2. The most frequently indicated procedure was esophago-gastrectomy in 36 patients; 1 patient underwent esophagectomy only. Associated surgical procedures included two cholecystectomies and two splenectomies.

In 6 patients, a second operation had to be performed in the hours following the first procedure: one spleno-pancreatectomy for necrosis, one laparotomy for peritonitis due to disruption of the duodenal stump, and four thoracotomies for necrosis of the trachea, bronchus, or both. The intrathoracic procedures were drainage of empyema on 1 occasion and 3 patch reinforcements of a bronchus—2 with right pulmonary parenchymal apposition, 1 with pedicled

Table 34-1. Agents Responsible for Caustic Burns in 37 Patients

Chemical Substance	n
Strong base plus wetting agent	24
Hydrochloric acid	6
Sulfuric acid	3
Nitric acid	1
Ammonia	1
Concentrated bleach	1
Iodized alcohol	1

muscle flap. Only 1 patient survived, after pulmonary apposition.

Esophagectomy was indicated in 1 patient after endoscopic disruption, although clinically the necrosis was not transmural. The pathologic examination, however, showed that panparietal necrosis had destroyed the esophageal wall in 36 localized areas.

TECHNIQUES

The abdomen is entered through a left or bilateral subcostal incision; the cervical esophagus is exposed through a left cervical incision along the anterior border of the sternomastoid muscle. The blackened appearance of the esophageal wall confirms a panparietal necrosis. If similar gastric wall changes are observed, a total gastrectomy is performed after division and closure of the duodenum with a stapling device (TA-55). The cervical esophagus is mobilized, preserving the recurrent laryngeal nerves. An attempt is made to save a cervical segment of esophagus for a satisfactory esophagostomy. A silicone tube is introduced into the lumen of the distal cervical esophagus and is advanced toward the pylorus (Fig. 34-1). The tube is sutured to the cervical esophagus with two transfixing U-shaped sutures. The esophageal mobilization is started by finger dissection through the hiatal orifice (assisted by gentle traction on the abdominal esophagus) and is facilitated by the inlaying tube so the intussusception of the esophagus occurs

Table 34-2. Time from Ingestion to Intervention

Interval	n
Not specified	2
6 hours	9
6 to 12 hours	8
12 to 24 hours	6
25 hours	6
Second day	3
Third day	1
Fourth day	2

from above along with stripping from below through the mediastinum (Fig. 34-1). Following esophagectomy, a mediastinal drain is brought out through the left hypochondrium. The right upper quadrant of the abdomen is also drained. A cervical esophagostomy and a feeding lateral jejunostomy complete the intervention (Fig. 34-2).

RESULTS

No patients died during the operation. Mediastinal hemorrhage was minimal, because of the thrombosis of peri-esophageal vessels from the caustic process and necrosis.

Thirteen patients died in the postoperative period. Causes of death were tracheo-bronchial necrosis in 10 patients, peritonitis in 2, and pancreatic necrosis in 1. The time that elapsed from ingestion to intervention is related to the mortality rate. Of the 7 patients who underwent operation within 6 to 12 hours after ingestion, 2 died, whereas of the 14 patients who underwent operation after 12 hours, 9 died.

Principal complications in surviving patients were pulmonary, with edema and bacterial pneumonia. Digestive tract continuity was restored within 3 to 4 months by retrosternal esophago-coloplasty. The right ileo-colon was used 23 times, and the transverse colon once.

DISCUSSION

Most authors accept the indications for emergency gastrectomy in cases of necrosis caused by the inges-

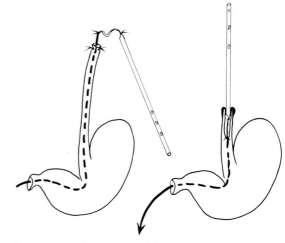

Fig. 34-1. *Left:* Insertion of the naso-gastric tube. *Right:* Traction on the tube provides esophageal intussusception. Placement of the mediastinal drainage tube follows the specimen.

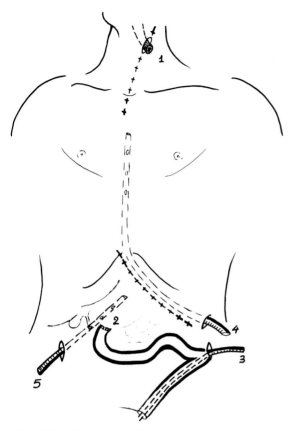

Fig. 34-2. Postoperative diagram. 1. Esophagostomy. 2. Duodenal closure. 3. Feeding jejunostomy. 4. Mediastinal drainage. 5. Drainage under the liver.

tion of caustic materials. Recently, success has been reported after an excision including part of the small intestine and the pancreas.[1,2]

Management of the necrotic esophagus remains controversial. Early excision of the esophagus could prevent potential perforation of the trachea from extension of the necrotic process. A contrary view by Burrington and Raffensperger suggests that the esophagus be left in situ, as it provides a natural patch over the tracheal defect.[3] The dilemma over early excision of the esophagus is governed by the degree of esophageal necrosis.

Serial histologic examinations after strong lye solutions had been experimentally introduced into the upper end of the esophagus revealed necrosis extending from the mucosa into the peri-esophageal areas.[4,5] Three of our patients had secondary tracheal necrosis after esophageal resection, although their bronchoscopic examinations were initially normal. Of 13 deaths after esophageal resection, 9 occurred in

patients who had undergone operation over 12 hours after the ingestion. Of these 9 patients, 8 died because of tracheo-bronchial necrosis.

Tracheo-bronchial lesions may be due to direct aspiration,[6] but are probably more often caused by extension of the esophageal necrosis into the tracheal wall. The technique of trans-hiatal blunt esophagectomy initially proposed by Denk[7] and successfully done in humans by Grey-Turner[8] had fallen into oblivion for three decades. The reason for discontinuing this technique were illustrations of vascular supply in textbooks of anatomy that suggested major arteries supplying the esophagus in the thorax. A recent study on blood supply of the esophagus made by Dorothea M.I. Liebermann-Meffert[9] shows that all major vascular branches divide into minute arterioles at some distance from the esophagus. It appears that such small extra-esophageal branches, when torn, will benefit from contractile hemostasis. Another fact is the early thrombosis of peri-esophageal vessels because of the caustic process and necrosis.

The technique of finger dissection appears very safe, as the progressive intussusception of the esophagus makes the blunt dissection as gentle as possible.[10,11] The average mediastinal bleeding was minimal, except in two cases in which 500 ml of blood was lost.

In severe caustic burns of the digestive tract with trans-mural parietal necrosis, aggressive management with a simplified technique has yielded an encouraging survival rate. The mortality rate depends primarily on the severity of the tracheo-bronchial necrosis. Pedicled muscle flap transplants conceivably could reduce the mortality from the localized tracheo-bronchial perforations.

REFERENCES

1. Ganepola GAP, Bhuta K: A case of total oesophago-gastro-duodeno-jejunostomy and partial pancreatectomy for lye burns, and reconstruction with colon interposition. J Trauma 24:913–916, 1984.

2. Mislawski R, Ghesquiere F: Exérèse large pour brûlure caustique gastro-duodenale. Presse Med 13:1742–1745, 1984.

3. Burrington JD, Raffensperger JG: Surgical management of tracheoesophageal fistula complicating caustic ingestion. Surgery 84:329–334, 1978.

4. Kirsh MM, Ritter F: Caustic ingestion and subsequent damage to the oropharyngeal and digestive passage. Ann Thorac Surg 21:74–82, 1976.

5. Haller JA, Bachman K: The comparative effect of current therapy on experimental caustic burn of the esophagus. Pediatrics 34:236–245, 1964.

6. Deneuville M, Andreassian B, Charbonnier JY, Assens P, Dubost C, Celerier M: Complications trachéo-bronchiques graves des ingestions de caustiques chez

l'adulte. Un cas de perforation guéri par patch pulmonaire. J Chir (Paris) 121:1–6, 1984.

7. Denk W: Zur radikaloperation des oesophaguskarzonoms. Zentralbl Chir 40:1065–1068, 1913.

8. Grey-Turner G: Carcinoma of the esophagus: the question of its treatment by surgery. Lancet 18:130–134, 1936.

9. Liebermann-Meffert DMI, Luescher U, Neff U, Ruedi TP, Allgower M: Esophagectomy without thoracotomy: is there a risk of intramediastinal bleeding? Ann Surg 206(2):184–192, 1987.

10. Brun JG, Celerier M, Besson JP, Ferry J, Dubost C: Oesophagectomie sans thoracotomie: 5 observations. Nouv Presse Med 10:2365–2367, 1981.

11. Gossot D, Sarfati E, Celerier M: Early blunt esophagectomy in severe caustic burns of the upper digestive tract. Report of 29 cases. J Thorac Cardiovasc Surg 94:188–191, 1987.

CHAPTER 35

THE VALUE OF AN INDWELLING TUBE THROUGH A STAPLED ESOPHAGEAL ANASTOMOSIS

Gustavo G.R. Kuster

The most common cause of an anastomotic stricture is considered to be the fibrosis and scar resulting from a leak. There have been cases of anastomotic stenosis in the rectum following the use of the circular stapler, without evidence of leak, when a temporary diverting colostomy had been done.[1] A membrane formation has been noted in these cases, and although the mechanism is not clear, it probably occurs as a result of the inverted live bowel edges touching together and adhering to each other.

We have observed the same type of membranous obstruction in some cases of circular stapled anastomosis after esophago-coloplasty.

MATERIALS AND METHODS

Forty-seven patients underwent esophagectomy with colon replacement in the last 10 years. In 4 of these patients, the operation was for benign strictures, and in 43 it was for adenocarcinoma of the mid or lower esophagus. The age of the patients ranged from 20 to 78 years. Most patients with carcinoma had a columnar lined or Barrett's esophagus that had developed with long-standing gastro-esophageal reflux.

Operation was performed through two separate incisions, starting by an upper midline laparotomy followed by right thoracotomy. The resection was done from at least 10 cm above any gross evidence of tumor in the esophagus to include a proximal portion of the stomach with the entire lesser curvature. The stomach was transected with a TA-90 stapler. The right or transverse colon was used for the replacement of the resected esophagus, in either isoperistaltic or antiperistaltic position. The colo-gastric anastomosis was placed on the posterior wall of the body of the stomach. This anastomosis was done with the EEA stapler, cartridge no. 31, introduced through a gastrotomy. A partial pylorectomy was done introducing a circular stapler no. 25 through the same gastrotomy. The end-to-end anastomosis to reconstruct the remaining colon was also done with the EEA stapler. The diaphragmatic hiatus was enlarged to accommodate the interposed colon with its mesocolon. The colon was placed in the posterior mediastinum and was anastomosed to the esophagus using the EEA stapler, cartridge no. 28 or 31.

In 27 cases a 16-French in-dwelling tube was placed through the nose and upper esophagus into the interposed colon; in 20 cases the tube was placed through the entire interposed colon into the stomach (Fig. 35-1).

RESULTS

No operative mortality or significant morbidity occurred in these patients. They were examined by water-soluble contrast swallow a week after the operation, before oral fluids were started. Solid food was not usually given until 3 weeks after the operation.

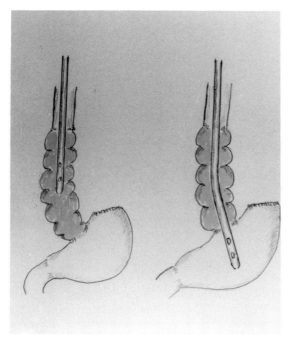

Fig. 35-1. *Left:* In 27 cases the in-dwelling tube was placed into the interposed colon only. *Right:* In 20 patients, the naso-gastric tube was advanced across two anastomoses into the stomach.

In 7 of 27 such approaches where the in-dwelling naso-gastric tube was not passed into the stomach, obstruction at the colo-gastric anastomosis developed. These patients complained of dysphagia when they started solid food; in one case the problem was not identified until 3 months after operation. Endoscopic examination revealed a membrane-like diaphragm partially occluding the anastomosis. A single dilatation disrupting this membrane was sufficient to solve the problem in all patients (Fig. 35-2).

This complication was not observed in any of the 20 patients in whom the naso-gastric tube was placed through the colo-gastric anastomosis at the time of the operation and left in place for 7 or more days. No patient developed a stricture at the esophago-colic anastomosis: all 47 patients had an in-dwelling tube at that level.

All patients were able to eat normal volumes of regular food after recuperation from the operation or after correcting the stricture. No patient complained of heartburn or reflux of gastric contents. One patient, however, developed a large asymptomatic peptic ulcer in the interposed colon, requiring an antrectomy that resulted in complete healing of the ulcer with no recurrence after followup of 6 years.

DISCUSSION

Replacement of the resected esophagus and cardiac end of the stomach for benign and malignant conditions can be accomplished by elongation of the residual stomach or through the use of an interposed segment of colon or jejunum. Colon interposition offers optimal functional results,[2,3] preventing disabling gastro-esophageal reflux,[4-7] esophagitis,[8] and stenosis.[2,3,6] It should be used when long survival is expected.[2,7,9,10]

Although some surgeons consider a tube through an anastomosis harmful, we have not seen any untoward effects from this. We have found that adherence of the inverted edges of the circular-staple anastomosis during the early period of healing should be prevented. Our observation indicates that presence of an in-dwelling tube may obviate stenosis of an anasto-

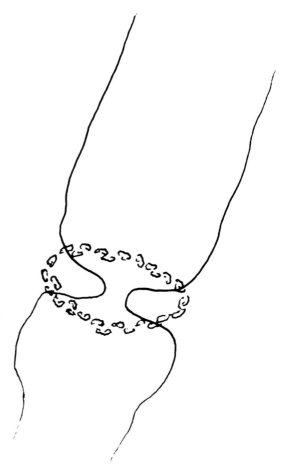

Fig. 35-2. Artistic representation of obstructing mucosal membrane in an otherwise intact, wide anastomosis, and preservation of the circular alignment and caliber.

mosis not given the benefit of early dilatation by food or intestinal contents.

Acknowledgment: This study was supported in part by the Harold and Daphne Oppenheimer Research Fund.

REFERENCES

1. Brain J, Lorber M, Fiddian-Green RG: Rectal membrane; An unusual complication following use of the circular stapling instrument for colorectal anastomosis. Surgery 89:271–274, 1981.

2. Skinner DB: Esophageal reconstruction. Am J Surg 139:810–814, 1980.

3. Wilkins EW: Long-segment colon substitution for the esophagus. Ann Surg 192:722–725, 1980.

4. Orel JJ, Erzen JJ, Hrabar BA: Results of resection of carcinoma of the esophagus and cardia in 196 patients. World J Surg 5:259–267, 1981.

5. Akiyama H. Surgery for carcinoma of the esophagus. Curr Probl Surg XVII:1980.

6. Molina JE, Lawton BR, Myers WO, Humphrey EW: Esophagogastrectomy for adenocarcinoma of the cardia. Ann Surg 195:146–151, 1982.

7. Orringer MB, Kirsh MM, Sloan H: Esophageal reconstruction for benign disease—Technical considerations. J Thorac Cardiovasc Surg 73:807–812, 1977.

8. Skinner DB, Belsey RHR: Surgical management of esophageal reflux and hiatus hernia; long term results with 1,030 patients. J Thorac Cardiovasc Surg 53:33–54, 1967.

9. Buntain WL, Payne WS, Lynn HB. Esophageal reconstruction for benign disease: A long-term appraisal. Am Surg 46:67–79, 1980.

10. Campbell JR, Webber BR, Harrison MW, Campbell TJ: Esophageal replacement in infants and children by colon interposition. Am J Surg 144:29–34, 1982.

Part VIII

Stapling in Operations at the
Esophago-gastric or
Esophago-jejunal Junction

CHAPTER 36

TRANS-HIATAL RESECTION FOR CARCINOMA OF THE DISTAL ESOPHAGUS AND ESOPHAGO-GASTRIC JUNCTION: ESOPHAGO-GASTROSTOMY AND ESOPHAGO-JEJUNOSTOMY WITH MANUAL AND MECHANICAL SUTURES

N. Kockel and B. Ulrich

For squamous cell carcinoma of the esophagus, we perform a subtotal esophagectomy with anterior or posterior mediastinal pull-through of an isoperistaltic greater curvature tube into the neck. In cases of carcinoma of the cardia, we prefer a trans-hiatal resection of the distal esophagus from the abdomen. This approach makes resection of the distal esophagus up to the tracheal bifurcation and stapled anastomosis possible. Since 1984, we have changed from proximal gastrectomy to total gastrectomy because of severe reflux symptoms and limited scope of tumor control with fundectomy only. The total gastrectomy is combined with a lymph node dissection of compartments I and II (nodes at the G-E junction, lesser and greater gastric curvatures, pylorus, celiac axis, and along the branches of its distribution). Continuity is reestablished with a Roux-en-Y jejunal loop and end-to-side stapled anastomosis.

TECHNIQUE

Through an upper midline laparotomy, the approach is maintained with a Rochard upper-arm retractor, and most of the left triangular ligament is divided to facilitate mobilization of the left liver lobe to the right. The transversely running inferior phrenic vein is ligated and divided together with the central tendon of the diaphragm. This incision is continued in a dorsal direction and—after gently dissecting the pericardium from the diaphragm—in a ventral direction. The esophagus can then be looped and cleared through the enlarged hiatus. By means of long narrow retractors (blood pressure and EKG monitoring is required because of possible compression of the heart), an optimal survey to the tracheal bifurcation is possible. After preparation of the distal esophagus together with total gastrectomy and lymph node dissection, a soft right-angle clamp is placed some 5 cm above the esophageal resection line. Following transection, a purse-string suture is run over all layers of the cut end of the esophagus. The food passage is reconstructed with a jejunal Roux-en-Y loop. The esophago-jejunostomy is performed as an end-to-side anastomosis with the circular stapling instrument.

A feeding tube is advanced across the anastomosis under digital control. The redundant jejunal stump is closed with the TA-55 and the excess jejunum is ex-

Table 36-1. Stapled Anastomoses of the Distal Esophagus

Indication	n	Procedure	n	Leakage Rate Radiologic	Clinical	Lethal	Stenosis
Gastric carcinoma	104						
Benign disease	2	Esophago-jejunostomy	129	7 (5.4%)	6 (4.7%)	1 (0.8%)	1 (0.8%)
Carcinome of the cardia	42						
Ulcer (benign)	1	Esophago-gastrostomy	35	3 (8.5%)	3 (8.5%)	1 (2.8%)	0
Adeno-carcinoma of distal esophagus	15						
Total	164		164	10 (6.1%)	9 (5.5%)	2 (1.2%)	1 (0.6%)

Table 36-2. Stapled Anastomoses After Resection of a Carcinoma at the Esophago-Gastric Junction

Procedure	n	Leakage Rate Clinical	Radiologic	Lethal	Stenosis
Esophago-gastric	35	3 (8.5%)	3 (8.5%)	1 (2.8%)	0
Esophago-jejunal	27	0	0	0	1 (3.6%)
Total	62	3 (4.8%)	3 (4.8%)	1 (1.6%)	1 (1.6%)

Table 36-3. Intra-Operative Instrument Complications in 62 Stapled Anastomoses After Resection of a Carcinoma of the Esophago-Gastric Junction

Complications	n	Therapy	n	Postoperative Leaks
Primary leaks	3	Reinforcement by handsewn suture	2	0
		New stapled anastomosis	1	0
Failure of cutting ring blade	1	New stapled anastomosis	1	0
Gastric tube stapled into anastomosis	1	New stapled anastomosis	1	0
Total	5 (8.1%)		5	0

Table 36-4. Pulmonary Complications After Resection of a Carcinoma of the Esophago-Gastric Junction and Stapled Anastomoses

Study Period	Approach	n	Pulmonary Complications	Lethal	Overall Mortality Rate
2/82–3/88	Trans-diaphragmatic	34	5 (14.7%)	1 (2.9%)	5 (14%)
2/79–1/82	Thoraco-abdominal	23	8 (35%)	6 (26%)	7 (30%)
2/79–2/86	Abdominal	5	2 (40%)	1 (20%)	1 (20%)
	Total	62	15 (24.2%)	8 (12.9%)	13 (21%)

Table 36-5. Complications in 34 Trans-Diaphragmatic Esophageal Resections

	n	Mortality Rate
Intra-Operative		
Gastric tube stapled into anastomosis	1	0
Pneumothorax, left side (thorax suction drainage)	12	0
Total	13	0
Postoperative		
Anastomotic leakage	2	2 (6.5%)
Stenosis	1	0
Pneumonia	2	1 (2.9%)
Pleural effusion, left side	2	0
Pericardial effusion	1	0
Cardiac arrest (infarction)	1	1 (2.9%)
Catheter sepsis	1	1 (2.9%)
Total	10	5 (14.7%)

cised. The integrity of the anastomosis is tested by injection of methylene blue into the feeding tube.

PATIENTS

Using this technique, 164 patients underwent operation from February 1979 to July 1984 in the Surgical Department of the University of Dusseldorf (Prof. Dr. K. Kremer); from August 1984 to September 1986 in the Surgical Department of the Juliusspital in Wurzburg (Prof. Dr. B. Ulrich); and from October 1986 to April 1988 in the Surgical Department of Dusseldorf-Gerresheim Hospital (Prof. Dr. B. Ulrich).

Indications were gastric cancer in 104 patients, carcinoma of the esophago-gastric junction in 42 patients, 15 adenocarcinomas of the distal esophagus (Barrett's carcinoma), and 3 benign lesions. We performed 129 esophago-jejunostomies and 35 esophago-gastrostomies (these only until 1984 and not thereafter because of severe reflux complications).

There were 62 carcinomas of the esophago-gastric junction. Until 1982, these patients underwent operation by an abdomino-thoracic approach (23); since 1982, the operation has been done by a trans-diaphragmatic approach (34). An abdominal approach without incision of the diaphragm was done in 5 cases.

The leakage rate of the stapled and manual anastomoses were compared and tested by the four-field test.

RESULTS

The clinical leakage rate of all stapled anastomoses in the distal esophagus was 5.5% (9 of 164); the mortality rate was 1.2%.

The esophago-gastrostomies resulted in a higher leakage rate (8.5%) than did the esophago-jejunostomies (4.7%) when both were done by stapling, although the difference is not statistically significant (Table 36-1).

Table 36-6. Evaluation of Stapled Esophago-Gastric Anastomoses in the Literature

Reference	Stapler	Number of Anastomoses	Leaks	Deaths
Dorsey et al.[2]	EEA	9	0	0
Kivelitz and Ulrich[11]	EEA	19	0	0
Shahinian et al.[14]	EEA	10	0	0
West et al.[21]	EEA	31	0	0
Wilson[22]	EEA	30	1	0
Behl et al.[1]	EEA	40	1	1
Hopkins et al.[7]	EEA	60	1	0
Féketé et al.[4]	EEA	127	7	0
	ILS	73	3	0
Spina[17]	EEA	17	1	0
Ulrich*[20]	EEA	35	3	1
Total		451	17 (3.8%)	2 (0.5%)

* Since February 1982: trans-diaphragmatic.

Table 36-7. Evaluation of Stapled Esophago-Jejunal Anastomoses in the Literature

Reference	Stapler	Number of Anastomoses	Leaks	Deaths
Fasching and Moritz[3]	SPTU/EEA	8	1	0
Hollender[6]	EEA	23	1	0
Molina and Lawton[12]	EEA	9	0	0
Sannohe et al.[13]	EEA	14	2	0
Huttunen et al.[8]	EEA	16	2	0
Jatzko and Redtenbacher[9]	EEA	25	1	0
Sugimachi[18]	SPTU/EEA	17/11	1	0
Ulatkowski et al.[19]	EEA	29	1	0
Junginger et al.[10]	EEA	31	4	1
Guerrera[5]	EEA	25	0	0
Spina[17]	EEA	26	1	1
Winter et al.[23]	EEA	54	4	1
Ulrich[20]	EEA	110	5	1
Total		398	23 (5.8%)	4 (1%)

After resection of a carcinoma of the esophago-gastric junction, the leakage rate was 8.5% (Table 36-2). Leaks occurred only after esophago-gastrostomies. There were 5 intra-operative instrument complications.

As shown in Table 36-3, postoperative leaks can be avoided by appropriate corrective steps intra-operatively. In followup examinations, we noticed only 1 stricture (1.6%), which could be dilated. Until 1982 we routinely used an abdomino-thoracic approach. The high mortality rate of 30.4% was mainly caused by pulmonary complications. After changing to the trans-diaphragmatic procedure, the pulmonary complication rate dropped from 34.8% to 14.7%, and the mortality rate from 26.1% to 2.9% (p < 0.01). The overall mortality rate decreased from 30.4% to 14.7% (Table 36-4). Intraoperative and postoperative complications of trans-hiatal esophageal resections are listed in Table 36-5.

DISCUSSION

During the pre-stapling period, anastomosis after resection of the distal esophagus was only possible through a thoracotomy, which can now be avoided with the help of stapling techniques. The dissection of the distal esophagus and corresponding lymph nodes is also possible by the trans-diaphragmatic approach, and does not require a thoracotomy to assure a more radical extirpation of neoplasm. The literature averages of anastomotic leakage rates of esophago-gastrostomies are 7.7% after hand-sewn[20] and 3.8% after stapled anastomoses (Table 36-6). Similar differences are noted after esophago-jejunostomies, with average leakage rates of 13.8% vs. 5.8% (Table 36-7).[20] These results are confirmed by our experience.

After the introduction of staplers, the leakage rates of the esophago-jejunostomies decreased particularly. By using the trans-diaphragmatic approach routinely since 1982, the overall mortality rate has decreased because of a significant lowering of deaths caused by pulmonary complications.

CONCLUSIONS

The trans-hiatal resection for carcinoma of the lower esophagus, GE junction, and proximal stomach has significantly reduced postoperative pulmonary complications as compared to a thoraco-abdominal approach, without compromising the radical nature of an operation for cancer. Since a majority of deaths were due to pulmonary causes, the overall mortality has been similarly reduced. In addition to resection, the reconstructive phase—previously requiring thoracotomy for anastomosis—is now possible through a trans-hiatal approach with the use of stapling instruments. A side benefit is the reduction in anastomotic leaks as compared to manual techniques.

REFERENCES

1. Behl P, Holden M, Brown A: Three years experience with esophageal stapling device. Ann Surg 198:134–136, 1983.
2. Dorsey JS, Esses S, Goldberg M, Stone R: Esophago-gastrectomy using the Auto Suture EEA surgical stapling instrument. Ann Thorac Surg 30:308, 1980.
3. Fasching W, Moritz E: Zirkuläre Klammeranastomosen im Magen-Darmtrakt mit den Klammernahtgeräten SPTU und EEA. Chirurg 30:308, 1980.
4. Fékéte W, Moritz E: Zirkuläre Klammeranastomosen im Magen-Darmtrakt mit den Klammernahtgeräten SPTU und EEA. Chirurg 51:644, 1980.
5. Guerrera C, Liboni A, Scalco GB, et al: La gastrectomia

totale con sutura meccanica: un reale progresso? Minerva Chir 39:13–18, 1984.

6. Hollender L, Blandiot P, Meyer C, et al: Erfahrungen mit der Anwendung von Nähapparaten in der Magen-Darm-Chirurgie. Zentralbl Chir 106:74, 1981.

7. Hopkins R, Alexander J, Postlethweit R: Stapled esophagogastric anastomosis. Am J Surg 147:283, 1984.

8. Huttunen R, Laitinen S, Staahlberg M, Mokka REM, Kairaluoma M, Larmi TKI: Experiences with the EEA stapling instrument for anastomoses of the upper gastrointestinal tract. Acta Chir Scand 148:179, 1982.

9. Jatzko G, Redtenbacher M: Anwendungsmöglichkeiten für Maschinenanastomosen in der Abdominalchirurgie. Acta Chir Austr 5/6:131–133, 1982.

10. Junginger Th, Walgenbach S, Pichlmaier H: Die zirkuläre Klammeranastomose (EEA) nach Gastrektomie. Chirurg 54:161–165, 1983.

11. Kivelitz H, Ulrich B: Klammernahtgeräte am Ösophagus. Langenbecks Arch Chir S:455–457, 1981.

12. Molina J, Lawton B: Use of circumferential stapler in reconstruction following resections of the cardia. Ann Thorac Surg 31:325–328, 1981.

13. Sannohe Y, Hiratsuka R, Doki K, Inutsuka S, Hirano M: Mechanical suture in esophagogastointestinal anastomosis. Jpn J Surg 9:313, 1979.

14. Shahinian TK, Bowen JR, Dorman BA, Soderberg CH, Thompson WR: Experience with EEA stapling device. Am J Surg 139:549, 1980.

15. Siewert JR, Hölscher AH, Becker K, Gössner W: Kardiacarcinom: Versuch einer therapeutisch relevanten Klassifikation. Chirurg 58:25, 1987.

16. Sombrowski J: Das Karzinom von Ösophagus und Kardia. Ergebnisse nach der Behandlung 1960–1980. Düsseldorf, Med Fakultät: Diss (1985).

17. Spina GP, Rosati R, Rebuffat C, Montorsi M, Zago M: La sututrice meccanica circulare EEA in chirrugia digestiva. Analisi di 76 casi. Minerva Chir 39:197–203, 1984.

18. Sugimachi K, Ikeda H, Ueo H, Kai H, Okudaira Y, Inokuchi K: Clinical efficacy of the stapled anastomosis in esophageal reconstruction. Ann Thorac Surg 33:374–378, 1982.

19. Ulatkowski L, Usmiani J, Kantarzis M: Maschinelle Ösophago-Jejunostomie: Moderner Trend oder Fortschritt? Chirurg 53:495, 1982.

20. Ulrich B, Kremer K, Kockel N: Chirurgie des Kardiakarzinoms. Akt Chir 23:110–115, 1988.

21. West PhN, Marbarger JP, Marzt MN, Roper ChL: Esophagogastrostomy with the EEA stapler. Ann Surg 193:76, 1981.

22. Wilson SE, Stone R, Scully M, Ozeran L, Benfield JR: Modern management of anastomotic leak after esophagogastrectomy. Am J Surg 144:95–101, 1982.

23. Winter J, Nier H, Ulrich B, et al: Ergebnisse der maschinellen Oesophagojejunostomie nach Gastrektomie. In: Häring R, ed: Therapie des Magenkarzinoms. Basel: Edition Medizin Weinheim, 1984.

CHAPTER 37

ESOPHAGO-GASTRECTOMY USING THE EEA STAPLER

Raymund J. Donnelly, David Kaplan, Richard I. Whyte, and Derek D. Muehrcke

Esophago-gastrectomy is an accepted treatment for resectable tumors of the esophagus and for undilatable peptic strictures of the esophagus. This procedure has traditionally carried appreciable morbidity and mortality rates, but recent advances in operative techniques and management have brought about an improvement in results. Stapling devices have contributed to this improvement and have proved to be reliable and safe.[1]

MATERIALS AND METHODS

Between January 1980 and December 1987, 195 patients underwent esophago-gastrectomy using stapling instruments at the Broadgreen Hospital. Of these, 178 (91.3%) were for malignant disease and 17 for benign undilatable peptic stricture. There were 121 males and 74 females. The mean age was 64.3 (range: 33–84) years, with 51 patients over the age of 70.

Preoperative assessment consisted of history and physical examination, barium studies, biochemical screen, esophagoscopy and, in case of mid-esophageal tumors, bronchoscopy. Isotope, ultrasound, and CT scans were obtained when indicated for evaluation of local or metastatic disease.

The operative technique has been previously described.[2] Early in the series all patients were explored either by a left thoraco-abdominal incision for lower third tumors and peptic strictures or by laparotomy and right thoracotomy for middle third tumors.

Since June 1983, however, we have employed a left thoracotomy with incision of the diaphragm through the chest as our preferred approach to all intrathoracic resections. During this period, it has been necessary in 12 patients to extend the incision across the costal margin because of limited exposure due either to intra-abdominal adhesions or a bulky tumor.

The anastomosis was carried out in all cases using the EEA stapling device (Autosuture, UK). TA, GIA, LDS, and Surgiclip instruments were used as previously described for mobilization and division of the stomach and for closure of the gastrotomy used for insertion of the EEA. Since January 1984, all linear gastric staple lines have been reinforced with a continuous, non-inverting layer of 3-0 Mersilene. Patients were normally extubated in the operating theater and returned to the general ward. Chest physiotherapy, antibiotics, and subcutaneous heparin were given, but parenteral nutrition was not routinely used. Chest tubes were removed on the first or second postoperative day, as was the naso-gastric tube when aspirates were minimal. Oral fluids were commenced on the fourth day and diet was advanced thereafter as tolerated. Radiologic examination of the anastomosis was only performed if a leak was suspected or if there had been undue difficulty in performing the anastomosis.

After discharge, all patients were seen at regular intervals in clinic and evaluated for evidence of tumor recurrence, anastomotic stricture, and metastatic spread. Patients complaining of dysphagia underwent esophagoscopy and biopsy or dilatation as indicated.

The incidence of anastomotic stricture was calculated after excluding patients who died in the postoperative period or who developed recurrent tumor at the anastomosis. In this way, only patients at risk were included in the analysis. Radiotherapy was only used for palliation of residual or recurrent disease.

RESULTS

Operative Mortality

Overall operative mortality, defined as death within 30 days or during the initial hospital stay, was 9.7% (Table 37-1). Mortality in 76 patients undergoing resection via the thoraco-abdominal approach occurred at a rate of 11.8%; in 103 patients with only a left thoracotomy incision, the mortality rate was 7.7%. This difference was not statistically significant. Fifty-one patients were over the age of 70 years; in this group the operative mortality rate was 12.7%. Of these patients, 16 were over 75 years of age and had an operative mortality rate of 6.3%.

In the overall group, one death was due to development of a leak at the anastomosis and one followed dehiscence of the gastrotomy staple line. The other causes of death were not staple-related, and are listed in Table 37-2.

Complications

The complication rates, excluding those patients who died in the postoperative period, was 16.4% with 29 complications occurring in 25 patients (Table 37-3).

In addition to the fatal anastomotic leak (vide supra), there were three non-fatal leaks for an overall incidence of 2.1%. Three patients developed leaks at the gastrotomy staple line (1.5%), of whom one patient died. Patients were discharged from the hospital at an average of 14 days (range: 6–99). The complication rate in the left thoracotomy subgroup was 18.6%, the anastomotic leak rate 2.0%, and the mean hospital stay 13 days.

Anastomotic Stricture

Postoperative dysphagia developed in 32 of 176 discharged patients (18.1%). Recurrent malignant disease occurred at the anastomosis in 6.25% of patients undergoing and surviving surgery for cancer.

Table 37-1. Operative Mortality—Incidence Within 30 Days or During First Hospital Stay

Overall	9.7%
Thoraco-abdominal	11.8%
Left thoracotomy	7.7%
Patients over 70	12.7%

Table 37-2. Operative Mortality

Case of Death	No. Patients	Post-Op Day
Anastomotic leak	1	35
Gastrotomy leak	1	18
Broncho-pneumonia	6	4, 4, 11, 12, 15, 19
Cardiac arrest	5	2, 3, 4, 12, 17
Pulmonary embolus	2	1, 32
Chylothorax	2	4, 15
Septicemia	2	6, 17
Total	19	

Patients were classified as having anastomotic stricture if they complained of dysphagia and benefitted from dilatation, regardless of the degree of anastomotic narrowing. Excluding postoperative deaths and patients developing recurrent malignant disease at the anastomosis, benign anastomotic narrowing occurred in 22 patients (13.2%). The highest rate was in patients undergoing operation for benign peptic stricture, with an incidence of 35.3% (6/17), compared to 10.6% (16/151) for resections in patients with malignant disease (p < 0.05). There appeared to be a trend toward a higher incidence of stricture with a smaller EEA: 17.4% for the 25-mm instrument, 14.3% for the 28-mm size, and 5.3% for the 31-mm size (Table 37-4). However, these differences did not reach statistical significance.

Strictures became evident 1 to 48 months postoperatively, with 82% of patients presenting with their first episode of dysphagia within 6 months of operation. Seventy-seven percent of patients with stricture responded completely to only one or, at most, two dilatations. The strictures were generally soft and localized, and "popped" readily with passage of the dilators. One patient developed a hard stricture and required revision of the anastomosis, but in this pa-

Table 37-3. Operative Morbidity (Excluding Post-Operative Deaths)

Anastomotic leak	3
Gastrotomy leak	2
Instrument failure	1
Atrial fibrillation	3
Bile peritonitis	1
Broncho-pneumonia	6
Congestive cardiac failure	3
Chylothorax	3
Deep vein thrombosis	2
Septicemia	1
Wound infection	4
Total	29

Table 37-4. Anastomotic Stricture: Incidence in Relation to Size of Stapler

EEA Stapler Size	Anastomoses at Risk	Strictures	%
25 mm	46	8	17.4
28 mm	84	12	14.3
31 mm	38	2	5.3

tient malfunction of the EEA was experienced at operation.

DISCUSSION

The use of mechanical stapling devices for restoring continuity of the gastro-intestinal tract after esophago-gastrectomy was pioneered in the West by Ravitch, Steichen, and Chassin before the advent of the circular end-to-end anastomotic device.[3–6] Following the introduction of the EEA instrument in 1979, stapling of the esophagus became widely accepted and proved to be simple, time-saving, and reliable.[7,8]

We previously reported no leaks in our first 100 patients using the EEA instrument[1] and have now performed 195 esophago-gastrectomies, with 4 anastomotic leaks for an incidence of 2.1%. Each of these leaks can be attributed to an identifiable technical error. In three patients the esophagus was traumatized by trying to insert too large an EEA into a noncompliant organ. In each instance the problem was recognized and an anastomosis carried out with a smaller instrument, but a postoperative leak still occurred. These patients were managed with drainage, antibiotics, and parenteral nutrition. Two survived and one died a month later of a massive bleed from an aorto-enteric fistula at the site of the anastomosis. A fourth patient was re-explored for a large leak: a mucosal gap was found on the gastric side of the anastomosis. A single stitch was all that was required, and the patient made a full recovery. There has always been debate on the surgical approach to esophagectomy, with more recent controversy regarding the trans-hiatal method. We used the traditional left thoraco-abdominal incision for lower-third tumors and laparotomy, and right thoracotomy (Ivor Lewis) for middle-third tumors until June 1983. Since then, however, we have preferred a simple left thoracotomy, stripping the upper border of the seventh rib and gaining access to the abdomen by an incision in the diaphragm through the chest. We have found that all resectable tumors can be adequately removed by this route and that stapling instruments have considerably facilitated the mobilization of the stomach from above and allowed a secure anastomosis to be performed high in the thorax with relative ease. The incision can readily be extended across the costal margin if exposure is restricted by abdominal adhesions or by the bulk of the tumor. Dark et al. advocated a similar approach;[9] we would agree with them that the smaller incision reduces operative time and, since it does not cross the costal margin, is less painful and allows for better coughing and respiratory effort, postoperatively.

Early in the series, three patients developed leaks at the gastrotomy staple line; one died. Since then we have oversewn all linear gastric staple lines with a continuous non-inverting suture. West reported a similar problem and also recommends oversewing the gastrotomy staple line.[10] An alleged disadvantage of the circular stapling device is the higher incidence of anastomotic stricture. We have found an overall incidence of 13.1%, although the incidence was 10.6% following resection for malignant disease. We were, however, very strict in our definition of stricture, and in many cases the stricture amounted to no more than some degree of narrowing of the anastomosis. If a patient complained of some dysphagia and this was relieved by dilatation of the anastomosis, the patient was categorized as having a stricture, although in most cases the lumen was still at least 1 cm wide. In only one instance did we find a tight, pinhole fibrotic stricture; this patient underwent revision of the anastomosis. Seventy-seven percent of patients responded to only one or two dilatations, with permanent relief of symptoms. The characteristics of an anastomotic stricture following a stapled anastomosis are that it usually appears within 6 months of operation; that it is localized, soft, and not severe; and that it readily opens up to the passage of the dilators. The incidence of anastomotic narrowing following resection for benign peptic stricture is known to be high. Bender and Walbaum reported a 39.5% incidence following hand-sewn anastomoses.[11] Our rate of 35.3% is similar to this.

Finally, our data suggest that age alone should not be a contraindication to esophageal resection. The hospital mortality rate in our series of 51 patients over the age of 70 years was 12.7%, and was 6.3% in those patients over 75 years of age. Stapling instruments have an advantage in this age group by virtue of the reduced operating time and the facility with which they allow resection through a single left thoracotomy incision. Overall, we feel that stapling devices have made a positive contribution to improvements in the morbidity and mortality rates following esophageal resection. They do not, of course, replace good judgement, attention to detail, and meticulous surgical technique.

SUMMARY

Since January 1980, the authors have used stapling instruments whenever possible for esophageal resection and esophago-gastric anastomosis. Standard approaches to the esophagus were used until June 1983; since then a left thoracotomy incision has been employed for lesions of the gastric cardia and lower or mid-esophagus. Stapling instruments have facilitated this more limited approach. Esophago-gastrectomy was performed on 195 patients, using stapling instruments during an 8-year period; 103 of these were via left thoracotomy. Fifty-one patients were over 70 years of age. The overall operative mortality rate was 9.7%, 12.7% in those patients over 70 years of age. Complications occurred in 19.1% of patients, with anastomotic leakage in 2.1% and anastomotic narrowing in 13.1%. The mean hospital stay was 14 days. In the left thoracotomy subgroup, the operative mortality rate was 7.7%, the complication rate 18.6%, the leak rate 2%, the anastomotic narrowing rate 13.8%, and the mean hospital stay 13 days.

REFERENCES

1. Donnelly RJ, Sastry MR, Wright CD: Oesophagogastrectomy using the end to end stapler: results of the first 100 patients. Thorax 40:958–959, 1985.
2. Fabri B, Donnelly RJ: Oesophagogastrectomy using the end to end stapler. Thorax 37:296–299, 1980.
3. Ravitch MM, Steichen FM: Technics of staple suturing in the gastrointestinal tract. Ann Surg 175:815–824, 1972.
4. Steichen FM: Clinical experience with autosuture instruments. Surgery 69:609–615, 1971.
5. Chassin JL: Stapling technic for esophagogastrotomy after esophagogastric resection. Am J Surg 136:399–404, 1978.
6. Steichen FM, Ravitch MM: Mechanical sutures in esophageal surgery. Ann Surg 191:373–381, 1980.
7. Hopkins RA, Alexander JC, Postlethwaite RW: Stapled esophagogastric anastomosis. Am J Surg 147:283–287, 1984.
8. Steichen FM, Ravitch MM: Operations on the esophagus. In: Stapling in Surgery. Chicago: Year Book, 1984:220–257.
9. Dark JF, Mousalli H, Vaughan R: Surgical treatment of carcinoma of the oesophagus. Thorax 36:891–895, 1981.
10. West PN, Marbargar JP, Martz MN, Roper CL: Esophagogastrectomy with the EEA stapler. Ann Surg 193:76–81, 1981.
11. Bender EM, Walbaum PR: Esophagogastrectomy for benign esophageal stricture. Fate of the esophagogastric anastomosis. Ann Surg 385–388, 1986.

CHAPTER 38

TOTAL GASTRECTOMY AND ESOPHAGO-JEJUNOSTOMY WITH LINEAR STAPLING DEVICES

Bruno S. Walther, Thomas Zilling, Folke Johnsson, Christer Stael Von Holstein, and Bo Joelsson

The main reason for postoperative mortality after total gastrectomy is anastomotic leakage.[1,2] With the introduction of circular stapling devices, the time required to perform the esophago-jejunal anastomosis has been reduced, which is of substantial benefit in this time-consuming operation.[3] As shown in a recent postoperative study, the outcome for patients with total gastrectomy was better after a stapled esophago-jejunostomy than after a hand-sewn one. Two disadvantages are inherent in the use of circular stapling devices:

1. Placement of a time-consuming purse-string suture is required.
2. Insertion of the instrument anvil into a narrow esophagus can be extremely difficult and can produce esophageal rupture.[3]

To eliminate these drawbacks, we have developed a technique using the two linear stapling devices for the esophago-jejunal anastomosis that parallels the earlier work of Welter, Patel, Charlier, Psalmon, and Moller with the "anastomose résection intégrée" in this area.[4] This article describes the surgical procedure in 14 consecutive patients undergoing total gastrectomy and randomly chosen for the new technique. The width of the esophago-jejunal anastomosis was measured 6 months postoperatively using a fiberendoscope and a Fogarty balloon. The results were compared to those obtained with a conventional end-to-side esophago-jejunostomy performed with a circular stapling device.[3]

PATIENTS

From May 1986 through April 1988, 8 men (median age of 68 years, range of 42 to 81 years) and 6 women (median age of 65 years, range of 38 to 74 years) underwent total gastrectomy for cancer (11 patients), lymphoma (2 patients), and gastrinoma (1 patient). Four of the cancer patients had previously had a Billroth-II resection for benign disease. Six of the 11 patients with cancer presented with tumor confined to the body of the stomach; in 1 patient it was limited to the cardia. Eight of the 11 adenocarcinomas penetrated the stomach wall, and lymph node metastases were present in 5 patients. The patient with cardia carcinoma had a liver metastasis.

METHODS

Operative Procedures

Total gastrectomy, along with omentectomy, splenectomy, and dissection of the lymph nodes around the celiac axis and hepato-duodenal ligament, were performed in all patients. An extended procedure was done in 7 patients, including resection of the pancreatic tail in 5, enucleation of a gastrinoma in the pancreatic head in 1, and a small bowel resection in another. Thirteen of the operations were performed via laparotomy alone; the remaining one was performed through a left thoraco-abdominal incision. All patients were given prophylactic antibiotics (400 mg of intravenous doxycycline hydrochloride—Vibramycin). Dextran 70 (Macrodex) was used as the anti-thrombotic drug.

At the end of the en-bloc resection, the specimen remains attached only to the esophagus and is brought up to the patient's chest (Fig. 38-1). A Roux-en-Y jejunal loop of 50 cm length is prepared and divided distal to the ligament of Treitz with a linear cutting and stapling device. A small incision is placed into the back wall of the esophagus proximal to the G-E junction, using the stomach for traction. A second stab-wound is placed anti-mesenterically some 6 cm distal to the closed end of the Roux-en-Y loop (Fig. 38-1B). The forks of the GIA or PLC-50 instrument are introduced into the esophagus and the jejunum respectively, and the two organs are brought together at the hiatus by matching and locking the instrument halves (Fig. 38-1C). The instrument is fired (Fig. 38-1D). After withdrawal of the instrument, the common opening is closed with a linear stapler, which also encircles the anterior wall of the esophagus (Fig. 38-1E). The esophagus and excess gastric tissue are transected; as the specimen is delivered, the esophago-jejunostomy is completed (Fig. 38-1F). To accomplish the same anastomosis in the left chest, the specimen is brought up into the thorax through the hiatus, and the anastomosis is completed in the same way as in the abdomen. When the common opening of the GIA or PLC-50 placement sites is closed with the TA-55 (US Surgical Corp) or RL-60 (Ethicon Inc.), care must be taken not to grasp the

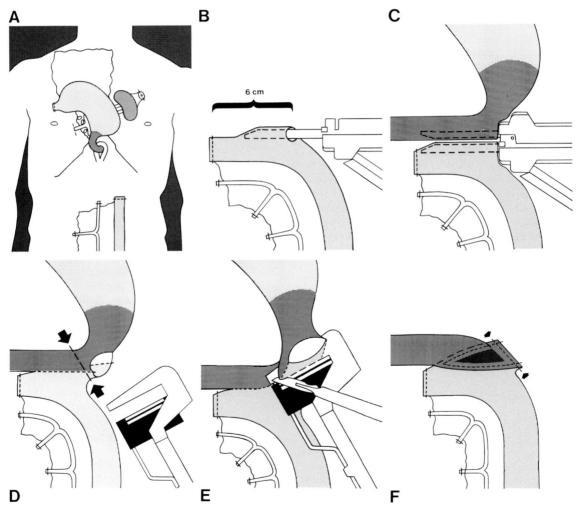

Fig. 38-1. End-to-side esophago-jejunal anastomosis after total gastrectomy with the PLC-50 or the GIA and the RL-60 or the TA-55 stapling instruments.

jejunal mucosa on the mesenteric side by pulling up too much of the jejunal lip (Fig. 38-1*E*).

To close the entire circumference of the common opening, the free ends of the linear GIA staple lines are pulled apart in a V-fashion. Linear TA closure of the anterior esophageal wall to the lower jejunal lip is performed and the specimen is excised peripheral to the stapler. The time to perform the anastomosis is measured by the anesthesiologist (that is, the time from the incisions in the esophagus and jejunum to the closure of the esophago-jejunal opening with a linear stapling device, including the time to locate and oversew a leak). Frozen sections of the resected margins are done intra-operatively to ensure tumor clearance.

Postoperative Regimen

The naso-gastric tube is left with its tip well below the anastomosis, and the patient is fed intravenously for 5 days, after which the anastomosis is checked for leakage by radiographic examination with water-soluble contrast medium. If no leakage is observed, the patient starts to drink fluids, which is followed by a soft diet. On the seventh day, a regular diet is served and intravenous therapy is discontinued.

Followup

Six months postoperatively, the patients were examined by endoscopy. The width of the anastomosis was calculated by inserting a Fogarty aortic occlusion catheter along with the endoscope. With a syringe connected to the catheter, air is inflated until the balloon in the distal end fills the anastomotic lumen (Fig. 38-2). The balloon is pulled up and down for a couple of centimeters to make sure that it is not getting caught, but slides smoothly and only fills the anastomotic lumen. The volume of inflated air is noted. This is repeated three times and the average calculated. The air is aspirated by pulling the piston of the syringe back without disconnecting the syringe. After withdrawal of the endoscope and the balloon catheter, the latter is filled to the volume recorded before and the diameter of the balloon is measured with a caliper. This method of measuring the esophago-jejunostomy has been in use since 1984 at our department in a prospective series of patients who underwent operation with total gastrectomy and end-to-side esophago-jejunostomy with the EEA stapler.

RESULTS

We succeeded with our preoperative plan in all patients in whom we attempted and accomplished

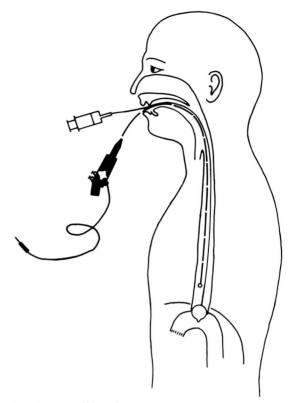

Fig. 38-2. A fiberendoscope and Fogarty aortic occlusion catheter are necessary for measuring the anastomotic width. For details see text.

the esophago-jejunostomy with the two linear stapling devices. The median operating time was 5 hours, 5 minutes (range: 205–505 minutes). The median time to perform the esophago-jejunal anastomosis was 12 minutes (range: 8–40 minutes).

The postoperative complications were small bowel obstruction (1), leak (1), empyema (1), and a fatal pulmonary embolus (1). This last patient was the only hospital death. The leaking anastomosis was found by radiographic examination to be confined on the fifth postoperative day, but sudden onset of abdominal pain the day after made us explore the patient. The leakage was in the angle between two crossing staple lines. It was oversewn and drained, and healed uneventfully in 2 weeks. The patient was discharged in good health after 28 days.

The median postoperative hospital stay was 10 days (range: 8–45). Nine patients are alive 3.7–21 months after the operation.

At endoscopic examination 6 months postoperatively, the width of the esophago-jejunostomy was equal or superior to the EEA-stapled anastomoses

(Fig. 38-3). Not a single patient complained of dysphagia.

DISCUSSION

Esophageal anastomosis with circular stapling devices is safe, as two large series report a leakage rate of 3.5%.[5,6] There are two main drawbacks, however: the need to construct a time-consuming purse-string suture and, in case of a narrow esophagus, the difficult and sometimes dangerous introduction of the circular instrument.

Wong found the stricture frequency to be inversely related to the size of the stapler.[6] This was confirmed by West in a series of patients with esophageal resection and esophago-gastrostomy.[7] We reported a higher leakage frequency in esophago-jejunal anastomoses when the smaller cartridges were used.[3] The size of the stapler follows the width of the esophagus, which is not controlled by the surgeon, unfortunately. With the GIA-TA method, however, the size of the esophagus is completely irrelevant, because even a narrow esophagus makes the insertion of the thin PLC-50 or GIA forks possible.

The time spent to perform the esophago-jejunal anastomosis with two linear staplers compares well with the circular anastomotic technique (12 minutes and 20 minutes, respectively).

The importance of the time-saving procedures must always be related to quality. That quality comes through standardization and is not controversial: stapling devices in this respect are unsurpassed. The type and rate of complications seen in this series is expected in this kind of surgery. What the leakage frequency (1/14) and mortality rate (1/14) will be in the long run cannot be predicted from this preliminary series, but it seems to correspond to the experience of others.[1,2,8]

The width of the esophago-jejunal anastomosis is promising. Since most operations for gastric carcinoma are palliative, postoperative morbidity and mortality rates should be low and the hospital stay short. Dysphagia should be absent for the rest of the patients' lives. We think the esophago-jejunostomy performed with two linear staplers fulfills these demands.

CONCLUSIONS

In performing total gastrectomies and esophago-jejunostomies with circular stapling devices, there are two disadvantages: (1) the need for purse-string suture, and (2) in case of a narrow esophagus, the introduction of the instrument can be nearly impossible, and the risk for rupture substantial. We therefore performed operations on 14 patients with the GIA or PLC-50 and TA-55 or RL-60 sequential anastomosis first, resection second technique. Fourteen patients with a median age of 65 years had a postoperative hospital stay of 10 days (range: 8–45). The leakage was 1/14. Hospital mortality was 1/14. Time to perform the anastomosis was 12 minutes (range: 8–20). Three re-operations were necessary (for intestinal obstruction, leakage, and a negative exploration). The width of the esophago-jejunal anastomosis 6 months postoperatively was an average of 32 cm (range: 27–41 cm). Esophago-jejunostomy performed with two linear staplers allows a quick and reliable anastomosis independent of esophageal lumen size and a time-consuming purse-string suture.

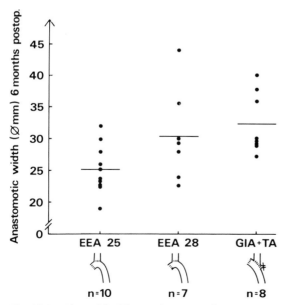

Fig. 38-3. The width of the esophago-jejunal anastomosis 6 months postoperatively in patients undergoing total gastrectomy with different anastomotic stapling techniques.

REFERENCES

1. Inberg MV, Heinonen R, Laurén P, Rantakokko V, Viikari SJ: Total and proximal gastrectomy in the treatment of gastric carcinoma: a series of 305 cases. World J Surg 5:249–257, 1981.
2. Lygidakis NJ: Total gastrectomy for gastric carcinoma: A retrospective study of different procedures and assessment of a new technique of gastric reconstruction. Br J Surg 68:649–655, 1981.
3. Walther BS, Oscarson JEA, Graffner HOL, Vallgren S, Evander A: Esophagojejunostomy with the EEA stapler. Surgery 99:598–603, 1986.
4. Welter R, Patel JCl, Charlier A: Chirurgie de l'estomac et du duodenum. In: Welter R, Patel JCl: *Chirurgie Mécanique Digestive—Techniques Raisonnées.* Paris: Masson, 1985:194–196.

5. Dorsey JS, Esses S, Goldberg M, Stone R: Esophago-gastrectomy using the autosuture EEA surgical stapling instrument. Ann Thorac Surg 30:308–312, 1980.

6. Wong J, Cheung H, Lui R, Fan YW, Smith A, Siu KF: Esophagogastric anastomosis performed with a stapler: the occurrence of leakage and stricture. Surgery 101:408–415, 1987.

7. West PN, Marbarger JP, Martz MN, Roper CL: Esophagogastrostomy with the EEA stapler. Ann Surg 193:76–81, 1981.

8. Huttunen R, Laitinen S, Stalberg M, Mokka RE, Kairaluoma M, Larmi TK: Experiences with the EEA stapling instrument for anastomoses of the upper gastro-intestinal tract. Acta Chir Scand 148:179–183, 1982.

ADDITIONAL READING

Moller E, Brun JG, Deliere Th, Patel JCl, Psalmon F, Welter R: Gastrectomie totale. Anastomose oeso-jejunale première pièce en place utilisant les pinces à suture mécanique linéaire. Presse Med 12:41, 1983.

CHAPTER 39

TECHNIQUE AND FUNCTIONAL RESULTS OF GASTRIC REPLACEMENT WITH JEJUNAL LOOP AND VENTRAL HEMI-JEJUNOPLICATION OF THE ESOPHAGO-JEJUNOSTOMY

J. Fass, V. Schumpelick, R. Bares, and U. Bull

At the end of the last century it was said that any surgeon who removed the stomach had no hesitation to kill two with a single blow: the patient and his own reputation. In 1943 Pack and McNeer wrote that a mortality rate of 37.6% after total gastrectomy was reason enough to give some optimism.[1] Today, total gastrectomy is the treatment of choice for some 70% of all gastric cancer cases, and the operative mortality rate is far below 10%. One main reason for this improvement is the lowered failure rate of esophago-jejunostomy. Stapling techniques and the development of sophisticated surgical procedures such as the different forms of jejunoplication have played an important role in this evolution.

Until 1985 we used the complete jejunoplication introduced by Schreiber[2] to protect the proximal anastomosis and prevent alkaline reflux. This procedure was performed in combination with jejunal interposition or Roux-en-Y gastric replacement with a jejunal loop. The jejunoplication covers the total circumference of the esophago-jejunostomy and is good protection against leakage. Complications such as stenosis or telescoping phenomenon are avoided by correct surgical technique. Nevertheless, in some of our patients, dysphagia with endoscopic proof of stenosis occurred. This complication led us to modify the method so that its benefits were preserved and a functional stenosis could not occur.

As a result we introduced an alternative technique to protect only the anterior or ventral portion of the anastomosis,[3] where all clinically significant anastomotic leaks occur, probably because of lack of coverage by adjacent organs. After performing the end-to-side EEA esophago-jejunostomy (Fig. 39-1), we leave intact an 8-cm long proximal portion of the jejunum. The open end is closed by the TA stapler and some inverting sutures (Fig. 39-2A).

The redundant end of bowel is placed around the anterior or ventral half of the circumference of the anastomosis (Fig. 39-2B) and is held with six sutures to the esophagus and jejunum (Fig. 39-2C). The plication should be under no tension to prevent a disruption or stenosis.

This technique can be combined with both jejunal interposition and Roux-en-Y reconstruction. Figure 39-3 shows both forms of gastric substitution with ventral jejunoplication. It is essential to choose long jejunal loops to provide a satisfactory substitute and sufficient length for the plication. To prove our new concept, we conducted a study in which we compared the clinical and functional results of the different forms of esophago-jejunostomy. In the last 6 years, the surgical technique of performing the esophago-jejunal anastomosis changed twice.

In 1982, stapling machines were introduced. In this study, only patients with stapled anastomoses us-

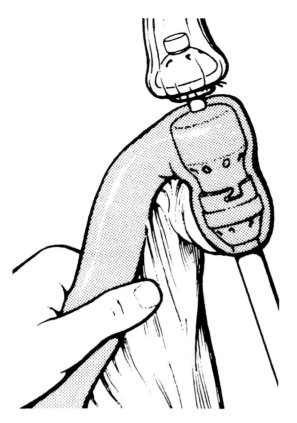

Fig. 39-1. Technique of stapled esophago-jejunostomy, end-to-side with circular anastomosing instrument.

ing a 25- or 28-mm magazine were considered; this provides comparable baseline conditions. In the first years, 53 end-to-end anastomoses were performed. In 1984 and 1985, a total of 21 complete jejunoplications were done (Schreiber type). Since the end of 1985, we changed to ventral hemi-jejunoplication as described above and performed operations in 65 gastric carcinoma patients in this way. The incidence of early complications showed no difference between the two jejunoplication groups (Table 39-1). The anastomotic leakage and mortality rates were nearly equal and ranged from 3.1% in ventral hemi-jejunoplications to 4.8% with complete jejunoplication. In the end-to-end anastomosis group, both complications occurred nearly twice as often. Three of the 5 postoperative deaths were traced to anastomotic insufficiency, resulting in a 9.4% mortality rate and a 7.1% rate of clinically relevant fistulae of the proximal anastomosis.

To evaluate the functional results of the different procedures, we performed a study at least 6 months after the operation. A total of 39 patients could be investigated. The group consisted of 15 patients with end-to-end anastomosis, 7 patients with complete jejunoplication, and 17 patients in whom ventral hemi-jejunoplication had been performed. After an interview to evaluate functional disturbances like reflux or dumping symptoms and dysphagia, an endoscopic and x-ray examination followed.

Only patients without proof of anastomotic stenosis, which means that the suture line could be passed by a GIF-P2 gastroscope, entered into the study. Local recurrence of carcinoma had to be excluded as well. All 39 patients complied with these criteria.

Clinically, symptoms were generally rare (Table 39-2). In the complete jejunoplication group, 3 patients complained of dysphagia. One patient in the hemi-jejunoplication group had disruption of the plication and suffered from reflux and dysphagia. Two cases of dumping with end-to-end anastomosis were correlated with too short an interposed jejunal loop— only 20 cm.

So that we could evaluate functional disturbances, all participants in the study were examined by scintigraphy. Emptying disorders were detected by a ^{99m}Tc-S-marked gruel meal. The regions of interest were the lower esophagus and the anastomotic area. The counts were detected by a gamma-camera as a function of time. Verification of reflux was done by hepato-biliary sequential scintigraphy with ^{99m}Tc-HIDA.

Only two patients experienced alkaline entero-esophageal reflux (Table 39-3). One had a short interposed jejunal loop and end-to-end anastomosis, and the other had a Roux-en-Y reconstruction and ventral hemi-jejunoplication. Here the cause can only be suspected, and may have been a distal stenosis of the small bowel.

In all other cases, the bile never reached the anastomosis because of long gastric substitutes. We could not find a difference in the esophageal clearance between end-to-end anastomosis and ventral hemi-jejunoplication. It was slightly below normal patterns, ranging around 90% in the first 10 seconds after swallowing. But there was a difference in patients with complete jejunoplication, four of which had an esophageal clearance comparable to the other two groups. But the three patients with dysphagia showed pathologic emptying studies.

In these studies we saw scintigraphically a functional stenosis, which we suspect was due to the jejunoplication. Typical was a normal passage in the beginning; then the jejunoplication loop filled up and caused an obstruction of the distal esophagus scintigraphically associated with proximal esophageal dilatation (Fig. 39-4). At the end of the delayed passage, the plication loop emptied itself and returned to the resting state. A graphic recording of esophageal emp-

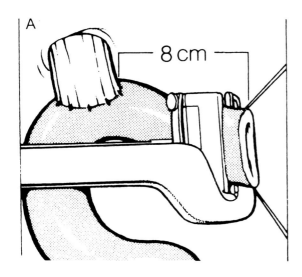

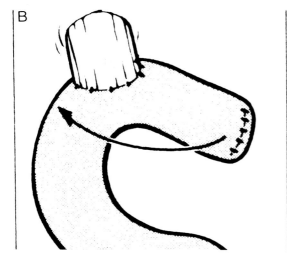

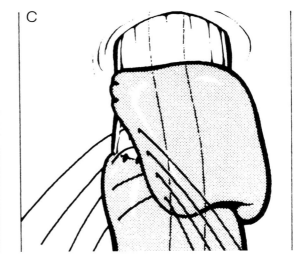

Fig. 39-2. Esophago-jejunostomy: surgical technique. *A*. Closure of the redundant jejunal loop with the TA stapler. *B*. Direction of the plication, from lateral to medial, ventral, or anterior. *C*. Fixation with six sutures to the esophagus and jejunum.

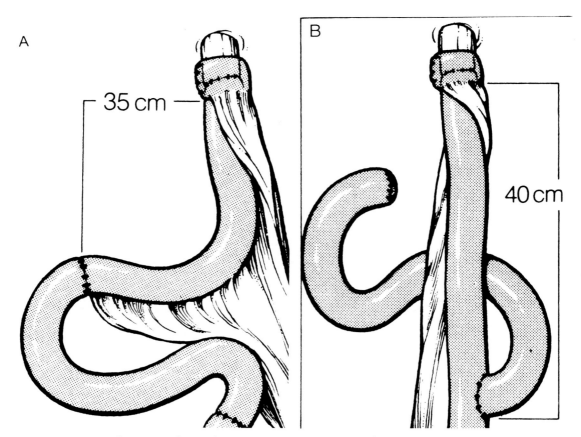

Fig. 39-3. Gastric replacement with jejunal interposition or Roux-en-Y procedure.

Table 39-1. Esophago-Jejunostomy in Gastric Replacement: Early Complications

Complication	End-to-End Anastomosis (n = 53)	Complete Jejunoplication (n = 21)	Ventral Hemi-Jejunoplication (n = 65)
Anastomotic leakage			
Clinically relevant	4 (7.1%)	1 (4.8%)	2 (3.1%)
Radiologic proof only	5 (9.4%)	1 (4.8%)	1 (1.5%)
Emptying of jejunoplication	–	1 (4.8%)	1 (1.5%)
Mortality	5 (9.4%)	1 (4.8%)	2 (3.1%)

Table 39-2. Esophago-Jejunostomy: Clinical Symptoms

Symptom	End-to-End Anastomosis (n = 15)	Complete Jejunoplication (n = 7)	Ventral Hemi-Jejunoplication (n = 17)
Reflux	1	–	1
Dysphagia	1	3	1
Dumping	2	–	–

Table 39-3. Esophago-Jejunostomy: Functional Results

Result	End-to-End Anastomosis (n = 15)	Complete Jejunoplication (n = 7)	Ventral Hemi-Jejunoplication (n = 17)
Esophageal clearance (mean ± SD)	68.1 ± 4.2	51.4 ± 23.2	71.7 ± 8.2
Entero-esophageal reflux (n)	1	–	1

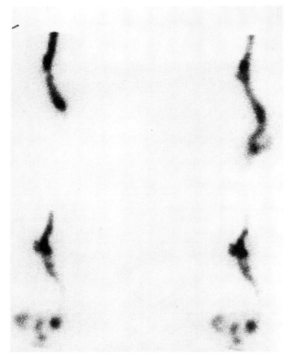

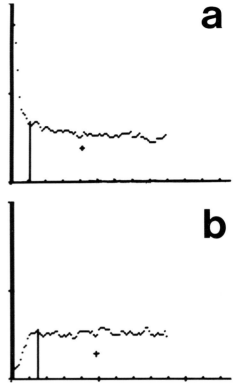

Fig. 39-4. Scintigraphical demonstration of functional stenosis after complete jejunoplication (^{99m}Tc-S marked gruel meal).

Fig. 39-5. Emptying curves of a patient with complete jejunoplication and functional stenosis (^{99m}Tc-S marked gruel meal). *A.* Proximal esophagus. *B.* Jejunoplication.

tying showed the same sequence of events (Fig. 39-5). After a quick initial passage of the bolus through the esophagus, the plication loop filled up and caused an obstruction, demonstrated by a flattening of the esophageal emptying curve.

CONCLUSIONS

A blind loop effect could be caused by complete jejunoplication. However, only 3 of 21 patients who underwent this procedure showed dysphagia, but we could not predict which patient would be afflicted because there were no differences in the surgical technique or the anatomic situation. Therefore, we think ventral hemi-jejunoplication to be a good alternative. It provides safety for the anastomosis comparable with total plication, but does not result in a functional stenosis.

REFERENCES

1. Pack GT, McNeer G: Total gastrectomy for cancer. Int Abst Surg 77(4):265–299.
2. Schreiber HW, van Ackeren H, Rehner M: Chirurgische Behandlung bösartiger Geschwulstkrankheiten des Magens. Chirurg 43:551, 1972.
3. Schumpelick V, Fass J: Magenersatz durch Dünndarm. Chirurg 59(3):125–132, 1988.

Part IX

Stapling in Gastric Surgery

CHAPTER 40

TOTAL GASTRECTOMY AND ESOPHAGO-DUODENAL JEJUNAL POUCH INTERPOSITION

A. Thiede, K.H. Fuchs, O. Stremme, and H. Hamelmann

Since 1984, we have used linear and circular stapling instruments (TA, GIA, and EEA) in the reconstruction of gastro-intestinal continuity after total gastrectomy. Our basic management concept is as follows: if the gastrectomy is palliative, the digestive tract is reconstructed by a simple Roux-en-Y jejunal loop with esophago-jejunostomy. If the total gastrectomy appears to be curative, continuity is established by a jejunal pouch and Roux-en-Y jejuno-jejunostomy[1] or by the interposition of a jejunal pouch between the esophagus and duodenum (Table 40-1).

The pouch interposition provides the patient with a substitute stomach and allows passage of food through the duodenum. The inverted J-jejunal reservoir is based on the same principles as a Hunt-Lawrence—Rodino pouch[2,3,4] created with stapling machines, similar to our previously described technique.[1]

The goal of this concept is to permit optimal quality of life for the patient with total gastrectomy. In the long run, it is reasonable to ask whether the magnitude of this operation and the increased cost of materials used are compensated by easier technical steps, diminished morbidity, and improved long-term quality of life associated with staplers.

MATERIAL AND METHODS

The extent of gastric resection depends on the type and location of the malignancy. A total gastrectomy is performed in all patients with carcinoma or lymphoma of the upper or middle thirds of the stomach. Distal gastrectomy is undertaken only in patients with carcinoma of the intestinal type; in all other malignancies of the lower third of the stomach, a total gastrectomy is performed also. A splenectomy is added only in the presence of metastatic lymph nodes in the splenic hilus or in the gastro-jejunal ligament, or because of the need for staging in lymphomas. Lymph node dissection is also performed in all anatomic areas that drain the tumor. The reconstruction is accomplished with the standard use of linear and circular stapling instruments.

Preoperatively, the patient is prepared with respiratory physiotherapy, irrigation of the stomach through a naso-gastric tube and, if indicated, correction of electrolyte imbalance, and administration of blood. Cefotaxim (2 g twice, perioperatively) is given as antibiotic prophylaxis.

Postoperatively, the patient is maintained on assisted ventilation for 24 hours and given low-dose heparin. The naso-gastric tube is removed on the first postoperative day; clear liquids by mouth are offered after that. The patient is moved out of bed on the first postoperative day, and from then on is encouraged and helped with increasing ambulation.

A radiologic contrast study using gastrografin is performed between the seventh and tenth postoperative days. Following discharge, the patient is seen four times in the first and second years, with monitoring of swallowing, weight, and function of the gastric substitute, as well as diligent searching for possible tumor recurrence or metastasis. Following this,

Table 40-1. Evaluation of Reconstructive Procedures

Aspect	Roux-en-Y	Roux-en-Y + Pouch	Jip + Pouch
Reservoir	−	+	+ +
Duodenal passage	−	−	+ +
Progressive emptying	−	(+)	(+)
Suitability	Always	Always	(80%)
Substitute function	−	−	?
Participation of bile and pancreas secretions	−	−	(+)
Technical ease	+ +	+	(+)
Duration (average and range)			
Total operation	3h 10m	4h 15m	4h 55m
	(2h 15m–4h 10m)	(3h 30m–5h 10m)	(3h 15m–6h)
Reconstruction	29m	50m	1h 30m
	(20m–43m)	(42m–1h 10m)	(45m–2h)

+ = positive or satisfactory; + + = very good to excellent; (+) = probable

the patient is seen once or twice yearly until the fifth year, often in cooperation with the referring physician.

Following our experience with some 700 major stapling procedures in the colon and rectum since 1978, we have extended the use of stapling instruments since 1982 to some 250 operations in the upper gastrointestinal tract. This report describes the use of Roux-en-Y reconstruction in 14 patients, jejunal pouch and Roux-en-Y in 57 patients, jejunal interposition in 1 patient, and jejunal pouch interposition in 31 patients, all following total gastrectomy. Three surgeons, well versed in the technique of total gastrectomy and reconstruction with manual methods, were responsible for the operations of jejunal pouch interposition.

OPERATIVE TECHNIQUE

Following total gastrectomy and lymphadectomy, a 65- to 70-cm jejunal loop (based on its corresponding vascular supply) is prepared beyond the duodeno-jejunal segment.

The preparation of the duodenal stump is accomplished with a 2-0 monofilament purse-string suture placed with the special purse-string instrument. Following transection beyond the previously liberated pylorus along the proximal edge of the special instrument, the purse-string is temporarily tightened with a tourniquet to avoid contamination of the operative field.

The preparation of the esophageal end follows the radical "en-bloc" dissection of the entire stomach, including all of the lymph nodes of compartment I in the greater and lesser omentum, as well as the lymph nodes of compartment II along the hepatic and splenic arteries together with the nodes of area 16 (Japanese node staging) along the upper border of the pancreas. The esophagus will be transected at a safe distance from the tumor by preserving as much of its abdominal portion as possible. A Satinsky clamp is placed proximal to the proposed site of transection, and the esophagus is then transected. An over-and-over purse-string suture of the esophageal circumference, carefully taking the mucosal and muscular layers of the organ, is then placed manually. Five stay sutures are also distributed around the circumference of the esophageal lumen to help with the introduction of the EEA anvil (Fig. 40-1).

The previously prepared 65- to 70-cm jejunal segment is now passed upward behind the transverse colon through a rent in the transverse mesocolon. The adequacy of the vascular supply and the length of the future pouch interposition are examined to assure a safe and tension-free anastomosis. Continuity below the transverse colon is established with a one-layer end-to-end manual jejuno-jejunostomy.

Following the intravenous administration of 2 ml of glucagon to facilitate the passage of the EEA-25 through the interposed jejunal segment, a classic end-to-end anastomosis is performed between the jejunal segment and the duodenum with the circular stapling instrument, as shown in Figure 40-2.

The jejunal reservoir, or pouch, is then constructed by returning the proximal end of the jejunal segment onto itself for some 15 cm in an inverted J-configuration. Through the open end of the inferiorly pointing bowel and an opposing stab-wound in the anti-mesenteric border of the mid-jejunal loop, the GIA-50 instrument is placed repeatedly to achieve a 15-cm pouch between the anti-mesenteric

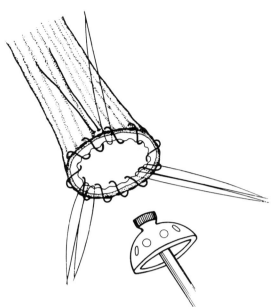

Fig. 40-1. Preparation of the abdominal segment of the esophagus with an over-and-over circular whip stitch and five stay sutures.

aspects of the juxtaposed bowel loops. With the newer GIA-90, two applications of this instrument will suffice, whereas with the smaller GIA-50 instrument, progressive eversion of the pouch becomes necessary to achieve the uppermost placements of the instrument. Careful hemostasis is performed while the pouch is everted. Superficial bleeding sites are controlled with electro-coagulation without touching the metal staples. More important bleeding is controlled with a manual suture.

Following hemostasis, the pouch is returned to its normal configuration and is then anastomosed with

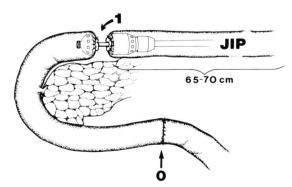

Fig. 40-2. Circular end-to-end anastomosis between the jejunal loop and the duodenal stump with the EEA-25 instrument. Manual one-layer end-to-end jejuno-jejunostomy (1) for the reconstruction of bowel continuity (0).

the EEA-25 or -28 to the esophagus. The use of the corresponding premium CEEA instruments will facilitate this anastomosis by allowing for separate placements of the instrument and its cartridge into the jejunal pouch and of the anvil into the esophageal end. In either approach, the instrument carrying the staple cartridge is placed through the now-common GIA introduction site from below upward; the central rod of the earlier (EEA) instrument or the trocart of the premium (CEEA) instrument is advanced through the apex of the jejunal pouch. If the earlier version of the EEA instrument is used, the cartridge is now attached to the central rod and advanced into the esophagus held open by the five previously placed stay sutures, and the purse-string is tied around the central rod. If the premium CEEA is used, the anvil with its rod has already been placed separately into the esophageal stump, and the purse-string suture has been tied around the notch in the rod. In this case, the rod of the anvil is then introduced into the hollow rod of the cartridge and the instrument is closed, which is also done if the technique with the regular version of the EEA is used. The stay sutures are removed prior to closing the instrument. The circular end-to-end anastomosis between esophagus and jejunal pouch is then accomplished, and the instrument is removed. Patency, hemostasis, and imperviousness of the anastomosis are examined (Fig. 40-3).

The common GIA opening of the pouch is closed with a linear row of the TA-90 stapler that encroaches sufficiently onto the efferent loop of the pouch to achieve a pseudo-pylorus, resulting in some emptying delay of the pouch (Fig. 40-6). This narrowing is moderate in character, so as to avoid stasis and reflux from the pouch into the esophagus. The tip of the nasal gastric tube is placed some 5 cm beyond the esophagus-to-pouch anastomosis. The rent in the mesocolon is closed around the jejunal mesentery (Fig. 40-4). Following removal of the naso-gastric tube, postoperatively the patient may have 100 to 150 ml of clear, lukewarm fluids by mouth. X-ray control is undertaken, at the earliest, on the seventh day; most often it is obtained between the seventh and tenth postoperative days (Fig. 40-5A, B).

PATIENTS AND RESULTS

The patients who underwent operations for carcinoma or localized lymphoma of the stomach averaged 61 years of age, with a range of 38 to 80 years. The prospective study, undertaken from May 8, 1985 to March 31, 1988, comprised 10 women and 21 men. Previous gastric disease was documented in 16 patients with 7 gastric ulcers, 2 duodenal ulcers, 2 cases

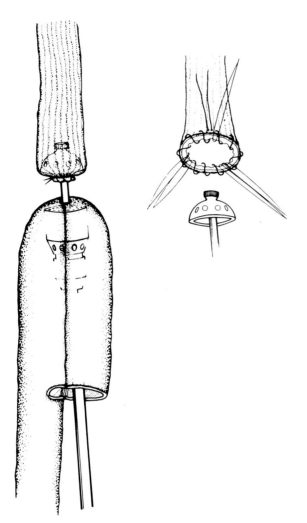

In almost 10% of our patients, a serosal split was seen with the EEA-25 instrument advanced through the jejunal loop for the end-to-end anastomosis with the duodenum. In all such cases, we used a manual suture to repair the serosal lacerations. In one case the anastomosis had to be done manually, since the spastic interposed jejunal loop did not allow the placement of the EEA-25 down to the level of the planned jejuno-duodenal anastomosis.

Postoperatively, one patient died in the hospital. In this 74-year-old patient, a nephrectomy for hypernephroma had been necessary along with the gastric resection for carcinoma. Postoperatively, the patient developed renal and respiratory failure and died from multi-organ failures.

Fig. 40-3. End-to-side anastomosis between the esophagus and the jejunum pouch with the EEA-25 or -28 instrument. The previously placed stay sutures are held apart to permit the introduction of the anvil. These stay sutures are removed once the purse-string suture is tied around the rod of the anvil and before the instrument is closed.

of gastritis, and 2 cases of gastro-esophageal reflux. Multi-organ disease, often related to age, was present in 18 patients.

Location, histologic definition, and staging of the various cancers are described in Table 40-2. Statistical analysis was done using the median-quartil system.

The intra-operative findings, tumor stages, and technical problems are shown in Tables 40-3 and 40-4. Based on our experience, we have found it important to examine the GIA staple lines carefully for bleeding and to perform supplementary hemostasis, which was necessary in some 13% of our cases.

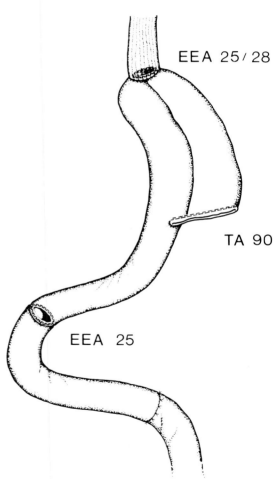

Fig. 40-4. The completed reconstruction with the jejunal reservoir anastomosed to the esophagus, the placement of the narrowing linear TA suture line on the jejunal loop from the pouch, the jejuno-duodenostomy with the EEA-25 instrument, and the manual jejuno-jejunostomy for reconstruction of bowel continuity.

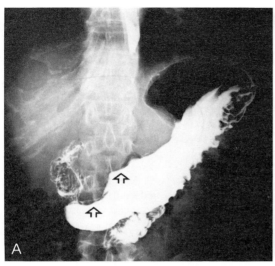
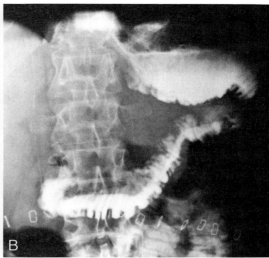

Fig. 40-5. *A.* A 64-year-old man with carcinoma of the antrum extending into the body of the stomach. *B.* X ray of the control jejunal pouch 8 days after operation.

Postoperative complications are shown in Table 40-5, and were as follows:

1. Broncho-pneumonia in 2 patients
2. Small dehiscence of the esophagus-to-pouch

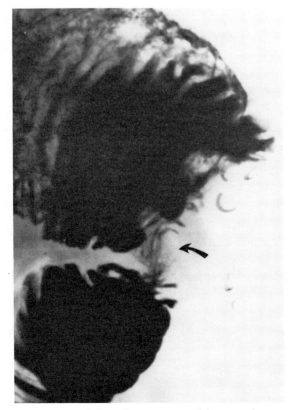

Fig. 40-6. Radiologic demonstration of the neo-pylorous.

anastomosis in one patient that healed spontaneously; subphrenic abscess in two patients; and delay in abdominal wound healing in one patient

POSTOPERATIVE EXAMINATIONS AND RESULTS

Endoscopic examination demonstrated anastomotic rings that were free of adverse reaction and inflammation. There were no signs of reflux esophagitis, although radiologic examination showed that the mixture of food, bile, and jejunal secretions remained in the pouch for some 20 minutes with a volume of 300 to 400 ml. From there it was evacuated progressively into the distal segment of the interposed jejunum through the narrowed exit area of the pouch that appeared to function like a neo-pylorus.

Table 40-2. Operative Data of Jip and Pouch (n = 31)

Number of surgeons: 3
Total operative time (mean and range): 4 hours 55 min (3:15–6:00)
Duration of reconstruction (mean and range): 90 min (45–120)
Blood loss (mean and range): 1500 ml (350–2700)
Blood transfusion (500-ml units) mean: 2.5 range: 0–5
Postoperative hospital stay (mean and range): 14 days (10–51)

Extended Operative Procedures (number of patients)
Resection of transverse colon: 2
Resection of tail of pancreas: 3
Resection of left lobe of liver: 1
Splenectomy: 14

Table 40-3. Tumor Analysis in Patients with Jip and Pouch (n = 31)

Location
  Cardia: 7
  Subcardia or fundus: 3
  Antrum: 11
  Body of stomach: 4
  Diffuse: 6
Histologic Classification
  Diffuse: 17
  Intestinal: 7
  Mixed type: 4
  Lymphoma: 3
Carcinoma Staging (n = 28)*
  T1, N0, M0: 4
  T2, N0–N1, M0: 10
  T3, N0–N3, M0: 9
  T4, N1–N3, M0–M1: 5

* T = tumor; N = nodes (0 = none, 1 = small, 2 = intermediate, 3 = large); M = metastases (0 = none, 1 = present)

The quality of life according to the criteria of Visick was examined in 18 patients anywhere from 6 to 34 months postoperatively, with an average postoperative observation period of some 14 months. This period averaged 18 months (8 to 34) in 12 surviving patients, twice as high as in 6 deceased patients, whose average observation period was 9 months (6 to 16). The Visick indices showed a good-to-very-good quality of life in 75% of the 12 patients with prolonged survival. In the 6 patients who died within the first 16 months after operation, the quality of life was significantly below that of the long-term survivors (Table 40-6).

DISCUSSION

The use of stapling instruments has significantly reduced the technical challenge of reconstructive procedures following total gastrectomy, especially in the area of the esophago-jejunal anastomosis, which until recently had been the "Achilles heel" of these reconstructive procedures. However, it should be acknowledged that surgeons who prefer manual anastomosing techniques have also observed a significant reduction in anastomotic complications with the use of atraumatic, resorbable suture material.[5] These observations concern the anastomosis to the abdominal segment of the esophagus. If the esophageal anastomosis is located above the diaphragm and a transabdominal, trans-diaphragmatic approach is possible, then the circular stapling instruments have a definitive advantage over manual techniques and may also avoid the necessity for a thoracotomy. Junginger and his associates[6] described, in 1983, the following advantages with stapled esophageal anastomosis:

1. Speed and therefore reduction of potential contamination from open bowel lumina
2. Symmetric anastomotic line with equal tissue compression by the individual staples
3. Preservation of the vascular supply through the B-shaped staples and excision of the esophageal rim that has been subjected to technical manipulations distal to the circular anastomotic line
4. Extension of the abdominal approach into the mediastinum, allowing for resection of a carcinoma of the cardia with intrathoracic anastomosis from the abdominal cavity

The vascular supply to the anastomotic line is superior with the use of staples, as shown by Smith and Wheeless.[7,8] There is a definite learning curve, however, so that with increasing experience the incidence of intraoperative and postoperative complications diminishes.

In the reconstruction following total gastrectomy, certain basic principles should be aimed for, such as a standard, reproducible, simple procedure providing optimal substitute function. The study of Troidl and Kusche[4] shows that the Hunt-Lawrence—Rodino pouch and the Roux-en-Y reconstruction fulfill the requirements for optimal functional substitu-

Table 40-4. Intra-Operative Technical Mishaps and Pouch Reconstruction (n = 31)*

Anastomotic Area	Technique	Complications		
		Bleeding	Serosal Tear	Anastomotic Dehiscence
End-to-end Jejuno-jejunostomy	Manual	–	–	–
Jejuno-duodenal anastomosis	EEA-25	1	3	1
Pouch	GIA	4	–	–
Esophagus-pouch anastomosis	EEA-25	1	–	–

* Treatment: primary control and repair of all of these intra-operative complications

Table 40-5. Postoperative In-Hospital Complications in Jip and Pouch (n = 31)

Mortality	Morbidity (n)	Re-Operation
Concomitant nephrectomy ↓	General:broncho-pneumonia (2)	–
Renal failure ↓	Local: fistula (1) of the esophago-pouch anastomosis; radiologic control only	–
Respiratory failure ↓	Subphrenic abscess (2)	2×
Death	Delay in abdominal wound healing (1)	–

Table 40-6. Quality of Life (Visick's Criteria) in 18 Patients with Jip and Pouch Reconstruction

Patients	n	Quality of Life Index	
Long-term survivor	12	3 × 1 6 × 2 2 × 3 1 × 4	Most recent follow-up
Deceased	6	1 × 2 1 × 3 4 × 4	Maximal observed index

tion. However, with the use of manual techniques, the other three requirements are not satisfied. Since the beginning of systematic use of linear and circular staplers, we have been able to satisfy the requirements of standardization, reproducability, and simplicity of these techniques.

In 1979 Barone proposed the creation of a Hunt-Lawrence pouch with the GIA instrument.[9] His technique had the following disadvantages:

1. Creation of additional stab wounds to place the GIA instrument in three or four applications. This resulted in a loss of time
2. Eversion of the pouch is impossible, and therefore complimentary hemostasis—if needed—cannot be achieved
3. Anastomosis of the esophagus to the pouch is done with a manual technique, which increases the potential for complications at this level

In the technique we have proposed, the use of stapling instruments at all levels eliminates the need for manual sutures and provides the patient with a substitute stomach in the most physiologically sound position. This is confirmed by Troidl's and Kusche's studies that demonstrated an improved nutritional status in patients with total gastrectomy and jejunal pouch and Roux-en-Y reconstruction, as opposed to the simple esophago-jejunostomy. Our concept of jejunal pouch interposition and creation of a neo-pylorus fulfills the requirement of a food reservoir, progressive emptying, and passage of the foodstuffs through the duodenum. The early postoperative analysis seems to show that quality of life is better than that obtained by us with jejunal pouch and Roux-en-Y

reconstruction.[1] However, these results are so far preliminary. Only a controlled prospective study can give the correct answer to the question of quality of life following the various principles of reconstruction, and only such a study can show if the interposed jejunal pouch is superior to the Roux-en-Y jejunal pouch.

Translated from the German by F.M. Steichen, M.D.

REFERENCES

1. Thiede A, Fuchs KH, Hamelmann H: Pouch and Roux-en-Y reconstruction after gastrectomy. Arch Surg 122: 838–842, 1987.
2. Hunt CJ: Construction of food pouch from segment of jejunum as substitute for stomach in total gastrectomy. Arch Surg 64:601–608, 1952.
3. Lawrence W Jr: Reservoir construction after total gastrectomy. Am J Surg 155:191–198, 1962.
4. Troidl H, Kusche J: Lebensqualität nach Gastrektomie: Ergebnisse einer randomisierten Studie zum Vergleich Oesophago-Jejunostomie nach Schlatter mit dem Hunt-Lawrence-Rodino-Pouch. In: Rohde H, Troidl H, eds: Das Magenkarzinom. Stuttgart, New York: Thieme-Verlag, 1984.
5. Bittner R, Berger HG: Esophago-jejunostomy: the importance of surgical technique. Nutrition 4:169–170, 1988.
6. Junginger Th, Walgenbach S, Pichlmaier H: Die zirkuläre Klammeranastomose (EEA) nach Gastrektomie. Chirurg 54:161–165, 1983.
7. Smith CR, Loklet GR, Adams BT, Schwartz SI: Vascularity of gastrointestinal staple lines demonstrated with silicone rubber injection. Am J Surg 142:563–566, 1981.
8. Wheeless CR, Smith JJ: A comparison of the flow of iodine 125 through three different intestinal anastomoses: standard, Gambee and stapler. Obstet Gynecol 62:513–518, 1983.
9. Barone RM: Reconstruction after total gastrectomy. construction of a Hunt-Lawrence Pouch using Auto Suture (R) staples. Am J Surg 137:578–584, 1979.
10. Thiede A, Fuchs KH, Hamelmann H: Esophagojejunostomy: new stapling techniques. Nutrition 4:171–173, 1988.
11. Visick AH: Measured radical gastrectomy. Lancet 254:505–510;551–555, 1948.

CHAPTER 41

STAPLING IN PROXIMAL AND DISTAL GASTRECTOMY

H.D. Becker

Surgical techniques for the resection of the proximal and distal stomach have been standardized during the last century. Reconstruction of food passages by intestinal anastomosis is usually achieved by a two-layer inverting technique, or a one-layer anastomosis if this method is preferred by the surgeon. The first layer includes the mucosa and submucosa for the control of bleeding, whereas the second layer is fashioned with an inverting seromuscular suture if the two-layer technique is chosen. For the single-layer technique, all components of the gastric and intestinal walls are included in the inverting suture line. After the development of mechanical stapling devices for the construction of gastro-intestinal anastomoses, several new techniques have been described. In this chapter we report the experiences with conventional and mechanical anastomotic techniques after proximal or distal gastrectomy.

MATERIAL

The results are based on a total of 965 abdominal operations in which manual or stapled anastomoses were performed from June 1985 through April 1988 (Table 41-1). In 102 operations for esophageal cancer we mostly performed intrathoracic esophago-gastric anastomoses. In a few cases, esophago-jejunal or esophago-colic anastomoses were done or we used interposition of a free small bowel transplant. Esophago-gastric anastomoses were performed almost exclusively by conventional manual anastomotic techniques.

Of 240 patients with resection of the stomach, hand-sewn anastomoses were done in 146 patients and stapled anastomoses in 94. Of small bowel resec-

Table 41-1. Gastro-Intestinal Anastomosis

Location	Total	Hand	Stapling
Esophagus	102	95	7
Stomach	240	146	94
Small intestine	207	89	118
Colon	212	152	60
Rectum	204	19	185
Totals	965	501	464

tions in 207 patients, stapled anastomoses were done in 118. Of 212 resections of the colon, hand-sewn anastomoses were performed in 152 patients, whereas in 204 resections of the recto-sigmoid, stapled anastomoses were preferred.

GASTRIC PROCEDURES

We performed 240 resections of the stomach, including 109 total gastrectomies with esophago-jejunostomy (Table 41-2). In 87 of these patients, the anastomosis was done by hand, whereas stapling was used in 22 patients. In Billroth-I resections, the ratio of hand-sewn anastomosis to stapling was 2:1. Of 89

Table 41-2. Gastro-Intestinal Anastomosis: Stomach

Type	Total	Hand	Stapling
Esophago-jejunostomy	109	87	22
Billroth I	18	12	6
Billroth II	89	35	54
Roux-en-Y	24	12	12
Totals	240	146	94

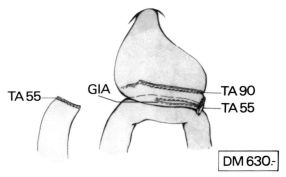

Fig. 41-1. Stapled Billroth-II gastro-jejunostomy.

patients with a Billroth-II resection, manual anastomosis was done in 35 cases, and stapling anastomosis was performed in 54 patients; stapling and hand-sewn anastomoses were done in 12 cases each with Roux-en-Y reconstruction.

BILLROTH-II GASTRO-JEJUNOSTOMY

The following stapling technique was applied: closure of the duodenal stump with the TA-55, closure of the gastric stump with the TA-90, construction of the anastomosis with GIA-50, and closure of the introduction site for the GIA with the TA-55 (Fig. 41-1).

In our 89 patients with Billroth-II resection, we performed a two-layer hand-sewn anastomosis in 35 cases. The technique with stapling only was used in 54 patients (Table 41-3).

Intra-operative complications consisted of difficulties in closure of the introduction opening for the GIA and bleeding from the gastro-jejunostomy immediately after construction of the anastomosis. Most problems could be solved by single manual sutures. The postoperative complications are shown in Table 41-3. There were no differences in complications after both types of reconstruction, except for postoperative bleeding of more than 1000 ml per 24 hours,

Table 41-3. Gastro-Intestinal Anastomosis: Stomach Billroth-II Gastro-Jejunostomy

Complication	Total	Hand	Stapling
No problems	76	31	45
Leakage	4	1/35	3/54
Bleeding	6*	1/35	5/54*
Stenosis	3	2/35	1/54
Intra-operative problems	4*	–	4/54*
Totals	13/89	4/35	9/54
Re-intervention	4	2	2

* Bleeding from the anastomosis was controlled intra-operatively in 4 patients

Table 41-4. Gastro-Intestinal Anastomosis: Stomach Duodenal Stump Closure

Complication	Total	Hand	Stapling
No problems	195	4/9	191/203
Leakage	4	2/9	2/203
Bleeding	4	2/9	2/203
Pancreatic fistula	3	–	3/203
Local infection	6	1/9	5/203
Totals	17/212	5/9	12/203
Re-intervention	5	2	3

which was seen more often in stapled anastomoses. Re-intervention was necessary in 4 patients, 2 in each one of the anastomotic groups.

DUODENAL STUMP CLOSURE

We performed a duodenal stump closure in 212 patients. Only in 9 patients was the closure done by hand suture; in 203 patients the closure was done with the TA-55. In 20 of these 203 patients, additional coverage with serosa or with pancreatic capsule was indicated mainly because of blood oozing. Leakage was observed in less than 2% of our 203 patients (Table 41-4). The very high percentage of leakage in hand-sutured duodenal stumps was caused by very difficult anatomic situations, which did not allow closure of the duodenal stump with the TA-55. Re-intervention had to be performed in 3 of our 203 patients with stapled duodenal closures.

BILLROTH-I ANASTOMOSIS

The following technique has been used for stapled anastomosis in Billroth-I patients (Fig. 41-2): resec-

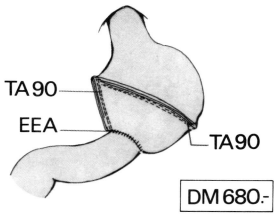

Fig. 41-2. Stapled Billroth-I gastro-duodenostomy.

Table 41-5. Gastro-Intestinal Anastomosis: Stomach Billroth I Gastro-Duodenostomy

Complication	Total	Hand	Stapling
No problems	15	9	6
Leakage	1	1	–
Bleeding	–	–	–
Stenosis	2	2	–
Intra-operative problems	–	–	–
Total	3/18	3/12	0/6
Re-intervention	–	–	–

Table 41-6. Gastro-Intestinal Anastomosis: Stomach Roux-en-Y

Complication	Total	Hand	Stapling
No problems	21	11	10
Leakage	1	1	–
Bleeding	2	–	2
Stenosis	(3)	(2)	(1)
Intra-operative problems	1	–	1
Total	3/24	1/12	2/12
Re-intervention	–	–	1

tion of the stomach along the lesser curvature with the TA-90 instrument and end-to-side gastro-duodenostomy with the EEA through the open remnant of gastric antrum. The excess gastric antrum along the greater curvature is then closed with the TA-90 and resected distal to this closure.

We performed a Billroth-I anastomosis in only 18 patients (Table 41-5). In 12 of these patients, a hand-sewn anastomosis was done. In 6 patients, a stapled anastomosis was performed.

No postoperative problems were observed in our stapled patients, but 2 of our 12 patients with hand-sewn anastomoses showed a delayed gastric emptying postoperatively. In 1 of these patients, a small fistula at the anastomosis was observed.

ROUX-EN-Y ANASTOMOSIS

The following technique has been developed for the construction of Roux-en-Y anastomosis exclusively by stapling. We used the GIA-50 twice (for gastro-enterostomy and jejuno-jejunostomy), the TA-55 three times (for closure of the duodenum and of both GIA introduction sites at the gastro-enterostomy

and the Roux-en-Y jejuno-jejunostomy), the TA-30 twice (for closure of both ends at the proximal jejunal transection), and the TA-90 once (for closure of gastric stump).

A Roux-en-Y anastomosis was done in 24 patients. In 2 of the 12 patients with stapled anastomosis, postoperative bleeding was observed, which caused re-intervention in 1 patient (Table 41-6). The postoperative delayed gastric emptying could not be traced either to anatomic problems of the anastomosis only or to pathophysiologic problems of the reconstruction procedure.

ENTERO-ENTEROANASTOMOSIS

The Braun enteroanastomosis with stapling was done using the GIA and TA-55 instruments. In this series, a Braun enteroanastomosis was done in 19 patients, using the stapling technique in 12 cases (Table 41-7). Postoperatively, in one case bleeding occurred, which was treated non-operatively.

CONSTRUCTION OF A GASTRIC TUBE AFTER ESOPHAGEAL RESECTION

In 100 patients we constructed a gastric tube to replace the resected esophagus. In 14 patients we used the TA-55 and TA-90 without additional reinforcing sutures of the resection line. In 1 patient a

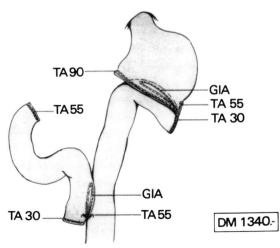

TA 90
TA 55
GIA
TA 55
TA 30
GIA
TA 30
TA 55

DM 1340.-

Fig. 41-3. Stapled Roux-en-Y gastro-jejunostomy.

Table 41-7. Gastro-Intestinal Anastomosis: Braun Enteroanastomosis

Complication	Total	Hand	Stapling
No problems	17	7	10
Leakage	–	–	–
Bleeding	1	–	1
Stenosis	–	–	–
Intra-operative problems	1	–	1
Total	2/19	0/7	2/12
Re-intervention	–	–	–

fistula occurred, which was treated non-operatively. In 12 patients we used the GIA-50 without additional serosal coverage. In 2 patients postoperative bleeding occurred, which led to a repeat thoracotomy. In the last 74 patients we used the GIA-50 and -90 for resection of the lesser curvature and transection of the proximal stomach, and additional sero-muscular coverage of the stapled resection line. No postoperative bleeding from the resection line has been observed.

CONCLUSIONS

Stapling anastomosis is a secure method in the reconstruction after distal gastrectomy. The major postoperative problem is bleeding from the stapled gastro-jejunostomy. The major advantage of using staples at the stomach is the closure procedure of the duodenal stump, which is much easier and very secure by this method.

CHAPTER 42

ISO-PERISTALTIC JEJUNAL INTERPOSITION FOR POST-GASTRECTOMY SYNDROME

G. Di Matteo, G. Palazzini, A. Cancrini Jr., E. De Antoni, and L. Boemi

The majority of patients undergoing partial gastrectomy for ulcer readjust well to the new anatomic and physiologic situation. A minority do not, and develop a single or complex late post-gastrectomy syndrome (PGS).[1,2,3] The word "post-gastrectomy" is inaccurate, because similar alimentary disorders may develop even after non-resective gastric operations.[4] In most cases, symptoms are mild to moderate and do not prevent patients from carrying on with their daily activities. Only a small fraction of these patients, whose symptoms are severe and refractory to diet and medications, are proper candidates for surgical treatment.

A series of 18 iso-peristaltic jejunal interpositions for PGS occurring after Billroth-II gastrectomy is reported here. Indications for operation are reviewed and a detailed description of techniques is given, together with analysis of early and late results.

INDICATIONS FOR OPERATIVE TREATMENT

Despite the alarming frequency of side effects after partial gastrectomy (5 to 35%), only a minority of patients, presenting with severe and invalidating symptoms refractory to non-operative management, need a remedial operation.[1,3-6] These patients suffer from reflux gastritis, afferent loop syndrome, or early or late dumping. Remarkable weight loss is nearly a constant additional finding.

Post-gastrectomy syndromes can develop several years after operation. A single patient can present with a single or a complex post-gastrectomy syndrome.

Reflux gastritis is, by far, the most common PGS. Histologic patterns of gastritis are quite common in patients who have undergone partial gastrectomy.[1,3-7] Atrophic gastritis is regarded as a premalignant condition when intestinal metaplasia and epithelial dysplasia are present. Only a small fraction of these patients have symptoms (epigastric pain and bilious vomiting, generally unrelated to meals; weight loss and anemia are additional findings). Endoscopy shows pancreato-biliary reflux with marked gastric stasis, gross findings of "tiger-striped gastritis," and sometimes, lower third esophagitis.[4,8-11]

Alkaline gastritis is promoted by pancreato-biliary reflux and high gastric pH, leading to bacterial overgrowth that yields oncogenic N-nitroso compounds and nitrosamine.[1,4,9,12,13,14]

The surgical management of the most severe cases should aim at eliminating reflux by interposing an iso-peristaltic jejunal loop between the gastric remnant and duodenum or by converting the Billroth-II procedure to a Roux-en-Y gastro-jejunostomy.[3,4,9,10,19-21]

Afferent loop syndrome refers to the onset immediately after meals of epigastric pain relieved by bilious vomiting. Following the widespread use of endoscopy and the recognition of reflux gastritis as a clearly defined pathologic and clinical entity, the incidence of afferent loop syndrome has decreased over the past decade so that some authors doubt its existence.[8]

Mechanical obstruction accounts for most of these cases; hypochlorhydria with bacterial colonization of the afferent loop is responsible for the remainder.[1,4]

Proper surgical treatment aims at removing the obstruction, which is achieved by a simple Braun's entero-enterostomy between afferent and efferent limbs or by conversion to a Roux-en-Y or a Billroth-I procedure or by a jejunal interposition.

Early and late dumping syndromes present with pronounced weakness improved by recumbency, following ingestion of food. Their pathophysiology is still controversial and multiple theories have been offered.[1,4,9,20,22–24]

The surgical treatment of dumping syndromes occurring after Billroth II gastrectomy aims at restoring the duodenal passage. Direct conversion of Billroth II to Billroth-I[4,12] and jejunal interposition[1,3–7,17,18] are adequate procedures.

It is easy to infer that all PGS amenable to surgical correction share common pathophysiologic events, which is proved by the frequent combination of two syndromes in a single patient. Alimentary disorders after Billroth-II gastrectomy are related to alkaline reflux and suppression of the duodenal transit, which alters the complex neuro-endocrine coordination of the digestion.

Operation should therefore aim at diverting the alkaline secretions from the gastric remnant together with restoring the duodenal passage. Various procedures have been suggested as adequate treatment for severe PGS following Billroth-II gastrectomy; side-to-side entero-enterostomy between afferent and efferent limbs; Roux-en-Y gastrojejunostomy; direct conversion to a Billroth-I procedure; and jejunal interposition. Only the latter is able to achieve restoration of the duodenal transit together with prevention of alkaline reflux. Jejunal interposition was therefore chosen for treatment of severe and intractable PGS after the Billroth-II procedure.

OPERATIVE TECHNIQUES

Jejunal interposition provides restoration of the duodenal passage with the efferent loop interposed between the gastric remnant and duodenum.[18]

It was suggested that antiperistaltic interposition is indicated in case of dumping syndrome, to prevent rapid gastric emptying. However, hormonal disorders[1,4,5,9,11,22–24] or peristaltic incoordination[11,20] are held responsible for dumping symptoms. Antiperistaltic interposition does not eliminate reflux of alkaline secretions and alters the endocrine continuity of the small bowel. Moreover, such a procedure requires intestinal transection at the level of the ligament of Treitz, which can result in a leak because of the relatively poor vascularization of the duodeno-jejunal angle.[1,5] These reasons explain our choice of an iso-peristaltic interposition.

Suppression of reflux requires a rather long (some 40 cm) interposition to keep bilio-pancreatic secretions away from the gastric remnant. On the other hand, both early and late dumping syndromes should benefit from a short interposition (approximately 10 cm), which is likely to restore the anatomy and physiology close to the original. Because of the common combination of reflux gastritis and dumping syndrome, we believe that a 20- to 30-cm jejunal interposition is a sensible compromise.

Gastro-jejunostomies of a Billroth-II procedure were mostly found in an antecolic position with the afferent limb at the lesser, more rarely at the greater, curvature (Fig. 42-1).

In the earlier cases of this series, the end-to-side jejuno-duodenostomies and the end-to-end entero-enterostomy of the remedial procedure were manually sutured as described by Soupault and Boucaille in 1955.[18] Later, stapling devices were adopted to facilitate anastomotic techniques, and jejuno-duodenostomies were accomplished either end-to-side or side-to-side; entero-enterostomies were always constructed in an end-to-side fashion (Fig. 42-2).

The afferent limb is divided in close proximity to the gastric remnant, between a purse-string device on the duodenal side and an intestinal clamp on the anastomotic side.

At 20 to 30 cm from the anastomosis, the efferent limb is transected between a proximal purse-string instrument and a distal intestinal clamp.

After wide duodeno-pancreatic mobilization, a purse-string suture is placed into the anterior wall of the second portion of the duodenum and a full-thickness nipple of duodenal wall, projecting beyond the arms of the purse-string device, is resected.

A circular anastomosing stapler is inserted into the anastomotic end of the afferent limb and advanced out through the proximal purse-stringed end of the efferent loop. This purse-string is tied over the cartridge, and the anvil is inserted into the duodenum. The duodenal purse-string is also tied, anvil and cartridge are closed, and end-to-side jejuno-duodenostomy is carried out (Fig. 42-3).

Proper positioning of the stapler requires rotation of the lesser curvature anteriorly and to the left. This moves the gastric remnant behind the instrument. If

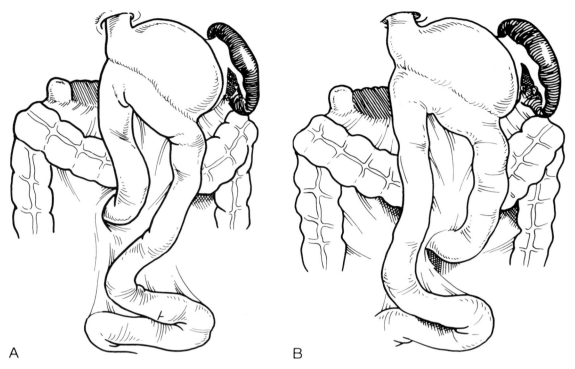

Fig. 42-1. Billroth-II gastrectomy with afferent limb of gastro-jejunostomy at the lesser (A) or greater (B) curvature.

such a maneuver turns out to be difficult, the lesser curvature should be rotated posteriorly and to the left, so that the gastric remnant lies before the instrument (Fig. 42-4). When the afferent limb is at the greater curvature, proper positioning of the stapling instrument does not require any rotation of the gastric remnant.

After withdrawal of the circular instrument, the anastomotic end of the afferent limb is sutured with a linear stapler (Fig. 42-5). If the performance of an end-to-side anastomosis turns out to be difficult or hazardous in spite of wide mobilization, side-to-side jejuno-duodenostomy should be carried out.

With this technique, after closing the anastomotic end of the afferent limb with a linear stapler (Fig. 42-5), a circular stapling device, devoid of its anvil, is inserted into the (initially purse-stringed) proximal open end of the efferent limb. The central rod is advanced through the jejunal wall on its antimesenteric aspect close to the open bowel end. The anvil is attached and inserted into the duodenum, the purse-string is tied, and after approximating anvil and cartridge, a side-to-side circular anastomosis is carried out. The open end of the interposition jejunum is sutured with a linear instrument (Fig. 42-6) after removal of the circular instrument.

Jejunal continuity is restored between the afferent duodeno-jejunal segment and the efferent distal jejunum with a stapled end-to-side anastomosis, using a circular stapler and a technique similar to the one just described (Fig. 42-7). The distal open end of the small bowel, used to place the EEA, is closed near the anstomosis to prevent the development of a cul-de-sac.

PATIENTS AND METHODS

Eighteen patients (13 males and 5 females with a mean age of 41 years) underwent iso-peristaltic jejunal interposition from June 1982 to February 1987. All patients had undergone Billroth-II gastrectomy for duodenal (14 cases) or gastric (4 cases) ulcer. All gastro-jejunal anastomoses lay before the transverse colon. In 3 patients the afferent limb was at the greater curve.

Symptoms occurred on an average of 2 years after operation (range: 3 to 75 months). All patients complained of epigastric pain, often exacerbated by meals, and frequent episodes of bilious vomiting. Two patients reported relief of epigastric pain after vomiting and were therefore considered affected by

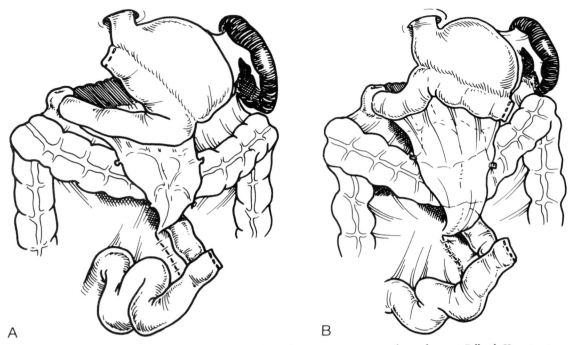

Fig. 42-2. Remedial operation using the anastomotic loop of jejunum in patients who underwent Billroth-II gastrectomy with afferent limb at the lesser *(A)* or greater *(B)* curvature.

both reflux gastritis (as proven by endoscopic findings) and afferent loop syndrome (as suggested by clinical data). Seven patients presented with reflux gastritis together with early (5) or late (2) dumping syndrome. Remarkable weight loss was reported by 13 patients, who had lost an average of 8 Kg after gastrectomy. Weight loss was less apparent in the remaining patients.

Prolonged non-operative management had proven to be unsuccessful; symptoms continued to be severe and invalidating. Admission at our institution was required on an average of 5 years after gastrectomy.

Radiographic contrast studies never showed any obstruction at the level of the gastro-jejunostomy.

Gross findings of gastritis were evident on endoscopy with marked reflux of bile and gastric stasis in all

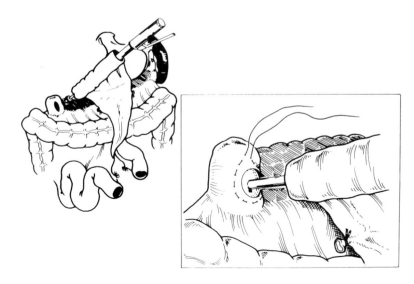

Fig. 42-3. End-to-side jejuno-duodenostomy.

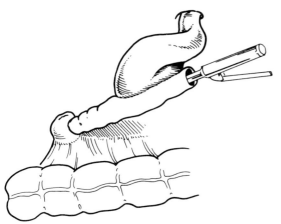

Fig. 42-4. Rotation of the gastric remnant allows proper positioning of the stapler.

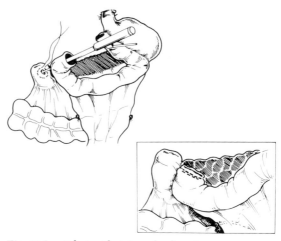

Fig. 42-6. Side-to-side jejuno-duodenostomy.

patients, 4 of whom were also affected by mild to moderate esophagitis.

Multiple biopsies were taken for histologic examination. Superficial gastritis was found in 8 cases; atrophic gastritis with intestinal metaplasia in 10, 4 of whom showed signs of mild to moderate epithelial dysplasia (Tables 42-1, 42-2).

Gastric pH sampling showed that patients with superficial gastritis had a slightly reduced acid-secreting capacity, whereas those with atrophic gastritis had a severely impaired acid output (Tables 42-1, 42-2).

All patients underwent either liver and pancreas sonography or endoscopic retrograde cholangio-pancreatography (ERCP), to rule out possible associated pathologic lesions.

Iso-peristaltic jejunal interposition was carried out in all 18 patients; concomitant cholecystectomy was performed in 2. Both anastomoses of the first 5 cases were sutured with manual techniques. In 3 additional

patients, manual and mechanical sutures were used. Both anastomoses of the last 10 cases were stapled: 7 end-to-side and 3 side-to-side jejuno-duodenostomies were performed; all the stapled jejuno-jejunostomies were constructed in an end-to-side fashion.

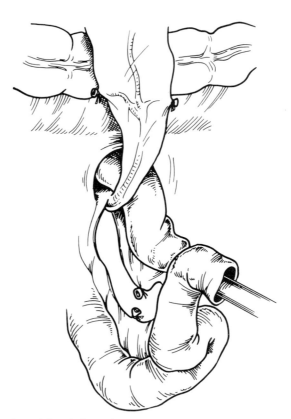

Fig. 42-7. End-to-side jejuno-jejunostomy.

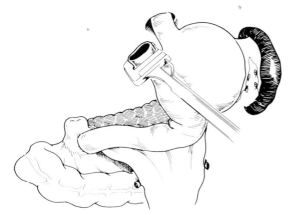

Fig. 42-5. The distal (anastomotic) end of the afferent limb is sutured with a linear stapler.

Table 42-1. Acid Output and Histology in Patients with Superficial Gastritis

| Patient | Sex | Preoperative | | | Postoperative | | | Histology (Regression of Superficial Gastritis) |
		BAO	PAO	MAO	BAO	PAO	MAO	
B.M.	M	2	8	13	2.7	8	15	Moderate
L.C.	F	1	7	12	1	7	12	Moderate
R.D.	M	0.8	5	10	1	6	11	Moderate
S.T.	M	2	9	11	2	9	12	None
R.B.	M	2.4	9	12	3	9	15	Advanced
A.I.	F	3	10	14	3	10	14	Moderate
A.S.	M	1.5	7	11	1.5	6	11	Moderate
Averages		1.8	7.8	11.8	2	7.8	12.8	

RESULTS

No operative morbidity or mortality related to the suture or staple techniques was recorded. One patient, however, developed obstructive jaundice 2 weeks postoperatively and died within a few days of hepato-renal syndrome. At autopsy, a small 1-cm cancer of the head of the pancreas was discovered. The tumor had not been detected intra-operatively or by sonography or ERCP preoperatively and postoperatively.

One patient developed cancer of the descending colon 2 years after remedial operation and underwent left colectomy. Recovery was uneventful and she is still doing well.

Sixteen patients were followed regularly over 1 year (range: 15 to 71 months). In addition to the patient who died, 1 patient was lost to followup.

No postoperative peptic ulcer was recorded. Ten patients (62%) experienced complete relief of their symptoms and gained weight; 5 (31%) were doing well but did not gain weight; and 1 (7%), who had improved after 6 months, complained of early dump-ing symptoms 6 months later: his symptoms, however, are not invalidating, and he is being managed with diet and medications.

Contrast radiography of the upper digestive tract never showed any anatomic or functional abnormality.

Endoscopic findings of reflux gastritis disappeared in all cases.

Histologic examination of biopsy specimens of the 7 patients with superficial gastritis showed that 1 returned to a nearly normal mucosal pattern, 5 showed regression of inflammation, and 1 had no change of preoperative findings. Among the 9 patients with atrophic gastritis, 3 had their preoperative pattern unchanged; 6 showed regression of inflammation, but in only 2 of them was a mild oxyntic and zymogenic cell repopulation apparent (Tables 42-1, 42-2).

At gastric pH sampling, no patient with superficial gastritis showed any improvement; 2 of those with atrophic gastritis (the same who had mild oxyntic and zymogenic cell repopulation) showed a moderate recovery of their acid-secreting capacity (Tables 42-1, 42-2).

Table 42-2. Acid Output and Histology in Patients with Atrophic Gastritis

| Patient | Sex | Preoperative | | | Postoperative | | | Histology | |
		BAO	PAO	MAO	BAO	PAO	MAO	Regression of Inflammation	Oxyntic and Zymogenic Cell Repopulation
G.M.	M	0.5	2	6	0.5	2	7	Yes	No
S.M.	F	1	5	9	1.3	6	10	Yes	No
E.L.	M	0.5	3	9	0.5	3	10	No	No
C.L.	M	0.7	5	8	1	6	9	No	No
S.T.	F	0.5	2	5	1	8	13	Yes	Yes
S.R.	M	0.9	4	10	0.9	5.2	10	Yes	No
B.D.	M	0.6	3	9	1	4	8	Yes	No
A.N.	M	1	5	10	1	5.3	11	No	No
M.L.	M	1.5	6	9	1.5	7	13	Yes	Yes
Averages		0.8	3.8	8.3	0.9	5.1	10.1		

DISCUSSION

Only a small percentage of patients presenting with PGS after Billroth-II gastrectomy need remedial surgery. In fact, symptoms are generally mild, episodic, and transient, and do not prevent patients from carrying on with their daily activities; moreover, in most cases a severe PGS can be managed with adequate diet and medications.[1,2,4] Surgical correction is indicated only in case of severe alkaline reflux gastritis, dumping, and afferent limb syndromes refractory to non-operative treatment.

Iso-peristaltic jejunal interposition is able to affect both main factors that promote a PGS occurring after Billroth-II gastrectomy. In fact, restoration of the duodenal passage is provided together with suppression of alkaline reflux. Direct conversion of Billroth-II to Billroth-I provides restoration of the duodenal passage but does not eliminate alkaline reflux; moreover, it often turns out to be a rather difficult procedure. Conversion to a Roux-en-Y gastro-jejunostomy is an effective procedure in case of reflux gastritis, but restoration of the duodenal transit is not provided. Construction of a side-to-side entero-enterostomy between afferent and efferent limbs is a simple operation but cannot provide restoration of the duodenal passage; effective diversion of bile and pancreatic juice is rarely achieved.

Jejunal interposition is always indicated when two or more postgastrectomy syndromes develop in the same patient; this occurred in nine of our patients.

Preoperative assessment should always include contrast radiographic studies of the upper digestive tract, endoscopy, histologic examination, and gastric pH sampling. The latter is advisable to detect those patients whose acid-secreting capacity is still normal or elevated. We believe that these patients are the only candidates for a complementary vagotomy, to prevent the occurrence of a postoperative ulcer.

It has been suggested that complementary vagotomy be routinely added to diverting procedures, because regression of gastritis with increased proliferation of oxyntic and zymogenic cells could promote development of a postoperative ulcer.[1,9,10,16,25] Most post-surgical ulcers, however, develop only if removal of the antral mucosa at the time of gastrectomy was incomplete;[9] proliferation of oxyntic and zymogenic cells after remedial surgery is seldom so dramatic as to promote a marked recovery of the acid-secreting capacity.[3,6,7,17,19,23]

In this series, the preoperative acid-secreting capacity was always below normal values; therefore, no patient was scheduled for complementary vagotomy. Patients with mild hypochlorhydria, however, were placed under a regular H_2-suppression regimen. No postoperative ulcers were recorded.

Echotomography or contrast radiologic studies and pancreatic ducts are advisable to rule out associated pathologic findings. Two patients in this series had asymptomatic gallbladder stones detected at sonography; they were scheduled for cholecystectomy together with jejunal interposition.

Jejunal interposition proved to be a safe procedure, which can be performed in the absence of any operative morbidity or mortality. The advent of stapling devices further simplifies the technique of suturing and shortens the operation. Radiology and endoscopy gave evidence of the excellent quality of stapled sutures: the anastomoses were wide and a thin and regular scar was visible a few months after surgery.

A late clinical followup showed that jejunal interposition yielded excellent results in 10 of 16 patients (62%) and good results in 5 of the 16 (31%). One patient (7%), however, who had been doing well 6 months after surgery, complained of early dumping symptoms 6 months later.

At late assessment there were no gross findings of alkaline reflux in any patient, and phlogistic infiltrates had regressed in 15 of the 16 patients. A mild oxyntic and zymogenic cell repopulation, however, was observed only in 2 of 8 patients with atrophic gastritis (25%), which is in accordance with the findings of gastric pH sampling, that most of these patients (6 of 8) do not recover a normal acid-secretion capacity (Tables 42-1 and 42-2).

On the grounds of a favorable experience (no operative morbidity or mortality; success rate of 93% in a group of 16 patients), we support iso-peristaltic jejunal interposition as a simple and safe procedure, highly effective in case of severe PGS occurring after Billroth-II partial gastrectomy.

SUMMARY

Eighteen patients (13 males and 5 females with a mean age of 41 years) underwent iso-peristaltic jejunal interposition between 1982 and 1987. All patients presented with severe post-gastrectomy syndromes (PGS): alkaline reflux gastritis, early or late dumping, or afferent loop syndrome. Symptoms developed an average of 2 years after Billroth-II partial gastrectomy. Half of these patients presented with 2 PGSs, one of which was alkaline reflux gastritis.

In the earlier cases, both the anastomoses were hand-sewn according to the original procedure described by Soupault and Boucaille in 1955. Later, autosuture devices were adopted to construct the anastomoses to simplify the procedure. Stapled jejuno-duodenostomies were done in either end-to-side or side-to-side fashion, while jejuno-jejunostomies were always performed as an end-to-side procedure. No operative morbidity or mortality was recorded.

Sixteen patients underwent a regular followup for more than 1 year (range: 15 to 70 months). Ten patients experienced complete relief of their symptoms and gained weight. One patient, who had been doing well 6 months after surgery, complained of early dumping symptoms 6 months later.

Iso-peristaltic jejunal interposition proved to be a safe and effective procedure in case of severe and intractable PGS occurring after Billroth-II gastrectomy.

REFERENCES

1. Campana FP, Raschellà GF, Marchesi M, et al: L'intervento di Soupault & Boucaille nella correzione delle sindromi da gastroresezione sec. Billroth II. Giorn Chir 5:415, 1984.
2. Di Matteo G, Campana FP, Zechini F: La gastro PH radiomanometria nello studio dei resecati gastrici a distanza dall'intervento. Il Progresso Medico 22:57, 1966.
3. Reber H, Way L: Surgical treatment of late postgastrectomy syndromes. Am J Surg 71:129, 1975.
4. Cooperman A: Postgastrectomy syndromes. Surg Annu 13:139, 1981.
5. Di Matteo G, Campana FP, Cancrini A Jr, et al: La gastrodigiunoduodenoplastica per la patologia da gastroresezione. 87 Congr Soc Ital Chir Torino, 1985.
6. Ramus N, Williamson R, Johnston D: The use of jejunal interposition for intractable symptoms complicating peptic ulcer surgery. Br J Surg 265:69, 1982.
7. Marchesi M, Raschellà GF, Redler A, et al: E' possibile la correzione chirurgica delle lesioni istologiche croniche dello stomaco dopo gastroresezione? 89 Congr Soc Ital Chir Napoli, 1987. Comunicazioni 483.
8. Alexander-Williams J, Hoare A: Alkaline reflux gastritis; a myth or disease? Am J Surg 143:17, 1982.
9. Di Gesù G, Fiasconaro G, Vetri G, Feo M: La gastrite alcalina. Fisiopatologia e prevenzione. Minerva Chir 42:683, 1987.
10. Ritchie WP: Alkaline reflux gastritis: late results on a controlled trial of diagnosis and treatment. Ann Surg 203:537, 1986.
11. Smout AJPM, Akkermans LMA, Roelofs JMM, Pasma FG, Oei HY, Wittebol P: Gastric emptying and postprandial symptoms after Billroth-II resection. Surgery 101:27, 1987.
12. Morgenstern L, Yamakawa T, Seltzer D: Carcinoma of the gastric stump. Am J Surg 29:125, 1973.
13. Orlando R, Welch JP: Carcinoma of the stomach after gastric operations. Am J Surg 487:141, 1981.
14. Ruddel WS, Bone E, Hill M, Blendis M, Walters C: Gastric juice nitrite: a risk factor for cancer in the hypochlorhydric stomach? Lancet 1037–1039, 1976.
15. Di Matteo G, Palazzini G, Cancrini A Jr, De Antoni E: La gastrodigiunoduodenoplastica (film). 87 Congr Soc Italy Chir Torino, 1985.
16. Jascalevich MC: Jejunal interposition gastroduodenostomy with automated suturing devices. Am J Surg 152:320, 1986.
17. Sawyers J, Herrington J: Superiority of antiperistaltic jejunal segments in management of severe dumping syndrome. Am J Surg 311:178, 1973.
18. Soupault R, Boucaille M: La transplantation de l'anse efferente au duodénum. Operation correctrice de certaines gastrectomies subtotales. Rev Chir 74:181, 1955.
19. Kennedy T, Green R: Roux diversion for bile reflux following gastric surgery. Br J Surg 323:65, 1978.
20. Labò G, Bortolot' M, Persani G: Effect of Billroth II operation on the i stiʌal motor activity. Digestion 31:194, 1985.
21. Van Heerden J, Phillips S, Adson M, McIllrath D: Postoperative reflux gastritis. Am J Surg 8:129, 1975.
22. Becker HD: Disorders of gastrointestinal hormones after surgery. Acta Hepatogastroenterol 26:516, 1979.
23. Bloom SR, Royston C, Thompson J: Enteroglucagon release in the dumping syndrome. Lancet 789–791, 1972.
24. Rehnfeldt J, Heding L, Holst J: Increased gut glucagon release as pathogenetic factor in reactive hypoglycaemia. Lancet 116–118, 1973.
25. Lawson H: The reversibility of postgastrectomy alkaline reflux gastritis by a Roux-en-Y loop. Br J Surg 13:59, 1972.

CHAPTER 43

ANTERIOR PYLORECTOMY (PYLOROPLASTY) WITH THE CIRCULAR STAPLING INSTRUMENT

Gustavo G.R. Kuster

Many procedures have been described to achieve incompetence of the pyloric sphincter. The classic pyloroplasty done by longitudinal incision with transverse closure requires sometimes extensive mobilization of the duodenum to avoid tension on the suture line. It may also produce significant deformity and distortion of the area. Several procedures of partial myectomy or partial pylorectomy have been developed.[1-5] They can be accomplished readily by a technique utilizing the circular stapler.

METHOD

The EEA-25 stapler device is introduced through a gastrotomy in the anterior wall of the stomach (Fig. 43-1), and the anvil is advanced through the pylorus into the first portion of the duodenum (Fig. 43-2). While closing the instrument and at the same time pushing the anterior half of the pylorus into the groove between the stapler and the anvil with a silk string (Figs. 43-3, 43-4), an anterior hemi-pylorectomy is accomplished.

CLINICAL EXPERIENCE

Anterior pylorectomy utilizing the EEA-25 circular stapler has been performed in 30 patients requiring esophageal and proximal gastric resections for benign or malignant conditions, and other various operations with associated vagotomy.

RESULTS

All of these pyloroplasties were effective and free of complications. An upper gastro-intestinal x-ray study

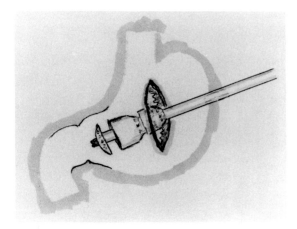

Fig. 43-1. The circular stapler is introduced through a gastrotomy; the anvil is separated from the cartridge while holding it firmly against the pyloric ring.

with contrast material was done between 5 and 7 days after the stapler pyloroplasty to check gastric emptying. Delay of gastric emptying was not observed, and all patients were able to take the food allowed. There was no evidence of pyloric leak or gastric retention.

DISCUSSION

This technique of anterior pylorectomy using the circular stapler is easy and fast to perform, and does not require mobilization of the duodenum since it does not produce traction between the antrum and the duodenum. It has become our procedure of

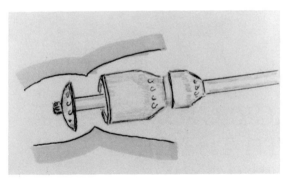

Fig. 43-2. The anvil is passed into the duodenum, and the cartridge remains proximal to the pylorus.

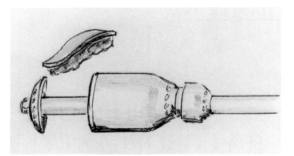

Fig. 43-4. As the stapler is activated, the full thickness anterior rim of the pylorus is excised; a transverse staple line is placed between the anterior gastric and duodenal walls. The instrument is disengaged as it would be for any entirely circular anastomosis. A full thickness anterior portion of pylorus should be recovered in lieu of the usual complete tissue circles.

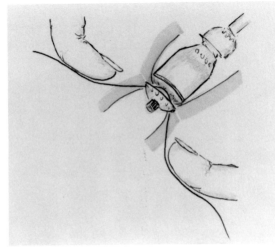

Fig. 43-3. The assistant pushes the anterior half of the pylorus into the cleft between anvil and cartridge with a silk string while the surgeon closes the anvil against the cartridge.

choice for pyloroplasty in cases without scarred, non-pliable pylorus.

Acknowledgment: This study was supported in part by the Harold and Daphne Oppenheimer Research Fund.

REFERENCES

1. Adams JT: Technique for anterior hemi-pylorectomy. Surg Gyn Ob 147:421–422, 1978.
2. Aust BA: New technique for pyloroplasty. Surgery 53:309, 1953.
3. Beattie AD: Vagotomy and partial pylorectomy—a new procedure for duodenal ulcer. Lancet, 1950, pp. 525–530.
4. Steichen FM: Vordere hemizirkuläre pylorektomic. *In* Kremer K, Liege W, Platzer W, Schrieber HW, and Weller S, eds, Chirurgische Operations lehre. Stuttgart, G. Thienne-Verlag, 1987.
5. Zakaria MAC: Anterior hemi-pylorectomy. J. Royal Coll Surg Edinb 29:367–369, 1984.

Part X

Stapling in Colo-rectal Surgery

CHAPTER 44

THE DIFFICULT ANTERIOR RESECTION

R.J. Heald

The "easy" anterior resection is confined to lesions 10 to 12 cm above the anus and higher, in persons of convenient shape with little extra-rectal spread of tumor. Such lesions in the upper third of the rectum can be mobilized without division of the lateral ligaments; the mesorectum may be divided with a generous 5-cm margin of mesorectum and bowel wall below the cancer; and either manual or stapled anastomosis presents no particular problem.

Below this level *no* anterior resection should be regarded as easy. Local recurrence of cancer, almost entirely preventable by good surgical technique, remains a common problem. Local recurrence rates in excess of 20% and sometimes as high as 40% are often observed when individual surgeons do not get enough practice.[1] It is difficult to follow planes that safely circumscribe the perirectal visceral mesentery properly and precisely. The dilemma can be likened to that of the boatman in the Straits of Messina: on one side is the cancer like a rocky headland—*Scylla*—with invisible outlying rocks; touch one of these and the craft will eventually sink, fast or slow. On the other side is the whirlpool—*Charybdis*—uncharted and subject to much argument by surgical pilots.[2] Should one clean the pelvic side wall and sacrifice the hypogastric plexuses, destroying potency and bladder function? There is little gain in doing so and much needless suffering caused thereby—but one is much better in the whirlpool than in touching one of those rocks! Nevertheless, the passage is never easy, certainly not for surgeons early in their training. The aim therefore of *low anterior resection*—for tumors from 4 to 12 cm in diameter—is total mesorectal excision with proper anterior clearance in the plane in front of Denonvillier's fascia, and wide lateral clearance. By using these principles, we have been able to achieve a local recurrence rate of 3.3% in curative cases.[2]

If these resections are all difficult, one must confess that some are indeed more difficult than others: what are the factors that make it so?

1. The flexibility of the pelvic floor
2. The width of the pelvis, depending on the sex of the patient
3. The upward push on the perineum by the assistant
4. Light and exposure
5. Height of the tumor

In all women (and in many men) the optimal use of upward pressure will make it possible to place the purse-string as low as 1 cm above the dentate line. Thus, a stapled colo-anal full-thickness internal-sphincter-to-colon anastomosis is possible in all but a few thick-set men.

Since we now regard a 2-cm clearance along the muscle tube as adequate, provided perirectal clearance is complete, this usually means that the separation point between anterior resection and abdomino-perineal excision is around 4 to 5 cm from the anal margin to the lower palpable edge of the tumor.

HISTOLOGIC TUMOR GRADE

The caveat against poorly differentiated tumors has largely been discarded, since the error in predicting the true behavior of the tumor is so great. In our own series, even the final grade of the carcinoma was not shown to have any predictive value in relation to 5-year survival, because the small number of extremely poorly differentiated tumors that spread viciously throughout the patient represents only a third of those identified initially by the pathologist as "poorly differentiated."

TUMOR STAGE

Wide local extension involving other organs introduces specific problems and influences the precise technical detail of the operation:

Extensive Spread into the Mesorectum

Even when this structure is almost completely replaced by tumor, the "Holy Plane" will usually clear it by 1 or 2 mm; such cases may even be cured, at least in terms of local disease. The planes along the edge of a tumor tear more easily than the body's healthy planes. Manual extraction is certain to lead to residual tumor cells on the side wall of the pelvis, as opposed to careful sharp dissection in the correct plane.

Invasion of the Lateral Pelvic Wall, Including Internal Iliac Vessels and Their Branches

While I do not believe in the routine clearance of the internal iliac lymph nodes, it is sometimes appropriate to ligate one or both sides of the internal iliac vessels when their major branches are invaded by tumor. This should only be on one side, although both internal iliacs can probably be safely ligated in many people.

Invasion of Genito-Urinary Structures

Upper-third lesions may invade the back of the bladder; middle-third lesions may invade the seminal vesicles. In the former, it is often helpful to enter the bladder initially and to excise a disc as required. In the latter, an extensive pelvic dissection to establish the precise anatomic relationships of the vital structures may be appropriate. The most commonly forgotten structures are the inferior hypogastric plexuses. Even during the most extensive pelvic clearance, these nerves can be preserved as shown by Walsh.[3] In radical prostatectomies, he succeeds in removing the prostate and vesicles and yet leave his patients capable of erection in almost 90% of cases.

The neurovascular bundle, formed by the confluence of the presacral and nervi erigentes, running across the back of the lateral edge of the vesicles, bladder neck, and prostate and entering the corpora cavernosa, is identified and preserved; everything else in the area can go. This is an example of Lockhart-Mummery's concept of "cutting the tops off the nerves."[4] There is a clear parallel in rectal excision;

Slack similarly looked carefully at the surface of excised anterior resection specimens for "tops" of nerves and correlated these with damaged function postoperatively.[5]

In extended rectal resections, opening Walsh's plane lateral to the prostate is very useful in establishing the course of the nerves. This is the plane opened bluntly by pushing a swab down on each side before performing a retro-pubic prostatectomy. Its lateral wall contains obturator internal muscle, vessels, and nerve. It may be easier to think of the surgical anatomy as two compartments created by a neurovascular diaphragm passing from lateral to medial at the level of the base of the prostate and carrying the entire genito-urinary supply line. In this diaphragm, from front to back, are the vas, the superior vesical artery, the ureter, and the inferior hypogastric plexus. Penetrating the latter in an irregular manner are the inferior hypogastric vesical and mid-rectal vessels.

In a difficult case or extended resection it may be valuable to find the nerves in the anterior compartment, visualize the ureter, divide the vas and the superior vesical artery to open up the pelvis, and thus see them throughout their course. Everything in the roof of the ureteric tunnels can be safely divided— and the vasa also mark a safe plane. Extended dissections in which positive identification of the nerves has not been performed almost invariably produce impotence and serious bladder dysfunction.

The ureters are not commonly involved in mid-rectal cancer, which is usually posterior to them. In upper-rectal carcinoma, however, invasion is not uncommon; therefore, an I.V.P. is appropriate. It is probably not a good idea to ligate the ureter after resection of the invading tumor and leave an obstructed kidney—re-implantation or cross anastomosis to the other ureter is the better course of action. If both ureters are involved, and after total exenteration, a Wallace-69 anastomosis with an ileal conduit is appropriate. The vesicles and bladder base between the ureters may be resected without sacrificing the whole bladder if this area is adherent to the front of a carcinoma. Erectile impotence only occurs if the nerves are damaged, which can be avoided by taking the trouble to identify them.

FOLDED-OVER SIGMOID COLON OR ILEUM

By impairing access to the rectum, a folded-over and adherent sigmoid colon or ileum can produce a prodigiously difficult operation. The principle must be to avoid peeling into actual tumor, and to clear the cancer by a margin of normal tissue—sometimes only achievable by total exenteration.

THE UTERUS AND VAGINAL VAULT

These usually present no special problem. The anastomosis, however, must be separated from the vaginal mucosa by placing it well down behind the distal remnant of posterior vaginal wall. Omentum may also be transposed to cover the anastomosis.

PELVIC EXENTERATION

Some rectal cancers and some uncontrolled cervical cancers may be offered a hope of cure by this formidable procedure. Once the principle of sacrificing the bladder is accepted, the planes around the whole block of pelvic organs are relatively easy. Urinary diversion is mandatory, but the anus need not be sacrificed, and so even this massive resection of tissue can still be termed "anterior" and a stapled colon-to-anus anastomosis effected in the usual way.

SELECTION OF CASES FOR RADIOTHERAPY

There can be no doubt that high doses of radiotherapy are effective in reducing the size of large rectal adenocarcinomas, and that their invasion of surrounding tissues within the pelvis may be forced to retreat so that excision becomes possible in a previously inoperable case. Radiotherapy should be restricted to those patients in whom an initial trial dissection has demonstrated that the dissection planes, required to circumscribe the tumor, would in fact go through tumor tissue. In such cases we perform a defunctioning colostomy and proceed to radical radiotherapy, to be followed 2 to 3 months later by a further attempt at an extended resection as just described.

DIAGNOSIS OF THE PELVIC MASS

In all cases it is desirable to have a histologic diagnosis pre-operatively, but this becomes even more important if extended surgery is being contemplated. One area of the management of pelvic disease that needs to advance is the precise pre-operative diagnosis of apparently malignant masses. No case should go forward to a mutilating operation without either a histologic confirmation of the malignant nature of the tumor or a full range of imaging techniques, including endoscopy, double-contrast radiology, CAT scan, ultrasound, and possibly NMR in the future. Endoluminal cytology may also be of considerable value when endoscopy does not provide the answer.

Despite all these techniques there are some cases in which definite diagnosis is still elusive; we are about to commence a trial of true-cut needle biopsy performed operatively in such cases.

STAPLING TECHNIQUES IN THE ULTRA-LOW ANTERIOR RESECTION

There is little doubt that circular stapling devices have had a profound impact on the performance of lower anastomoses in many of these difficult cases. The double-stapling technique using a TA plus a circular device saves time in the intermediate and low cases. Nevertheless, it is crucial to cross-clamp the rectum beyond the cancer and to wash out the lumen below this clamp; in the ultra-low case, there is often no room to insert a standard TA device beyond the first clamp. In these ultra-low cases, therefore, the roticulator TA linear stapler is a major step forward, allowing placement of a staple line below the clamp.

SUMMARY

The various problems and specific difficulties of extended anterior resections have been reviewed. The most important of these relate to the height of the tumor in relation to the build of the patient and to the techniques used in low stapling. Further specific difficulties are created by local extension of the tumor into surrounding structures.

REFERENCES

1. Phillips RKS, Hittinger R, Blesovsky L, Fry JS, Fielding LP: Local recurrence after curative surgery for large bowel cancer (1). The overall picture. Br J Surg 71:12–16, 1983.
2. Heald RJ: The holy plane of rectal surgery. J R Soc Med 81(9):503–508, 1988.
3. Lepor H, Gregerman M, Crosby R, Mostofi FK, Walsh PC: Precise localization of autonomic nerves from pelvic plexus to corpora cavernosa: detailed anatomical study of adult male pelvis. J Urol 133:207–212, 1985.
4. Lockhart-Mummery, Sir HE: Personal communication.
5. Williams JT, Slack WW: A prospective study of sexual function after major colorectal surgery. Br J Surg 67:772–774, 1980.

CHAPTER 45

EXPERIENCE WITH 140 STAPLED COLO-RECTAL ANASTOMOSES

K.W. Steegmuller and S. Broun

METHODS AND CLINICAL EXPERIENCE

Between 1 January 1980 and 15 February 1988, a total of 341 resections of the left colon and rectum were performed in our department. All elective operations were done as one-stage procedures. The EEA-31 or -28 instrument was used for all but two patients. The use of the circular stapling instrument was mandatory in all operations for anterior resection of the rectum. For all other anastomoses, this decision was left to the discretion of the surgeon and resulted in the use of manual sutures in one or two layers as an alternative technique. The EEA stapler was advanced transanally with one exception. The purse-string was placed at times with the special purse-string instrument, at other times by a manual over-and-over whipstitch, depending on the technical ease with which either maneuver could be executed. Up to this point we have used the double-stapling technique, consisting of the closure of the rectal stump with the linear TA-55 Roticulator and the intersection by this line with the circular anastomosing instrument, on three occasions.

The patient population (Table 45-1) comprised a total of 140 elective operations on the left colon and rectum and reconstruction of bowel continuity by mechanical circular anastomosis without protecting colostomy. Besides carcinoma, the recto-sigmoid group counts 2 patients with advanced ovarian cancer, 1 patient with Crohn's disease, and 2 patients with benign polyps, whereas in the group of patients with anterior resection of the rectum, operation was performed in 8 patients for benign tubulovillous adenoma, and for cancer in all other patients. Because of intra-abdominal tumor status, palliative sigmoid resection only was possible in 20% of patients and in 10% of the patients with anterior resection. In the overall group, 14 patients with colo-rectal carcinoma had a very extensive radical dissection and resection consisting in mobilization of the splenic flexure, radical lymphadenectomy from the level of the left renal vein into the pelvis beyond the tumor, and ligation of the inferior mesenteric vein at the lower border of the pancreas and of the inferior mesenteric artery directly on the aorta. All peri-aortic nodes were included in the dissection.

RESULTS

Of the 140 planned resections of the left colon and rectum using the mechanical anastomotic instruments without colostomy, the operation was accomplished in 133 patients (Table 45-1). A total of 24 (17%) intra-operative mishaps occurred with the use of the instruments (Tables 45-2 through 45-5), such as incomplete tissue rings and resistance to the placement of the instrument because of spastic colon. It is possible to correct such intra-operative complications in those operations where the anastomosis is situated above the peritoneal reflection, but corrective maneuvers are at best a problem of diagnosis and management when they are situated deep in the pelvis. For this reason, a temporary colostomy was created in 4 patients and a manual anastomosis in another 3 because of intra-operative problems with stapling.

A technically perfect stapled circular anastomosis was accomplished in 116 (83%) of all left-colon and rectal resections. In this group, 2 patients (1.7%) developed a clinically apparent anastomotic leak. In the group of 24 patients with intra-operative mishaps, 17

Table 45-1. EEA-Stapled Anastomoses in Sigmoid Colon and Rectum: Elective Operations Without Colostomy

Operation	Done	Planned
Sigmoid resection for carcinoma	22	24
Sigmoid resection for diverticulitis	13	14
Anterior rectal resection	90	94
Subtotal colectomy and ileo-rectostomy	2	2
Left hemicolectomy and transverse colon to rectum anastomosis	6	6
Total	133	140

received a stapled anastomosis without colostomy; of these, 2 patients (12%) developed a clinically anastomotic leak.

No intra-operative or postoperative problems were recognized in 6 patients with left hemi-colectomy (radical lymph node dissection and transverse colon-to-rectum anastomosis in 5 patients, transverse colon-to-sigmoid anastomosis in 1 patient), or in 2 patients with ileo-rectostomy after subtotal colectomy for multiple carcinomas or rectal cancer with polyposis of the remaining colon.

POSTOPERATIVE COMPLICATIONS AND MORTALITY

Two patients developed a fecal fistula that closed spontaneously within a few days; 1 patient suffered from pelvic abscess with sepsis that was drained transanally without laparotomy. A fourth patient de-

Table 45-2. Intra-Operative Problems with the Circular EEA Stapler in Elective Sigmoid Resections Without Colostomy

Spasm of colon at anastomotic site: 1
   Solution: Manual anastomosis
Questionable appearance of anastomosis: 2
   Solution: Repeat EEA anastomoses
Incomplete tissue rings: 3
   Solution: Reinforcing manual sutures
Unsafe EEA anastomosis: 1
   Solution: Proximal colostomy
Technical mishap: 1
   Solution: Manual anastomosis
Poor closure of EEA stapler: 1
   Solution: Circular manual reinforcement

Nine intra-operative problems in 38 EEA applications (23%)
Solutions: 2 manually sutured anastomoses, 1 diverting colostomy

There were no clinical manifestations of anastomotic insufficiency postoperatively

Table 45-3. Intra-Operative Problems with Circular EEA Anastomosis in Anterior Resections of the Rectum: Tumor Location at 13 to 16 cm; Elective Operations Without Colostomy (n = 40)

Incomplete tissue ring: 1
   Solution: Reinforcing manual sutures
Postoperative fistula: 1
   Solution: Non-operative treatment and spontaneous healing
One postoperative complication was encountered in 14 anastomoses, all considered to be safe at operation (2.3%)

veloped a recto-vaginal fistula 4 weeks after operation, which was treated with a Hartmann procedure for exclusion of the fistula site. Therefore, the incidence of clinically obvious anastomotic leaks was 3%. No patients died because of any of these complications.

There were 18 patients (14%) of the 133 patients overall who suffered from postoperative complications not related to the choice of the anastomotic technique: wound abscess and healing by secondary intention in 6%, injury to the bladder or ureter in 1.5%. Re-operation was indicated to control bleeding in 1 patient, and drainage of a subphrenic abscess in a second patient. In this patient, resection of the tail of the pancreas and of the spleen had been performed for cystadenoma of the pancreas during a left hemi-colectomy for sigmoid diverticulitis. Complications with the central venous catheter were observed in 3 patients (thrombosis, sepsis, pneumothorax); 2 patients suffered postoperative pulmonary embolism; and 1 patient had a myocardial infarction. Two pa-

Table 45-4. Intra-Operative Problems with Circular EEA Anastomosis in Anterior Resections of the Rectum (n = 47)*

Problem	n	Solution
Incomplete tissue rings	9	Manual reinforcing sutures (7) *Complications:* 1 fecal fistula, 1 pelvic abscess Proximal diverting colostomy (2)
Mechanical mishap	1	Repeat EEA anastomosis
Severe colon spasm	1	Manually sutured anastomosis

Total number of intra-operative technical problems: 11
Note: Of a total of 36 intra-operatively perfect anastomoses, 1 patient developed a recto-vaginal fistula (2.7%); the solution was to perform a Hartmann operation.

* Tumor location at 8 to 12 cm; elective operations; no colostomy

Table 45-5. Intra-Operative Problems with EEA Stapled Anastomosis in Anterior Resections of the Rectum (n = 7)*

Problem	n	Solution
Incomplete tissue rings	3	Manual reinforcing sutures (1)
		Proximal diverting colostomy (2)

Note: Four anastomoses at this level were perfect. No clinically obvious anastomotic insufficiency was observed in any patients.

* Tumor location below 8 cm; elective operations; no colostomy

tients died from cardio-respiratory insufficiency in the group of patients over 80 years old, and 1 patient, 70 years old, died from cardiogenic shock due to myocardial infarction. This resulted in an operative mortality rate of 2.2%. The surgical complications did not result in any mortality.

CONCLUSIONS

The condition for success with stapling techniques is a perfect understanding of the limits of their usefulness together with absolute competence in both mechanical and manual suture techniques.

If the tissue rings obtained with the mechanical anastomosing technique are incomplete, the anastomotic defect can be oversewn manually, if it is small. Following such repairs, the competence of the anastomosis should be re-examined with intraluminal injection of air, and the anastomosis covered with water. We do not consider this to be absolutely indicated in those patients in whom the tissue rings were complete at the first examination. If the surgeon is not satisfied after placing reinforcing sutures, or if the bowel had not been satisfactorily prepared preoperatively, then a temporary decompressing colostomy is indicated. We have observed spasm of the colon resisting the introduction of even the EEA-28 only when the operation is performed under epidural block. We have never succeeded in breaking these spasms with the injection of a spasmolytic agent, although the intraluminal placement of a sponge soaked in warm saline solution can be effective in these cases.

In conclusion, optimal preoperative preparation of the entire patient and, more specifically, the large bowel; perioperative antibiotic prophylaxis; a gentle operative technique respecting all of the principles of bowel anastomosis; and complete understanding of the stapling techniques, as well as potential intra-operative mishaps, make a one-stage sigmoid or rectal resection possible with minimal postoperative complications and avoidance of a decompressing colostomy.

Translated from the German by F.M. Steichen, M.D.

BIBLIOGRAPHY

1. Öhman U, Svenberg T: EEA stapler for midrectum carcinoma. Dis Colon Rectum 26:775–784, 1983.
2. Thiede A, Schubert G, Poser HL, Jostarndt L: Zur Technik der Rectumanastomosen bei Rectumresektionen. Chirurg 55:326–335, 1984.
3. Beart RW, Kelly KA: Randomized prospective evaluation of the EEA-stapler for colorectal anastomosis. Am J Surg 141:143–147, 1981.
4. Everett WG, Friend PJ, Forty J: Comparison of stapling and hand-suture for leftsided large bowel anastomosis. Br J Surg 73:345–348, 1986.

CHAPTER 46

CIRCULAR STAPLING TECHNIQUES FOR LOW RECTAL AND ANAL ANASTOMOSIS

Victor W. Fazio

The purpose of this chapter is to provide not only a general overview, but also a personally preferred choice of techniques available to the surgeon for restoring intestinal continuity following deep pelvic surgery. Since the focus is on anastomotic technique, there is relatively little discussion on bowel preparation and technique of resection.

INDICATIONS AND CONTRAINDICATIONS FOR USE OF THE CIRCULAR STAPLER

The ability to do an anastomosis is not, per se, an indication for doing so. The elderly patient with poor sphincters, the patient with rectal cancer and extensive peritoneal deposits of metastases, and the patient with co-existent radiation injury to the rectum and perineum are better off with a Hartmann operation following rectal resection. Patients with even advanced liver metastases may fare reasonably well with a primary anastomosis following resection of their rectal cancer.[1] The rigid-walled, non-distensible, and especially contracted rectum does not lend itself to transit of the instrument, and fracture or perforation is a distinct possibility with the introduction of the stapler. However, with a non-irradiated anal canal, a stapled anastomosis can still be done safely.[2]

Most surgeons agree that anastomotic integrity rates are similar to those of hand-sewn and stapled anastomoses of the intraperitoneal rectum. Many, however, choose to use the circular stapler in that situation, for a speedier anastomosis. My own view is that the hand-sewn technique is preferable when one is dealing with a narrowed distal rectal aperture that will not accept a 28-mm caliber instrument, or when

the proximal segment is similarly narrowed, or when there is inadequate distal tissue for placement of a purse-string in colo-anal anastomosis. Otherwise, stapled techniques are preferred.

OPERATIVE TECHNIQUE

The patient is placed in Lloyd-Davies stirrups with a slight head-down tilt. Povidone iodine, approximately 100 ml, is instilled in the rectum. Rectal resection follows the principles of surgery established for the condition—notably wide clearance of a cancer-bearing segment, or dissection close to the rectal wall in its lower third, for benign conditions. Assurance of an excellent blood supply to bowel ends, especially the proximal segment, is obtained by observance of arterial bleeding from the cut end of the colon (or ileum) or an adjacent appendix epiploica. Ideally, this bleeding should be enough to require cautery or ligation for control. For absence of tension in the anastomosis, mobilization of the splenic flexure and high ligation of the inferior mesenteric vessels are usually required.

Preparation of Bowel Ends

The colon or ileal contents adjacent to the proximal end are contained by placement of a loosely tied linen tape around the bowel. A purse-string suture, using a 1-0 Prolene stitch, is made by hand, employing an over-and-over stitch. These are placed in the sero-muscular layer, excluding mucosa, about 8 to 10 mm apart, starting and finishing on the anterior surface. A modified Furniss clamp can be used as a purse-string device on the proximal thin-walled bowel. Success is unpredictable; often, reinforcement sutures, especially posteriorly, are required. Techniques using the distal purse-string are discussed below. The purse-string suture should be placed sufficiently widely so that the suture can "run"; that is, with traction on both ends, the suture completely gathers the end of bowel to the point of occlusion. Otherwise, when tying the proximal purse-string in the distal pelvis, the surgeon is relatively blind to the "gathering" effects of traction on the suture prior to tying (Fig. 46-1). This can lead to a portion of the sutured tissue lying extraneous to the anvil/cartridge complex when the instrument is in the firing position. This in turn will lead to a posterior defect in the proximal tissue ring after firing (Fig. 46-2).

Insertion of the Instrument

After placing the distal purse-string, the bowel is assessed visually or with sizers to decide the optimal caliber of the instrument. Most anastomoses will ac-

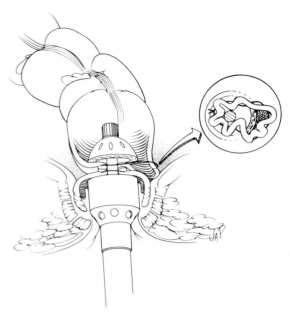

Fig. 46-2. If the proximal purse-string is not secured against the shaft posteriorly, this can lead to extension of the posterior edge of the proximal colon end and, after stapler firing, lead to an incomplete proximal donut. The detachable anvil/shaft complex of the CEEA allows excellent visibility and prevents this problem.

cept a 28- or 31-mm diameter instrument, and anastomosis can be made without difficulty. If the proximal or distal end is snug or just under 28 mm, I prefer to use rubber dilators to serially stretch the ends of the bowel. Care is taken to avoid fracturing or lacer-

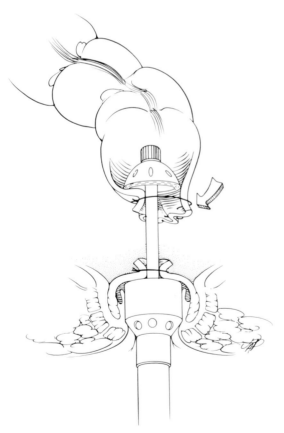

Fig. 46-1. The proximal purse-string may not be secured against the shaft posterior (arrow) when an anastomosis in the deep pelvis is being done. Posteriorly, visibility is poor, so that checking the tie is not easy.

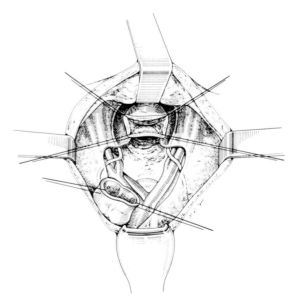

Fig. 46-3. Stay sutures on the cut end of the rectum facilitate placement of the purse-string suture.

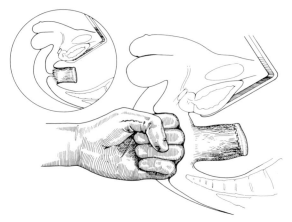

Fig. 46-4. Perineal pressure will "elevate" the low rectal segment to facilitate construction of the anastomosis.

ating the serosa. Provided the anastomosis is completed expeditiously, the lumen will not contract; insertion of the instrument, tying of the purse-strings, and extraction can be done quickly and efficiently. This also reduces the tendency of the anastomosis to prolapse and create tension on the anastomosis during the extraction process. Counter-traction with stay sutures placed through the anastomosis also facilitates extraction.

Checking the Anastomosis

This is done visually, but with low anastomoses this is usually inadequate. The tissue rings are carefully oriented on the removed instrument and checked for defects. This will provide a clue as to where reinforcement of the anastomosis is required. An apparently intact doughnut may be incomplete when the Prolene suture is removed. The anastomosis is then tested by transanal instillation of Povidine iodine until visible distension of the proximal colon segment is

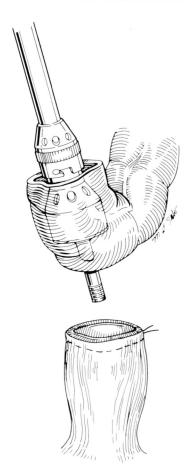

Fig. 46-6. The shaft is placed through the antimesenteric aspect of the proximal colon.

seen. Some slight oozing through the staple line itself is of no moment and requires no reinforcement. However, a defect, if present, will become painfully obvious, and attempts at correction are appropriate. For high anastomoses, or in a thin patient with a

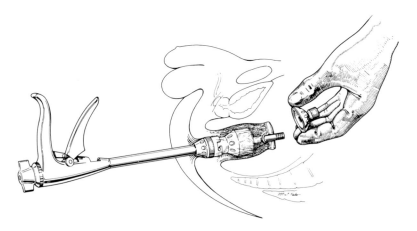

Fig. 46-5. If the double-stapled technique is used, the shaft should traverse the staple line itself or in its *immediate* proximity.

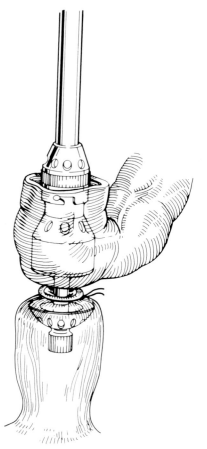

Fig. 46-7. The anvil is reattached and secured into the rectal stump with a purse-string tie.

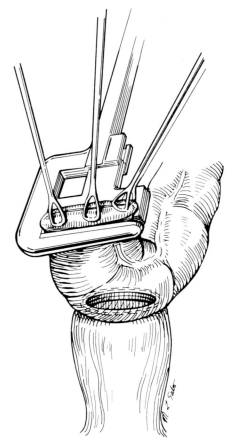

Fig. 46-8. After the stapler is fired, the open end of the proximal colon is stapled across.

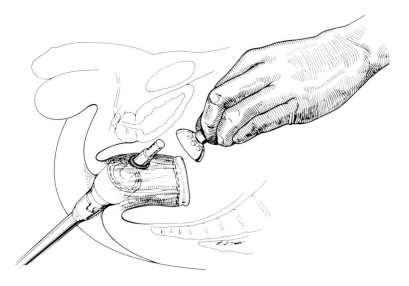

Fig. 46-9. End-to-side rectal anastomosis is potentially hazardous.

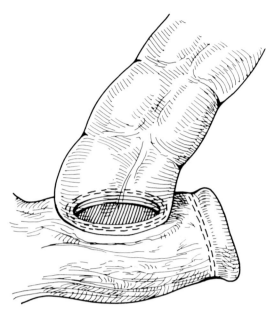

Fig. 46-10. The proximity of the two staple lines could produce ischemic necrosis of the intervening segment.

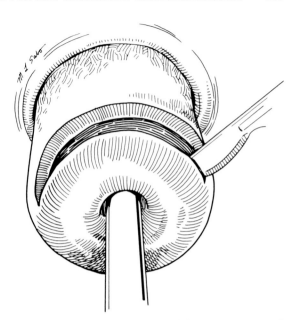

Fig. 46-12. The incision is carried down to non-everted, prolapsed rectum.

capacious pelvis, this poses few problems. For the ultra-low anastomosis, transanal reinforcement is attempted. For small leaks where local circumstances are forbidding—in obese men, or in patients with a narrow pelvis, a long anal canal, or an anastomosis located behind the prostate gland—sump drainage of the presacral space and diverting colostomy is indicated.

Protection of the Anastomosis

Omental wrap of the anastomosis is rarely possible for the very low anastomosis. However, placement of

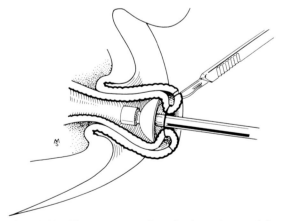

Fig. 46-11. The rectum is prolapsed using a tie around the obturator. The anterior rectal wall is incised.

an omental pedicle to occupy presacral dead space, placed in juxtaposition to the anastomosis, is probably a valuable maneuver.[3] Sump suction of the presacral space reduces the volume of exudate and blood that might otherwise nurture a bacterial inoculum, and so helps prevent a pelvic abscess. Contrary to my former views, combining irrigation with suction (to dilute the inoculum and to help eradicate blood clot) does not confer any added benefit, according to a recently conducted prospective study.[4] Temporary colostomy is used when intra-operative anastomotic leak is found and attempts at repair are unsatisfactory, the colonic bowel preparation was inadequate, or local or systemic factors are deemed unfavorable by the surgeon (e.g., excessive blood loss, gross pelvic contamination, high-risk cardiac patient, previous pelvic irradiation). In recent years, Ravo has shown the value of suturing a plastic or latex rubber tube to quarantine the anastomosis from the fecal stream.[5] The proximal end is sutured circumferentially with absorbable sutures on the inside of the proximal colon segment just beyond the anastomosis. The sleeve is delivered beyond the anastomosis and through the anus. This obviates the need for colostomy altogether. Studies in both animals and man so far have shown considerable success. I have no personal experience with this.

Methods to Facilitate Anastomosis Construction

The commonly encountered difficulties are exposure of the distal segment and, therefore, adequate

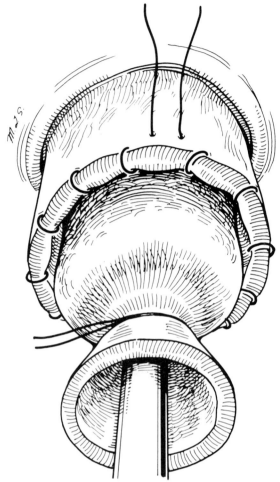

Fig. 46-13. A Prolene over-and-over suture is used for the rectal purse-string.

placement of the distal purse-string suture. Consequently, most maneuvers or technical variations are designed to facilitate this aspect. However, other difficulties may arise in "getting a good look" while tying the purse-strings, or in maneuvering the proximal

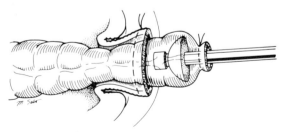

Fig. 46-14. The specimen is removed. The stapler anvil is inserted into the prolapsed colon and its purse-string is tied.

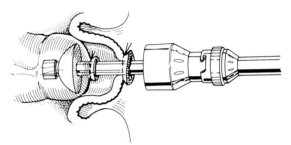

Fig. 46-15. The colon is withdrawn with the anvil into the pelvis. The rectal purse-string is tied.

bowel segment onto the anvil in preparation for tying the purse-string. A generous xiphoid-to-pubic-bone incision is used, if needed. Placement of stay sutures or clamps on the cut end of the rectum allow for positioning the edge in preparation of taking the stitch of the hand-sewn purse-string (Fig. 46-3). (I prefer three long Babcock clamps, as these can be adjusted as needed, and also provide excellent posterior traction.) A lighted Deaver or Goligher retractor, as well as one or two brawny assistants, are invaluable. Perineal pressure by an assistant positioned between the patient's legs will elevate the rectal stump into view in almost all cases (Fig. 46-4). For non-cancer cases, I prefer to use traction on the recto-sigmoid specimen, section the anterior half of the rectum at the site chosen for anastomosis, and place the anterior row of sutures starting in the left anterior aspect. Then half of the right posterior wall of rectum is incised; further sutures are placed until 90% of all sutures are in position. Perineal pressure and judicious use of Babcock clamps provide the final exposure needed to complete the purse-string. For anastomoses in the mid-pelvis, I have had a favorable experience with the double-armed Prolene suture placed through the Furniss clamp.[6] With two Keith

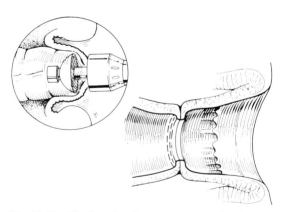

Fig. 46-16. The bowel ends are approximated and the stapler is fired, completing the anastomosis.

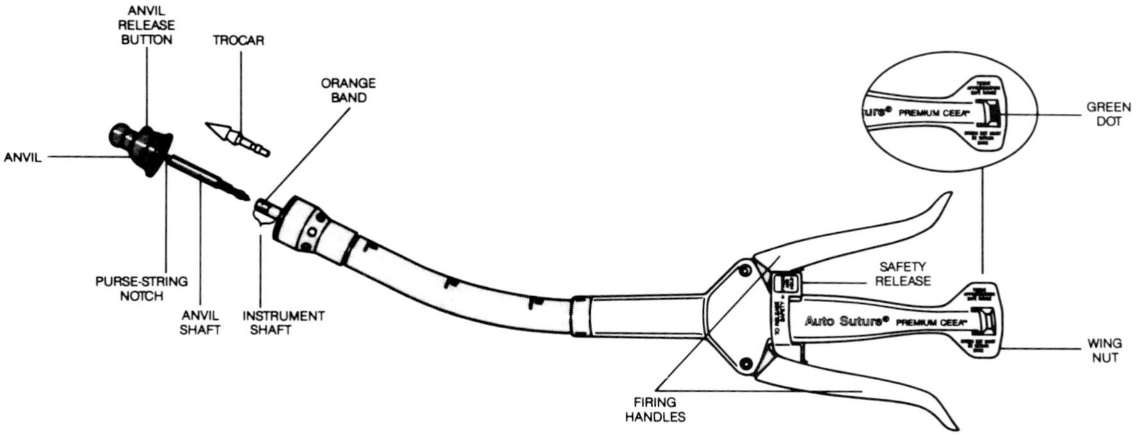

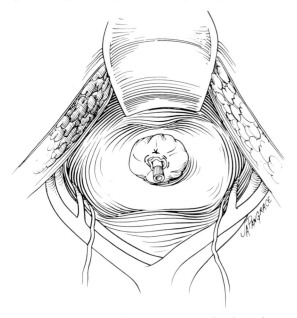

Fig. 46-17. The premium CEEA features the detachable anvil/shaft complex.

needles traversing the slots of the clamp, there is no concern about bending or twisting the needles on extraction. A metal retractor is used to protect the left iliac vessels as the needles are passed and removed from the clamp.

THE DOUBLE STAPLING TECHNIQUE

Knight and Griffen[7] described a technique of circular stapled anastomosis that obviated the need for a distal purse-string (Fig. 46-5). The rectal segment is stapled across with a linear stapler. The circular stapler is inserted transanally without the anvil. The shaft is then punched through the staple line or close to it. The anvil is reapplied and the proximal colon is manipulated over it. The purse-string is tied; the bowel ends are opposed and the instrument is fired. Cohen reported a favorable experience with this

technique.[8] For cancer cases, the rectal stump must be irrigated prior to application of the linear stapler to avoid entrapment of cancer cells that might produce later suture-line recurrence. A further concern is that the circular blade has to cut across a row of staples, although this may be more apparent than real. Julian and Ravitch found that staples were rarely cut: mostly the staples were bent by the EEA knife.[9] They concluded in their animal study that the practice was a safe one.

The side-to-end anastomosis has two main advantages. There is no need for special stirrups, and the patient is placed supine on the operating table. Sec-

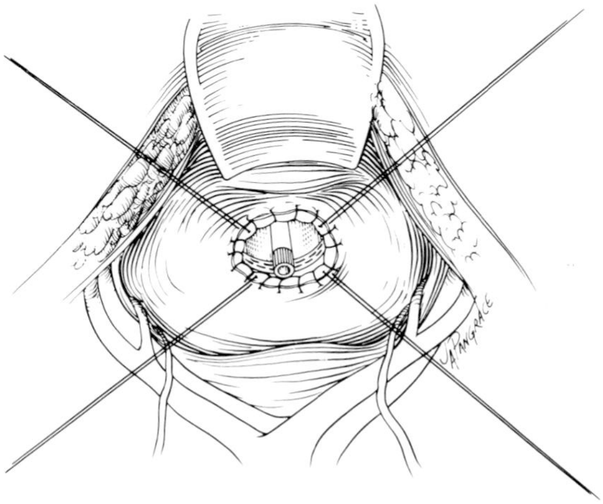

Fig. 46-18. After transanal insertion, the anvil/shaft is removed.

Fig. 46-19. The rectal purse-string is tied with good visibility.

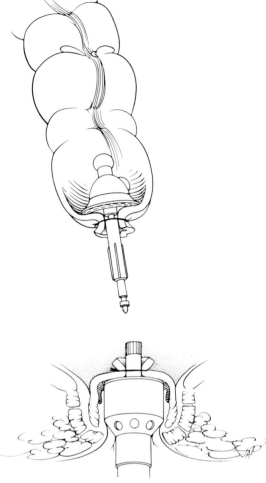

Fig. 46-20. The proximal purse-string tie is made over the detachable shaft with good visibility and the anvil shaft is then maneuvered to mate with the distal shaft.

ondly, for patients with a large-caliber proximal segment, the purse-string suture for an end-to-end anastomosis may produce a very large bulk of tissue. The side-to-end anastomosis, where no purse-string is needed on the proximal segment, overcomes this problem (Figs. 46-6, 46-7, 46-8).

End-to-side colo-rectal anastomosis is not recommended under ordinary circumstances. Performed originally for reconstruction after the Hartmann operation, a basic flaw in the principle of its use is that an ischemic necrosis may occur between the rectal cuff staple line and the cephalad aspect of the circular anastomosis (Figs. 46-9, 46-10).

Transanal placement of the purse-string is a valuable maneuver for stapled ileal pouch-anal anastomo-

sis or for colo-anal anastomosis when the anal canal is not excessively long. One or two Gelpi retractors or a lighted Ferguson retractor are very helpful.

The pull-through technique has been applied for stapled end-to-end anastomosis in both cancer and rectal prolapse cases. After full mobilization of the rectum, an obturator is passed transanally and a stout ligature applied just below the expanded end. Retraction produces a prolapse (Fig. 46-11) and a circumferential incision through full-thickness rectal wall is made (Fig. 46-12). The purse-string is easily applied under direct vision (Fig. 46-13). The mobilized sigmoid and rectum are delivered transanally and resected, and a purse-string is applied to the pulled-down proximal colon segment. The anastomosis is then easily carried out (Figs. 46-14, 46-15, 46-16). My colleague, Dr. Weakley, has enjoyed considerable success with this technique. Although this technique is innovative, I generally prefer others.

The curved end-to-end anastomosis stapler (CEEA) has recently been modified (Fig. 46-17). This major advance addresses one of the common difficulties encountered in performing circular stapled anastomoses. In the patient with a narrow pelvis, a bulky colon, and a poorly visible rectal stump, the surgeon will have (with the regular instruments) good visibility to tie one of the purse-strings and poor visibility for the other. Usually the surgeon will choose to tie the rectal (distal) purse-string under good vision (Figs. 46-18, 46-19), but then has to manipulate a bulky colon deep into the pelvis, maneuver the colon end over the anvil, and hope that the proximal purse-string tie is secure. Earlier, it was pointed out that this can leave part of the purse-string *outside* of the future staple line, resulting in an incomplete doughnut and leakage.

This new device allows detachment of the anvil *and shaft*. Consequently, the proximal purse-string can be tied in the upper abdomen, with excellent visibility and the ability to check the security of the purse-string (Fig. 46-20). Furthermore, it is relatively simple to maneuver the anvil/shaft complex and proximal colon into the deep pelvis, where the proximal shaft can easily "mate" with the shaft emerging from the cartridge. The perineal operator must maintain constant, steady pressure throughout. Too much pressure and the previously tied rectal purse-string may disrupt; too little pressure and the shaft of the cartridge may disappear distally from the rectal purse-string. The device is expensive, but for difficult low end-to-end anastomoses, it is the instrument of choice, in my view. In ten ultra-low colo-rectal anastomoses, I have had intact doughnuts, no leaks, and no need for temporary colostomy.

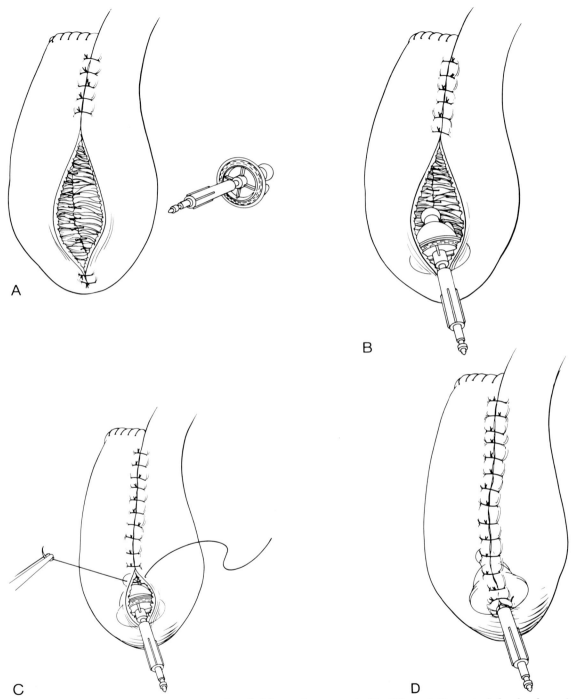

Fig. 46-21. *A–D*. The ileal pelvic reservoir and stapled ileo-anal anastomosis. The "J" pouch (linear stapled or hand-sewn) or "S" pouch can be used. The illustrations show a handsewn "J" pouch. The detachable anvil/shaft complex is placed in the dependent part of the pouch as the anterior layer is completed.

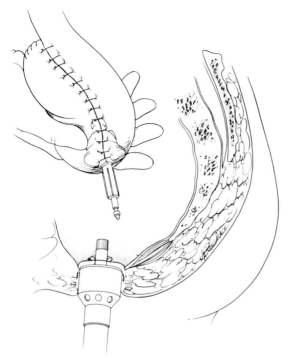

Fig. 46-22. The stapled pouch-anal anastomosis using the "J" pouch. The pouch is passed into the pelvis.

The instrument has been used for pelvic pouch anal anastomoses, both J- and S-pouches, as well. The techniques are illustrated in Figs. 46-21 through 46-24. Several centers (including the Mayo Clinic and St. Mark's Hospital, London) are presently evaluating the J-shaped colonic pouch, following its anastomosis to the upper anal canal or low rectum (Fig. 46-25).

PROBLEMS AND SOLUTIONS

Incomplete Tissue Rings

The key to management is prevention; I have alluded to several of the points already. Use the largest caliber instrument that the anastomosis will accommodate. Place the purse-strings so that excessive bulk of tissue does not appear around the shaft. Ensure that the purse-string can be snugged up close to the shaft. Reinforce the purse-string if in doubt about a slight gap. Use the detachable anvil/shaft of the CEEA if faced with a formidable pelvis. In the event that a defect is found, attempt reinforcement abdominally or transanally. If unsuccessful, drain the pelvis and cover with a colostomy.

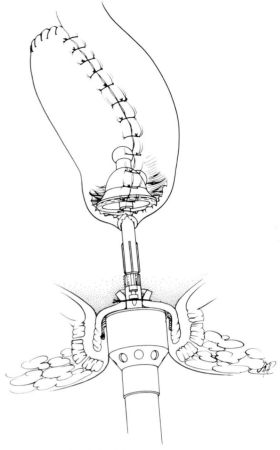

Fig. 46-23. The shaft of the anvil is mated with the shaft of the cartridge.

Perforated Distal Segment

This may occur with the introduction of the instrument minus its anvil. This is one reason why the anastomosis should be insufflated *even when there are intact tissue rings.* The defect should be repaired with or without covering stoma. If not possible, a *very* low redone anastomosis may be required, possibly a Parks' transanal anastomosis.

Immediate Anastomotic Dehiscence

This occurs because of faulty gap setting. The perineal operator may think that the bowel edges are accurately opposed, but has failed to check the indicator button. In that case, the staples are driven upward but fail to make a B-form. The circular blade, however, still cuts through, severing the bowel ends. Prevention is the key to management. Otherwise, a

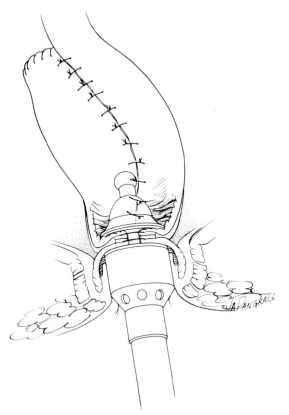

Fig. 46-24. The anvil and cartridge are approximated into firing range and the anastomosis is made.

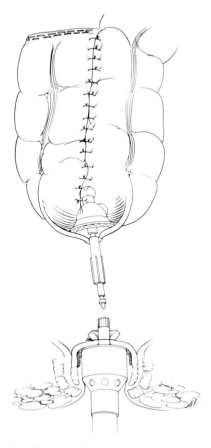

Fig. 46-25. The stapled colo-anal anastomosis using the "J" colon pouch.

new anastomosis has to be fashioned. A similar problem will occur if the anvil is not secured fully into place on the shaft.

POSTOPERATIVE COMPLICATIONS

Anastomotic Leak

In a poll of the members of the American Society of Colon and Rectal Surgeons (ASCRS),[10] approximately 10% of patients with circular stapled anastomoses had a clinical leak. I had previously reported a personal series[11] of 67 patients having a high colorectal anastomosis with radiologic and clinical leak rates of 1.5% and 0%, respectively; in 95 patients with a low colo-rectal anastomosis, the rates were 8.4% and 5.3%, respectively. Subsequently, we reviewed our department's results in 744 patients undergoing stapled colo-rectal anastomoses.[12] Clinical leak rates for high anterior resection, low anterior resection, and very low (under 5 cm) resection were 0.6%, 3.2%, and 5.8%, respectively. Gordon, in re-

viewing the literature, found three series comprising 100 patients or more in which there were clinical leak rates of 3%, 8%, and 13%.[13]

Bleeding

This is rarely of moment and is relatively easy to deal with in rectal anastomoses.

Stenosis

Some narrowing is found in practically all stapled anastomoses. Almost all dilate over a period of months, but some remain problematic. In the ASCRS report, stenosis was the commonest late complication, amounting to 8.8% of cases. Gordon reported rates of 1% ranging to 50% in his review; it would seem that most authors cite a 5 to 20% range. It is probable that the *problem* stricture is due to ischemia, resulting from vigorous clearing of the mesentery of the bowel ends. We deliberately avoid clearance of the proximal colon in preparing the bowel end. We observed 24 stenoses (inability to pass a 19-mm proctoscope) in 744 patients. One patient required re-anastomosis. The others responded to either time or dilatation.

Recurrence

There are only a few reports on the frequency of recurrence after stapled anastomoses. Most surgeons, including myself, feel that staple use, per se, does not influence recurrence rates; our own series bears this out.[14] Still, there is at least one report challenging this view. Reid et al. found pelvic recurrence in 8 of 29 patients, occurring between 5 and 45 months after stapled colo-rectal anastomosis.[15] This may be representative of margins of clearance, although in that study average cuff length was 4.8 cm (surgeon's assessment) and 3 cm (pathologist's measurement). There was no difference in cuff length between those with a local recurrence and those without recurrence.

My only comment on this subject is that one should first perform a good cancer operation; if there is then left an anal sphincter apparatus, the secondary consideration is that of restoring intestinal continuity.

SUMMARY

The techniques of restoring intestinal continuity after rectal resection for cancer have evolved throughout this century. For the most part, circular staplers have displaced the other pioneering and innovative techniques that our mentors and predecessors devised to improve the quality of life for our patients; with new technology, so also emerge new problems of the application of that technology. Although the future likely will render many of our present techniques obsolete (e.g., with refining of tissue adhesives), it is incumbent upon us to recognize the limits of our present array of weapons, and the limits placed on us by the biology of the tumor. About the latter, this means maintaining intellectual honesty in conducting a good cancer operation; about

the former, we have to recognize that most of the pitfalls of stapling use are preventable or correctable.

Acknowledgement: The author thanks Joseph Pangrace, Department of Medical Illustrations, The Cleveland Clinic Foundation, for the illustrations.

REFERENCES

1. Rothenberger D: Personal communication.
2. Robertson S, Heron H, Kerman HD, Bloom T: Is anterior resection of the rectosigmoid safe after preoperative radiation? Dis Colon Rectum 28(4):254–259, 1985.
3. McLachlin AD, Olsson LS, Pitt DF: Anterior anastomosis of the rectosigmoid colon: an experimental study. Surgery 80:306–311, 1976.
4. Galandiuk S, Fazio VW: Poster presentation: Annual Meeting of the American Society of Colon and Rectal Surgeons, Anaheim CA, June 1988.
5. Ravo B, Michrick A, Addei K, et al: The treatment of perforated diverticulitis by one-stage intracolonic bypass procedure. Surgery 102(5):771–776, 1987.
6. Last MD, Fazio VW: The rational use of the pursestring device in constructing anastomoses with circular stapler. Dis Colon Rectum 28(12):979–980, 1985.
7. Knight CD, Griffen FD: An improved technique for low anterior resection of the rectum using the EEA stapler. Surgery 88:710, 1980.
8. Cohen Z, Myers E, Langer B, et al: Double-stapling technique for low anterior resection. Dis Colon Rectum 26:231, 1983.
9. Julian TB, Ravitch MM: Evaluation of the safety of end-to-end (EEA) stapling anastomoses across linear stapled closures. Surg Clin North Am 64(3):567–577, 1984.
10. Smith LE: Anastomosis with EEA stapler after anterior colonic resection. Dis Colon Rectum 24:236, 1981.
11. Fazio VW: Advances in the surgery of rectal carcinoma utilizing the surgical stapler. In: Spratt JS, ed: Neoplasms of the Colon, Rectum & Anus: Mucosal and Epithelial. Philadelphia: WB Saunders, 1984:268–288.
12. Jagelman D, Fazio VW, Lavery IC, Weakley FL, Matana C: Results of stapled anastomoses to rectum. Dis Colon Rectum (in press).
13. Gordon PH, Vasilevsky CA: Experience with stapling in rectal surgery. Surg Clin North Am 64(3):555–566, 1984.
14. Ravitch MM: Varieties of stapled anastomosis in rectal resection. Surg Clin North Am 64(3):543–554, 1984.
15. Reid JD, Robins RE, Atkinson KG: Pelvic recurrence after anterior resection and EEA stapling anastomosis with potentially curable carcinoma of the rectum. Am J Surg 147:629–632, 1984.

CHAPTER 47

SUBTOTAL COLECTOMY FOLLOWED BY STAPLED CECO-RECTAL ANASTOMOSIS

J. Mouiel, N. Katkhouda, J. Gugenheim, P. Fabiani, D. Le Goff, E. Benizri, and B. Gouboux

Subtotal colectomy with ceco-rectal anastomosis saves the cecum, the ileo-cecal valve, and the terminal ileum. The advantage lies in avoiding diarrhea and malabsorption of biliary salts usually observed after subtotal colectomy. We have used this method in 30 patients with good results.

OPERATIVE TECHNIQUE

The first step of the operation is the large bowel resection. A limited elevation of the mesocolon is used and vascular ligatures are placed near the bowel border if the operation is for benign disease. Complete mobilization is necessary in case of a malignant tumor where blood vessels have to be secured near their origin. Only the ileo-cecal pedicle is carefully kept and protected (Fig. 47-1).

The reestablishment of bowel continuity is done by ceco-rectal anastomosis using a circular (EEA or ILS) and a linear stapling instrument (TA or LS). Usually the cecum lies in contact with the rectal ampulla. If this is not the case, mobilization of the mesocecum is completed. An end-to-end anastomosis using the largest-diameter stapler (EEA-31 or ILS-33) is performed. The central rod and cartridge without the anvil are placed through an ascending colotomy, and the central rod is brought through the appendicular stump. The position of the ileo-cecal valve is checked to avoid including it in the anastomosis. The anvil is attached and inserted into the purse-stringed rectal ampulla, which is kept open with three stay sutures (Fig. 47-2). The purse-string is tied down against the central rod. The instrument is closed, fired, opened, and withdrawn by spiral twisting. The double rings of the excised bowel are carefully inspected. The cecum is closed above the ileo-cecal valve with a linear stapler that also excludes the EEA introduction colotomy. The specimen is removed distal to this linear closure (Figs. 47-3, 47-4). The anastomotic integrity is tested by transanal injection of air or methylene blue (or both), using a double catheter placed prior to the operation.

INDICATIONS

From 1984 to 1988, 30 patients (17 women and 13 men) underwent operations by this method. The mean age was 71 years (ages ranged from 42 to 91 years). These patients had lesions of the left colon associated with lesions of the transverse colon, leaving the cecum intact.

Twelve patients presented with diffuse diverticulosis complicated by stenosis (9) or by hemorrhage (3)—among these last 3, 1 was associated with a villous tumor.

Eight patients had carcinoma: 4 of the transverse colon (1 associated with sigmoiditis, another associated with multiple polyps) and 4 of the left side of the large bowel (2 recurrences after initial segmental colectomy and 2 carcinomas associated with multiple polyps).

Four patients had acquired megacolon and failure of medical treatment; among them, 3 had occlusive complications.

Three patients had anastomotic stenoses after left colectomy.

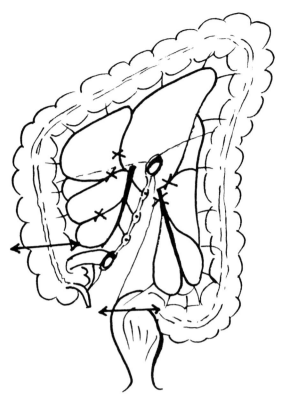

Fig. 47-1. The extent of colon resection.

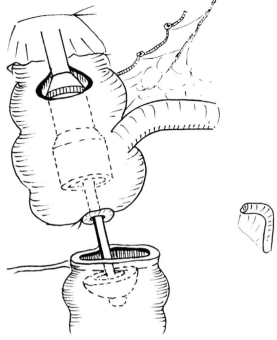

Fig. 47-2. Placement of the circular instrument, without anvil, through a lateral ascending colotomy, advancing the central rod through the base of the amputated appendix. The anvil is attached and placed into the purse-string-sutured rectum.

Two patients had non-familiar multiple polyposis, and 1 had reestablishment of continuity after left colectomy for sigmoiditis done in another institution and complicated by anastomotic leakage and peritonitis.

RESULTS

Considering the age of the patients and the presence of important and multiple risks (8 patients were ASA-III, 9 were ASA-II), immediate results were excellent, since we did not record any deaths.

Immediate followup showed 3 complications that were resolved by non-operative treatment. One patient with severe rectal bleeding, confirmed by endoscopy, required 3 units of blood postoperatively. One patient developed phlebitis while on anticoagulants, and 1 small anastomotic fistula was resolved without re-operation. In the long-term followup, we observed 1 anastomotic stricture, although a 31-mm diameter stapler was used. Operative correction was accomplished by using the same method, but with a 33-mm diameter stapler. Physiologic results 6 months after operation were promising, with 1 to 4 solid or fragmented stools per day (average was 2.1).

Some patients had diarrhea related to bad eating habits; these patients responded to dietetic rules and medical treatment. We did not notice persisting diarrhea, signs of malabsorption, or lithiasis.[1]

Endoscopic examination, performed in all cases after the operation, showed perfect permeability of the anastomosis with a well functioning cecal pouch with good compliance and emptying. Radiologic controls (with barium opacification carried out in 30% of patients) showed a reflux into the last jejunal loop. For this reason, we now prefer barium studies under low pressure.

DISCUSSION

Colo-rectal anastomosis using the right transverse colon mobilized and brought into the pelvis by a trans-mesenteric route (Toupet)[2] may be difficult in the case of a thick meso-colon. Other methods have been used: mobilization and swinging of the right colon (Courriade)[3] or freeing and turning over of the right colon (Deloyers).[4] Use of these methods is restricted by the size of the right colic artery. The ceco-rectal anastomosis, described for the first time in 1955 by Lillehei and Wangensteen, comprises the

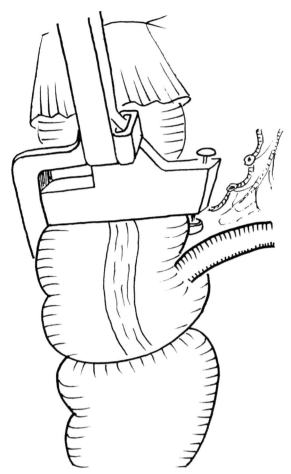

Fig. 47-3. Closure of the cecum above the ileo-cecal valve (linear stapler), excluding colotomy and specimen (if left attached).

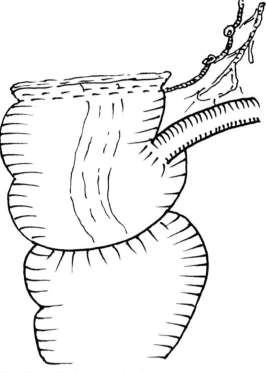

Fig. 47-4. Final aspect of end-to-end ceco-rectal anastomosis.

mobilization of the cecum and its swinging toward the opening rectal stump to perform a manual end-to-end anastomosis.[5] This method was successful for 13 patients with cancer, polyps, and diverticula. Rosi and Cahill used this technique in 1962 for 15 patients presenting with multiple polyps, and obtained good results.[6] Ryan and Oakley, in 1984, described a combined ceco-rectal side-to-side anastomosis that was mechanical for the closing of the cecum, manual for the ceco-rectal anastomosis.[7]

Since 1977, 21 patients have undergone operations with this procedure for cancer, polyps, diverticula, and angio-dysplasia. Ryan and Oakley noticed excellent results, without mortality, considering the age of the patients and the risk factors. The method described in this chapter,[8] with a mechanical ceco-rectal end-to-end anastomosis, is easy to perform. After mobilization of the cecum, we can slide it down

into the pelvis. The ileo-ceco-appendicular artery, which runs in the mesocolon, provides good vascularization of the last jejunal loop and of the cecum. We used the largest circular stapler admitted by the bowel lumina to avoid stenosis (e.g., we used the 33-, 31-, 29-, and 28-mm ILS and EEA and observed only one stricture (EEA-31), due probably to an asymptomatic leak with temporary blind fistula.

In preserving the cecum and the ileo-cecal valve, diarrhea and malabsorption, usually observed after total colectomy, are prevented. Experimentally, Kelley demonstrated in dogs that the ileo-cecal valve behaves like a sphincter.[9] Similar findings were demonstrated in man by Cohen.[10] Manometric pressures were measured on 5 patients; the ileo-rectal pressure barrier was 4 cm. The sphincter seems to play a role in the prevention of malabsorption, diarrhea, and retrograde flow. In the case of a high colon pressure (enema, for example), the ileo-cecal valve is incompetent in 90% of patients. Gazet studied the surgical importance of the ileo-cecal valve in 175 patients with right or left colectomy.[1] Diarrhea seemed to be related to the resection of the valve and extent of the resection.

It is well known that the terminal ileum absorbs

water, electrolytes, biliary salts, and vitamin B12.[11] The colon, and more so the cecum, play an important role in this absorption of water. In normal patients, 95% of the water goes through the colon; 1.5 l per day are reabsorbed.[12] We frequently observed diarrhea after total colectomy with ileo-rectal anastomosis (even with a proper diet and medical treatment). The subtotal colectomy with mechanical ceco-rectal anastomosis is a simple and effective procedure to treat benign or malignant tumors and to avoid diarrhea, malabsorption, and lithiasis. During 7 years, Ottinger studied 43 patients who had total colectomy (excluding inflammatory disease).[13] Fifty-six percent of them had more than 3 stools per day; 16% had more than 6. These facts confirm the advantage of preserving the last ileal loop and the ileo-cecal valve, pathologic findings permitting, to avoid diarrhea and malabsorption. The elective absorption of biliary salts by the terminal ileum maintains the entero-hepatic cycle and prevents lithiasis.

REFERENCES

1. Gazet JC: The surgical significance of the ileo-cecal junction. Ann R Coll Surg Engl 48:19–38, 1968.
2. Toupet A: Quelques considérations sur la vascularisation des colons et leurs abaissements dans la chirurgie du colon gauche et du rectum. Rev Chir 70:79–92, 1951.
3. Courriade S: La bascule de l'hémicolon droit dans la chirurgie du colon gauche et du rectum. Mem Acad Chir 84:545–548, 1958.
4. Deloyers L: La bascule du colon droit permet sans exception de connecter le sphincter anal après colectomie étendue du transverse et du colon gauche. Techniques. Indications. Résultats. Lyon Chir 60:404–413, 1964.
5. Lillehei RC, Wangensteen OH: Bowel junction after colectomy for cancer, polyps and diverticulitis. JAMA 159:163–170, 1955.
6. Rosi PA, Cahill WJ: Subtotal colectomy with cecorectal anastomosis for multiple adenomas of the colon. Am J Surg 103:75–80, 1962.
7. Ryan JA, Oakley WC: Cecoproctostomy. Am J Surg 144:636–639, 1985.
8. Mouiel J: Anastomose caeco-rectale et colectomie presque totale. In: Welter R, Patel JC, eds: Chirurgie Mécanique Digestive. Paris: Masson, 1985:252.
9. Kelley ML, Gordon EA, Deweese JA: Pressure responses of canine ileocotomic junctional zone to intestinal distension. Am J Physiol 211:43–56, 1966.
10. Cohen S, Harris D, Levitan R: Manometric characteristic of the human ileo-caecal junctional zone. Gastroenterology 54:72–75, 1968.
11. Levitan R, Fordtran JS, Burrows BA, Ingelfinger FJ: Water and salt absorption in the human colon. J Clin Invest 41:1754–1759, 1962.
12. Philips SF, Giller J: The contribution of the colon to electrolyte and water conservation in man. J Lab Clin Med 81:733–746, 1973.
13. Ottinger LW: Frequency of bowel movements after colectomy with ileo-rectal anastomosis. Am Surg 113:1048–1049, 1978.

ABDOMINAL SIDE-TO-END COLO-RECTAL ANASTOMOSIS WITH CIRCULAR STAPLING INSTRUMENTS

J.Cl. Ollier, M. Gavioli-Ferrari, and M. Adloff

Between January 1977 and December 1987, 280 operations were performed in our department using the side-to-end colo-rectal anastomosis after rectosigmoid resections. Since we first described this technique,[1,2,3] indications and technique have become well defined.

OPERATIVE TECHNIQUE

With the patient positioned in dorsal decubitus, the colo-rectal anastomosis is accomplished through a lower midline incision (Fig. 48-1). The dissection of the specimen is curative in intent, as it would be with any other plan of colo-rectal reconstruction, and the dissection is always carried to the floor of the pelvis to assure a radical cancer excision and to allow maximum elevation of the rectum to facilitate anastomosis.

A clamp is applied transversely at a safe distance beyond the tumor. The rectum is transected progressively below this clamp, using stay sutures to keep the open rectum exposed in the operative site and to allow additional intraluminal rectal Betadine irrigation. The purse-string suture is placed manually using a monofilament suture in a whip-stitch over-and-over fashion. The size of the rectal lumen is measured with Heggar dilators.

After selection of an anastomotic site on the proximal colon, at a safe distance proximal to the tumor, a colotomy is performed at a point that will be part of the specimen. Following injection of 2 ampules of glucagon intravenously, the colon is dilated with Heggar bougies. The size of the largest bougie safely accepted by the bowel lumen will decide the size of the EEA instrument to be used. The circular stapler without its anvil is then placed into the lumen of the colon through the colotomy and the central rod is pushed against the antimesenteric surface of the colon, proximal to the colotomy site. The central rod is then advanced through a small stab wound in the antimesenteric bowel wall, and the anvil is attached and advanced into the rectum. After tying the purse-string around the central rod, the instrument is closed and the anastomosis is accomplished.

Note: This procedure is greatly facilitated by the recent availability of the CEEA stapler, in which the cartridge can be placed—as described here—with perforation of the bowel wall by the central rod made easier with the newly available trocart. In addition, the detachable anvil with its own rod can be placed separately into the distal rectum and the purse-string suture tied around it. The rod of the anvil is then anchored into the hollow rod of the cartridge, after removal of its trocart. The instrument is closed just as with the original technique, and anastomosis is achieved. After removal of the circular instrument and examination of the anastomosis and tissue rings, the excess colon (representing the specimen) is closed flush with the circular anastomosis by a transverse application of the linear TA-55 instrument. Transection along the TA instrument on the specimen side yields the tumor and the temporary colotomy as one

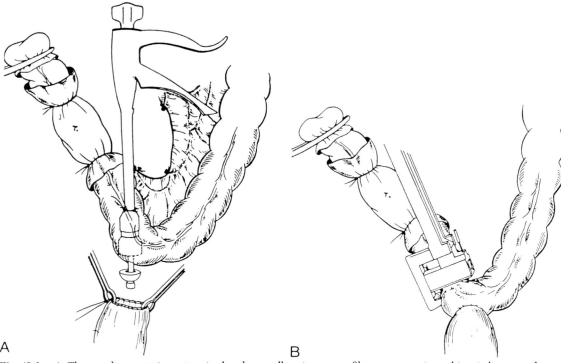

A   B

Fig. 48-1. *A.* The rectal purse-string suture is placed manually using a monofilament suture in a whip-stitch over-and-over fashion. The size of the rectal lumen is measured with Heggar dilators. Following the selection of an anastomotic site on the proximal colon at a safe distance proximal to the tumor, a colotomy is performed at a point that will be part of the specimen. The circular stapler without its anvil is then placed into the lumen of the colon through the colotomy. The central rod is pushed against the antimesenteric surface of the colon, somewhat proximal to the colotomy site. The central rod is then advanced through a small stab wound in the antimesenteric bowel wall. The anvil is attached and advanced into the rectum. After tying the pursestring around the central rod, the instrument is closed andthe anastomosis is accomplished. *B.* After removal of the circular instrument and examination of anastomosis and tissue rings, the excess colon, representing the specimen, is closed flush with the circular anastomosis by a transverse application of the linear TA–55 instrument. Transection along the TA-instrument on the specimen side yields the tumor and the temporary colotomy as one piece.

piece. We do not use a decompressing temporary proximal colostomy, nor do we examine intra-operatively the competence of the anastomosis with the injection of fluid or air. Retro-rectal drainage is usually but not routinely established.

This technique has the advantage of exposing the abdominal cavity to the open bowel lumen for a very short duration, and permits total visual control of all of the technical details of anastomosis.

CLINICAL EXPERIENCE

In 280 patients, colo-rectal anastomosis using circular instruments was performed through a transanal approach in 199 patients, and through an abdominal approach in only 89 patients. Among the 89 abdominal anastomoses, 8 were with the end-to-end triangulating method, 6 were side-to-side anastomoses using the GIA-TA technique, and 75 were achieved with the side-to-end anastomosis described in this

chapter. The results of the 75 operations will now be analyzed (Table 48-1).

Intra-operatively, the anastomosis appeared to be incomplete in 7 patients, requiring the placement of

Table 48-1. Analysis of Side-to-End Colo-Rectal Anastomoses

	Side-to-End (75)	Overall (280)
Sex		
Male	38	156
Female	37	124
Age (average	66.2	64.6
and range)	(25–85)	(30–83)
Etiology		
Cancer	78.6%	83.6%
Stage D	20.3%	19.2%
Sigmoid	18.6%	14.0%
Diverticulitis	57.1%	56.4%
Other	2.6%	2.5%

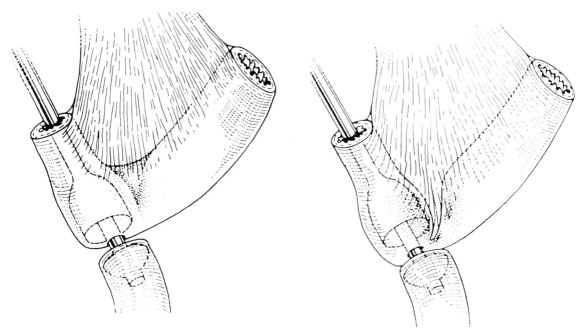

Fig. 48-2. Re-operation was necessary because of the accidental inclusion of a spur of proximal colon wall along its mesocolic border as the instrument was placed into position and closed. Re-operation took place on the eighth day and showed that this complication can only happen if the caliber of the bowel is too small for the cartridge chosen in a given case. In all of these anastomoses, it is important for the cartridge to slide with ease inside the lumen of the colon.

corrective individual manual sutures. On 3 occasions, the anastomotic deficiency was of a degree that mandated its protection after manual repair by a proximal temporary decompressing colostomy.

The postoperative course as it relates to the operative technique was uncomplicated in 64 patients (85.3%), with no complications related to the anastomotic technique or to the abdominal operative procedure. Average hospital stay was 12.3 days postoperatively.

Postoperative fecal leakage occurred through the retro-rectal drainage site and was observed on 8 occasions. All of these episodes were benign, never complicated by peritonitis or abscess formation in the cul-de-sac of Douglas. Seven of these complications subsided spontaneously, 3 of them under the protec-

tion of a primary proximal colostomy. The remaining patient required re-operation with colostomy for a total separation of the anastomosis produced by the operative extraction of an inspissated calcified fecaloma.

One patient with postoperative bleeding required blood transfusions, and in another re-operation was necessary because of the accidental inclusion of a spur of proximal colon wall along its mesocolic border, as the instrument was placed into position and closed. Re-operation took place on the eighth day and showed that this complication can only happen if the caliber of the bowel is too small for the cartridge chosen in a given case. In all of these anastomoses it is important for the cartridge to slide with ease inside the lumen of the colon (Fig. 48-2).

Table 48-2. Colo-Rectal Anastomoses: Comparison of Results

Type of Anastomosis	n	Average Hospital Stay	Primary Colostomy	Benign Postop. Course	Clinical Fistula	Secondary Colostomy
Manual						
Interrupted sutures	97	13.2	2	87 (89.7%)	3 (3.1%)	0
Running sutures	27	12.3	0	27 (100%)	0	0
End-to-side	75	12.3	3	64 (85.3%)	8 (10.7%)	1
End-to-end	119	15.3	2	95 (79.8%)	18 (15.1%)	1
Double stapling technique (Knight)	72	15.1	7	66 (91.7%)	4 (5.6%)	2

Table 48-3. Colo-Rectal Anastomosis: Comparison of Complications

Type of Anastomosis	n	Strictures	Hemorrhages	Miscellaneous	Mortality Overall	Staple-Related
Manual						
Interrupted sutures	97	0	0	2 (2.1%)	4 (4.1%)	–
Running sutures	27	0	0	0	0	–
End-to-side	75	0	1 (1.3%)	1 (1.3%)	5 (6.7%)	2 (2.7%)
End-to-end	119	6 (5.0%)	3 (2.5%)	2 (1.7%)	3 (2.5%)	1 (0.8%)
Double stapling technique (Knight)	72	2 (2.8%)	1 (1.4%)	0	3 (2.5%)	2 (1.7%)

Three patients died, 1 from other causes and 2 with an anastomotic leak and fistula. Of these, 1 patient died on the sixth postoperative day from renal insufficiency following postoperative septic shock, and the second patient died on the twentieth day from progressive liver failure due to cirrhosis.

DISCUSSION

The group of patients benefiting from a side-to-end abdominal colo-rectal anastomosis is comparable to the overall group of patients receiving stapled colo-rectal anastomoses, with respect to age, tumor stage, other existing diseases, and incidence of diverticulitis. The only difference was the level of rectal transection, which was slightly higher in the side-to-end anastomoses than in the end-to-end anastomoses.

We will therefore compare these results with those obtained in 191 original stapled transanal anastomoses (end-to-end technique 119, double stapling technique 72) and those of 124 anastomoses performed manually (interrupted sutures 97, running sutures 27) (Tables 48-2, 48-3). The abdominal side-to-end anastomoses are compared to these two groups to reach some conclusions about our preference in operative technique (Tables 48-2, 48-3).

The duration of postoperative hospitalization of

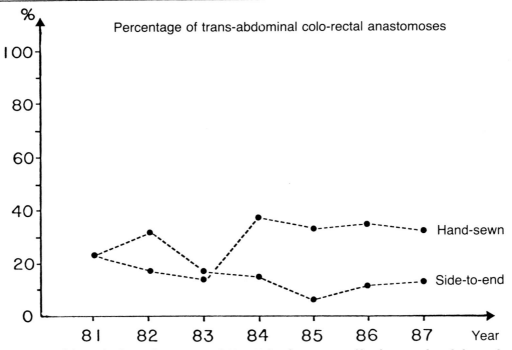

Fig. 48-3. Trans-abdominal colo-rectal anastomoses (1981–1987) and percentage of hand-sewn and stapled procedures.

COLO-RECTAL ANASTOMOSES

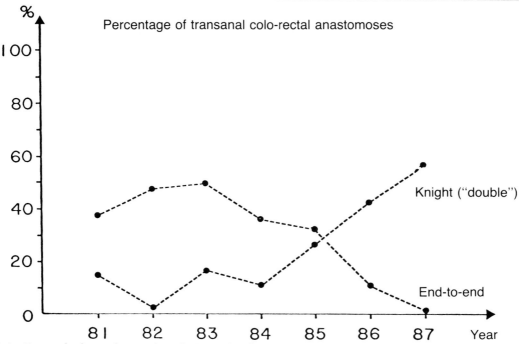

Fig. 48-4. Transanal colo-rectal anastomoses (1981–1987) and percentage of "double" (Knight) stapling technique, as compared to end-to-end EEA anastomoses using two purse-string sutures.

12.3 days with end-to-side abdominal anastomoses is comparable to the 12.3 and 13.2 days of the manual anastomoses. Both are significantly shorter (p < 0.01) then the postoperative hospitalization following transanal anastomosis (15.3 and 15.1 days). This is almost certainly due to the fact that if the operative status is allowing for an abdominal anastomosis, the dissection is less traumatic and the postoperative course much smoother.

However, the incidence of anastomotic leaks and fistula formation, similar between the various stapled anastomoses, is definitely higher than with the manual anastomosis (p < 0.05). This frequency resembles that obtained with anastomoses placed to the distal third of the rectum. However, our study is flawed in that it compares successive or non-randomized cases and describes the first years of the learning curve with mechanical sutures. During this time, the indi-

Table 48-4. Colo-Rectal Anastomosis: Comparison of Results (1985–1987)

Type of Anastomosis	n	Average Hosp. Stay	Benign Postop. Course	Primary Colostomy	Clinically Apparent Leak	Secondary Colostomy	Morbidity	Mortality Overall	Staple-Related
Manual									
Interrupted sutures	49	13.1	44 (89.8%)	0	1 (2.0%)	0	2 (4.1%)	2 (4.1%)	–
Running sutures	24	11.9	23 (95.8%)	0	0	0	1 (4.2%)	0	–
End-to-side	15	12.5	15 (100%)	0	0	0	0	0	0
End-to-end	17	14.8	14 (82.4%)	0	3 (17.6%)	1 (5.9%)	0	0	0
Double stapling technique									
(Knight)	54	15.3	51 (94.4%)	5 (9.3%)	3 (5.6%)	1 (1.9%)	0	1 (1.9%)	1 (1.9%)

cations for each individual technique evolved, and some of them were abandoned (Figs. 48-3, 48-4).

It seems therefore more logical to compare the results with colo-rectal anastomoses that were obtained in our department between 1 January 1985 and 31 December 1987. These cases were done using alternate techniques but without randomization. Of 159 colo-rectal anastomoses, 73 were done by hand (24 by running sutures, 49 by interrupted sutures), 71 were done with circular staples transanally (17 by end-to-end anastomosis, 54 by the double stapling technique of Knight), and 15 were of the side-to-end type described in this chapter. All 15 side-to-end anastomoses had uncomplicated postoperative courses, without the need for a primary or secondary protecting colostomy, or for the placement of corrective sutures intra-operatively (Table 48-4). This improvement, much superior to our overall results, is due to the fact that the technical indications and details were more clearly established, thanks to our previous experience, and because the decision of the level of the rectal transection and the caliber of the colon lumen was based on a better understanding of the requirements for success in this operation—in spite of the fact that this type of anastomosis was more often performed under less favorable circumstances by younger surgeons, operating on higher-risk patients with poorly prepared bowels.

CONCLUSIONS

The trans-abdominal side-to-end colo-rectal anastomosis with staplers is reliable and technically simple, provided these conditions are respected:

1. The caliber of the colon lumen equals or surpasses 30 mm in diameter, allowing the placement of a cartridge of sufficient size that can slide with ease inside the colic lumen.
2. The underlying disease, whether cancer or diverticulitis, permits the transection of the rectum at its upper or middle third, with a sufficiently large pelvis to allow complete and satisfactory visual inspection of the anastomosis during its different stages of construction. The indication for this type of anastomosis exists following anterior recto-sigmoid resection. The result compares favorably to that of manual anastomosis at the same level; the latter is obtained, however, at lesser cost.

Translated from the French by F.M. Steichen, M.D.

REFERENCES

1. Adloff M, Arnaud JP, Beeharry S, Turbelin JM: Side-to-end anastomosis in low anterior resection with the EEA stapler. Dis Colon Rectum 23(7):456–458, 1980.
2. Adloff M, Arnaud JP, Ollier JC: Place des anastomoses mécaniques circulaires dans la résection rectale pour néoplasme. Chirurgie 106(6):393–399, 1980.
3. Adloff M, Psalmon F, Welter R: Chirurgie du côlon et du rectum. In Welter R, Patel JCl: Chirurgie Mécanique Digestive. Paris: Masson, 1985:274–275.
4. Adloff M, Ollier JCl, Arnaud JP: Pièce de l'anastomose termino-latérale à la pince à suture mécanique. Presse Méd 12(21):1359–1361, 1983.

CHAPTER 49

STAPLED COLO-RECTAL ANASTOMOSIS THROUGH STAPLED DISTAL RECTUM

C.D. Knight Sr., F.D. Griffen, J.M. Whitaker, and C.D. Knight, Jr.

The original technique for low rectal anastomosis with the EEA stapler was described by Ravitch and Steichen in 1979.[1] In 1980, we reported our modification in which the lower rectal segment is closed with a linear stapler (TA-55), and the anastomosis with the EEA stapler is performed across the linear staple line (combined or double-stapling technique).[2] Our experience in 64 patients with such stapled colo-rectal anastomoses is the basis of this chapter.

MATERIALS AND METHODS

From June 1979 to December 1987, 64 patients had colo-rectal anastomoses using the combined or double-stapling technique. There were 28 men and 36 women, with a mean age of 65 years (range: 28 to 83 years); two thirds of these patients were in the seventh and eighth decades of life. Indications for operations are shown in Table 49-1. Forty-four patients had carcinoma of the recto-sigmoid colon, 15 had diverticulitis, 3 had carcinoma of the ovary, 1 had volvulus, and 1 had rectal prolapse. Among the 44 patients with carcinoma of the recto-sigmoid, preoperative location of tumors measured by rigid proctos-

Table 49-1. Indications for Operation

Diagnosis	n
Carcinoma recto-sigmoid colon	44
Diverticular disease	15
Carcinoma ovary	3
Volvulus sigmoid colon	1
Prolapse rectum	1

copy from the anal verge is shown in Table 49-2. Seventeen patients had tumors at 8 cm or below. Levels of anastomosis are shown in Table 49-3. Eighteen were below 6 cm.

TECHNIQUE

We have previously described the technique for low rectal reconstruction after extended low anterior resection using the combined stapler technique with the standard EEA instrument. The recent modifications by the United States Surgical Corporation of the circular stapling device (premium CEEA TM) and TA-55 stapler (Roticulator 55 TM) makes them even better-suited for this technique. Although surgeons using the traditional EEA and TA-55 staplers can still gain technical advantage using the technique previously described, the following description utilizes the new instruments, which further facilitate the procedure.

With the patient in the lithotomy-Trendelenburg position, providing for the simultaneous exposure of abdomen and perineum, the abdomen is entered through a low midline incision and the abdominal cavity is explored. The recto-sigmoid colon is mobilized as in any other anterior resection and, if it is determined that a low anterior resection is feasible, the mesorectum is divided. The 4.8-mm Roticulator 55 TM, a TA-55 stapler with a cartridge that can rotate and swivel on the instrument's shaft, is placed across the rectum at the distal margin of resection. The cartridge is placed at the proper angle to maximize exposure and resection margin, closed, and activated (Fig. 49-1). Pressure, applied to the perineum

Table 49-2. Distance of Tumor from Anal Verge

Distance (cm)	n
6–8	17
9–10	10
11–15	17

Table 49-3. Distance of Anastomosis from Anal Verge

Distance (cm)	n
3–6	18
7–9	16
10–13	30

by an assistant to elevate the region of dissection, aids in exposure for lower lesions. A long right-angle clamp placed proximal to the staple line prevents soilage. The rectum is divided along the proximal edge of the roticulator (Fig. 49-2). The purse-string instrument is applied to the colon at the proximal resection margin. The purse-string is placed by passing a 2-0 monofilament suture on a Keith needle through the purse-string instrument. An Ochsner clamp is placed

distal to the purse-string, the colon is transected, and the specimen is removed. A non-crushing clamp is applied across the proximal colon, and the purse-string instrument is removed. Sizers are passed proximally into the sigmoid lumen. If only the small sizer will enter, the middle-sized cartridge can be used; if the middle-sized sizer will enter the lumen, the large cartridge is chosen. We caution against the use of the small cartridge for this anastomosis. It may be too

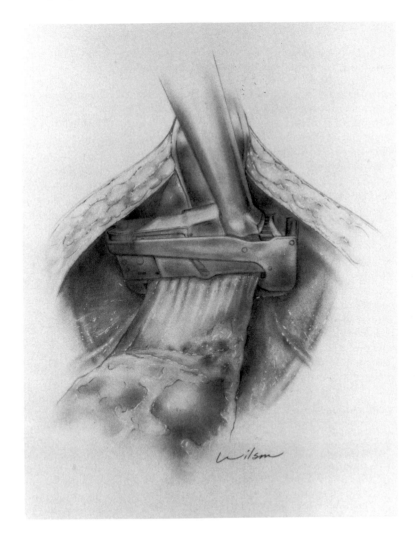

Fig. 49-1. After the recto-sigmoid colon has been mobilized, the Roticulator-55 stapler is applied at the lower limit of the resection and a double row of staples is placed.

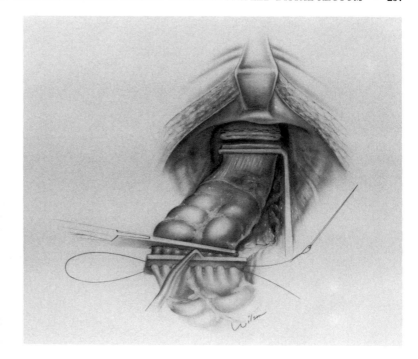

Fig. 49-2. A long right-angle clamp is placed proximal to the staple line, and the rectum is divided along the edge of the stapler. After the upper limit of resection is selected, the mesentery is divided and the colon is incised between the purse-string instrument proximally and an Ochsner clamp. (From Knight CD, Griffen FD: An improved technique for low anterior resection of the rectum using the EEA stapler. Surgery 88:710, 1980; with permission.)

small to accommodate the purse-stringed ring of bowel from the thick-walled rectum.

The anvil shaft assembly is then placed in the proximal bowel through the purse-string (Fig. 49-3) and the purse-string is tied into the groove on the shaft. The intestinal clamp can then be removed. Using the edge of the anvil as the proximal extent of dissection, the fatty appendices and mesentery are removed, allowing for the approximation of bowel wall rather than fat at the anastomosis.

Attention is then turned to the perineum. The instrument tray is moved to allow the assisting surgeon access to the anus. The rectal segment is irrigated transanally with sterile water under pressure from an irrigating syringe to examine for possible leaks or staple failures in the TA closure (Fig. 49-4). If in high anterior resections the distal pouch is too large to distend with 50 ml of fluid, a Foley catheter can be used through the anus to facilitate the injection of larger quantities of water. Any leaks detected are repaired with sutures.

The Premium CEEA TM stapler is introduced into the rectal segment with the anvil shaft assembly removed and the center rod retracted within the cartridge. The cartridge is centered at the Roticulator 55 TM staple line, and the hollow rod of the cartridge is advanced superiorly to allow its transmural visualization anterior or posterior to the staple row. Through

a stab wound in the bowel at that site, the rod is extended through the rectal wall adjacent to the staple line (Figs. 49-5, 49-6). The anvil shaft is anchored into the hollow cartridge rod. The premium CEEA TM is closed and activated to make a circular end-to-end inverting anastomosis (Fig. 49-7). No attempt is made to include the entire circumference of the rectal segment; only that part that matches the proximal colon is made part of the anastomosis.

We have used the trocart provided with the Premium CEEA TM for puncture of the rectal stump below. However, we prefer to make the stab wound after its site is chosen by the extended blunt hollow rod, thus eliminating the risk of penetration by the trocart at an imperfect site.

Two or three partial thickness mattress sutures of 3-0 silk are placed across the anastomosis, when it is technically feasible. The premium CEEA TM is then opened no more than three complete turns and the instrument is removed, using the mattress sutures for counter traction. The tissue in the chamber is checked to ensure that two complete rings, or doughnuts, are present. A shoe-string clamp is placed across the colon above the staple row, and the integrity of the anastomosis is checked by irrigating the rectum with water under pressure (Fig. 49-8). The bowel inflates and deflates with pressure changes; any leaks detected are repaired with silk sutures. A

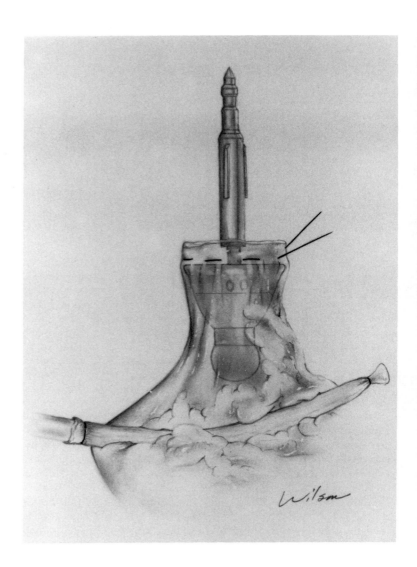

Fig. 49-3. After selection of the proper cartridge, the anvil shaft assembly is detached from the central rod and placed in the proximal bowel through the purse-string, and the suture is tied into the groove on the shaft.

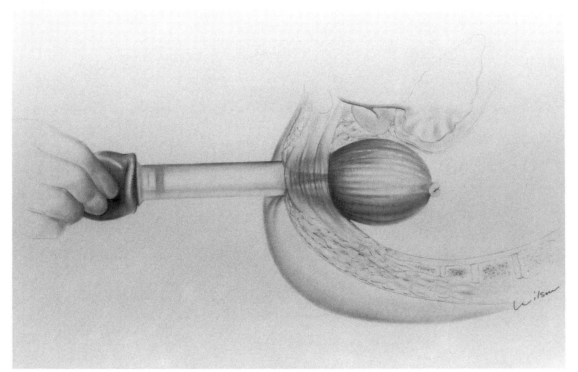

Fig. 49-4. The rectal segment is irrigated with water under pressure from an irrigating syringe to ascertain leaks or staple failures. (From Knight CD, Griffen FD: An improved technique for low anterior resection of the rectum using the EEA stapler. Surgery 88:710, 1980; with permission.)

sump drain, covered with a Penrose drain, is placed deep within the pelvis and is brought through a stab wound in the left lower quadrant. The pelvic peritoneum is not sutured, and the abdomen is closed in the usual manner.

RESULTS

Intra-operative complications were infrequent and usually minor. All doughnuts were intact circumferentially, although several were not full-thickness and others had mucosal tails. There were minor intra-operative water leaks in two anastomoses, which were easily repaired with sutures. There was no intra-operative anastomotic disruption, and protective colostomy was not performed in this series.

Postoperative complications were also rare. One patient developed a clinical anastomotic leak, which healed with non-operative treatment. Neither surgical drainage nor colostomy was required. Two patients had stenosis and stricture of the anastomosis that required treatment. One of these patients, with carcinoma of the rectum, developed a benign anasto-

motic stricture at 10 cm. Digital dilatation under anaesthesia was successful after the fibrous ring was fractured with the biopsy forceps. A second patient developed a high stricture after resection for diverticulitis and required reoperation and resection using the EEA stapler. Although 18 patients had anastomoses within 6 cm of the anal verge, no patient has been permanently incontinent. There were no deaths in this series. The followup of patients with malignant disease has not been adequate for statistical evaluation of recurrence.

DISCUSSION

The chief attraction of the EEA stapler is that it permits most surgeons to perform a low anterior anastomosis safely at a lower level than was feasible with other intra-abdominal techniques.

The double-stapling technique described here offers several advantages: (1) it obviates the technical frustration involved in placing the lower purse-string suture and permits a lower anastomosis in some pa-

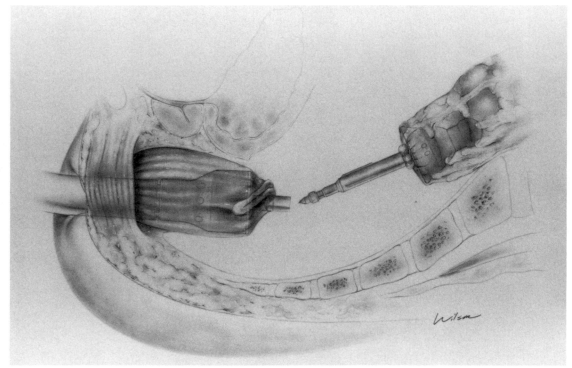

Fig. 49-5. The Premium CEEA stapler is introduced into the rectal segment with the anvil shaft assembly removed and the center rod retracted within the cartridge. The center rod is passed through a stab wound adjacent to the staple line.

tients; (2) the rectal segment is not opened, which minimizes intra-operative contamination; (3) it avoids problems of joining segments of bowel of disparate size (wide rectal ampulla to normal or smaller sigmoid colon), which may cause anastomotic complications.

There has been some concern that the intersecting staple lines that result from this procedure might increase the risk of anastomotic leak. In theory, this concern might seem justified. However, Julian and Ravitch addressed this problem in experimental studies in dogs and showed that although the linear staples are usually removed with the doughnuts and are deformed, cut, or squeezed out, no leaks occurred.[3] Reports of increasing clinical experience also attest to the safety of stapling across staple lines.[4,5,6]

Although we have found the original instrumentation introduced for end-to-end rectal reconstruction satisfactory for the double-stapling procedure, recent innovations in the staplers have made the technique easier and safer. The Roticulator 55 TM, with its adjustable cartridge, allows the rectum to be stapled at a lower level in some patients. Two changes in the EEA instrument facilitate the anastomosis. The ability to recess the naked center rod within the cartridge

allows safer passage of the instrument, especially if the pouch is long. The chief improvement, however, results from maintaining a shaft on the anvil so that the anvil can be introduced into the proximal bowel prior to connecting it to the hollow rod of the cartridge. Thus, the proximal purse-string can be observed circumferentially as it is tied. The anvil shaft with the purse-string already tied can be easily attached to the Premium CEEA TM deep in the pelvis. This eliminates one of the difficult steps in the procedure—placing the proximal bowel over the anvil in the pelvis.

Anastomotic leak is the most feared complication of gastro-intestinal surgery and is the chief parameter by which success of rectal reconstruction is measured. The incidence of clinical leaks in stapled colorectal anastomoses varies in reported series, but historic controls with handsewn techniques indicate that 10% is an acceptable rate. In 1982, when the EEA instrument was relatively new and most reported series included 50 patients or less, we reviewed 23 reports, which included 919 patients with stapled anastomoses.[7] Clinical leaks occurred in 8%. A recently collected series of 10 reports since 1982

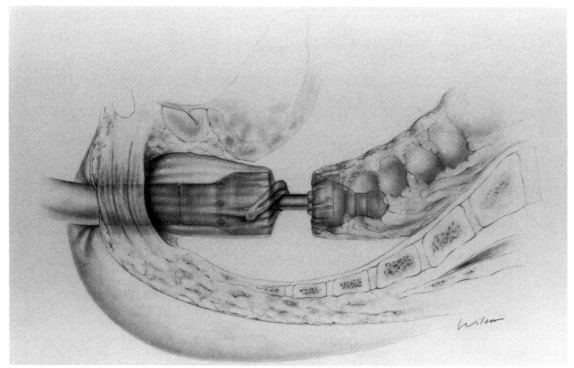

Fig. 49-6. The anvil shaft is inserted into the center rod and the instrument closure is begun.

yielded 1472 stapled colo-rectal anastomoses with 64 leaks, a rate of 4.3% (Table 49-4). The complication rate with the double-stapling technique is also encouraging. We have had 1 leak in 64 patients, no sepsis, and no protective colostomy was needed. Feinberg and associates have reported the results of the double-stapling method in 79 patients with carcinoma of the rectum and found 6 leaks, or a rate of 7.6%, with a mean level of anastomosis 5 cm above the dentate line.[4]

One of the criticisms of the EEA instrument concerns stenosis or stricture following its use. The incidence of this complication is difficult to determine, because the definition of stenosis is not standardized. In some series, stenosis is reported as occurring when the anastomosis will not permit the passage of the proctoscope, even though the patient is without symptoms. We believe that stenosis should be reported only when symptomatic, because asymptomatic "stenoses" are self-limiting, as demonstrated by followup endoscopy, which shows them to have disappeared.

In the 1982 review of 919 patients with stapled colo-rectal anastomoses, 31 had symptomatic stenoses, an incidence of 3%.[7] A review of the reports since 1982 is summarized in Table 49-5. Gordon and Dalrymple[8] reported an incidence of 17 to 20%, but a review of their data shows symptomatic stricture requiring treatment in only 1.4% of these. The overall stenosis rate in this collected series is 1.6%. Symptomatic stenosis following the double-stapling technique also occurs infrequently. Two patients of the 64 in our series required treatment for stenosis; Feinburg et al. noted no significant stenosis in 79 patients who had a similar procedure.

The cause of anastomotic stenosis is not completely understood. It is generally agreed that anastomotic leak may result in failure to heal by first intention, causing granulation, fibrosis, and stricture. Experimental studies[9,10] and clinical experience[11] indicate that stapled anastomoses heal by second intention, since the mucosa of the bowel segments is not in apposition but is separated by the muscular and serosal layers. Therefore, the precise stapled anastomosis predictably forms a perfect circular scar that results in narrowing of the intestinal lumen. Fortunately, this stenosis is almost always subclinical, and dilatation by the passage of feces ultimately provides for widely patent anastomoses, as observed at followup endoscopy. We have noted this process may

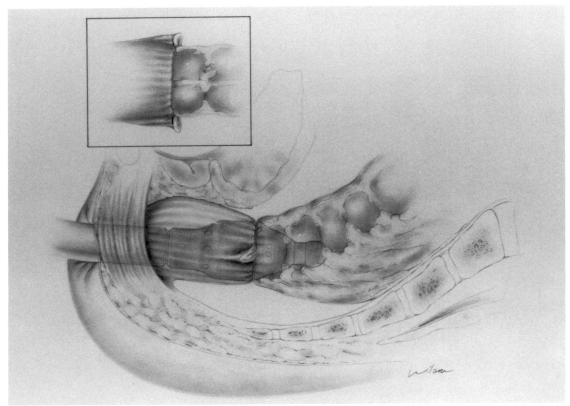

Fig. 49-7. The Premium CEEA stapler is closed and activated to make the circular end-to-end inverting anastomosis. No attempt is made to include the entire circumference of the rectal segment; only that part that matches the proximal colon is included.

take several months to 2 years. Postoperative stenosis is likely best prevented by avoiding both anastomotic leaks and protective colostomy, which prevents normal dilatation by passage of feces. We believe that the largest suitable cartridge should be used, because the smaller the circumference of the circular scar, the more likely it is to be symptomatic.

We have used this combined stapler technique at all levels of the rectum and sigmoid for anastomosis following resection for cancer and diverticulitis, but we find that it has its greatest applicability for low rectal reconstruction following resection for cancer. It is in these procedures that hand suturing or placement of a low purse-string suture becomes increasingly difficult, if not impossible, and the disparity in size of the bowel segments increases the hazards of the anastomosis.

Since the EEA-stapled anastomosis has been successfully used for rectal reconstruction at any level above the dentate line, the technique may replace other sphincter-saving procedures. These include ab-

domino-sacral resection, abdomino-transanal resection with colo-anal anastomosis, and trans-sacral and trans-sphincteric resections. It is probably not correct to say that the EEA stapler will make any procedure obsolete, because the stapler only offers another technique for rectal reconstruction following extended low anterior resection. A few surgeons will likely continue to be more comfortable with the abdomino-sacral and abdomino-anal procedures, yet many surgeons may use the EEA stapler to extend low anterior resection to lower levels using exposure, dissections, and concepts with which they are already familiar.

With improved techniques for sphincter preservation after rectal resection, there is an inclination to compromise the lower margin of resection for low anterior resection in patients with carcinoma of the rectum. This should be avoided. If the same strict criteria are observed in selecting candidates for extended low anterior resection with staple anastomosis that have been followed for low anterior resection

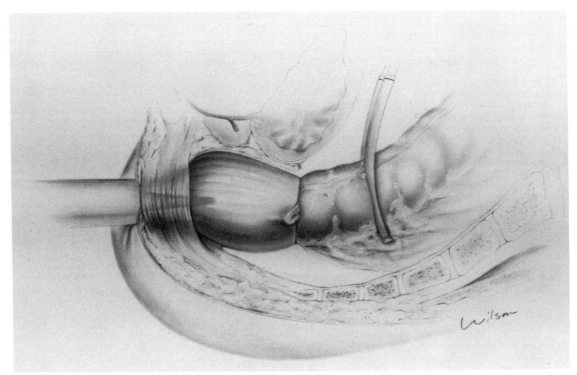

Fig. 49-8. After the stapler is removed, a shoestring clamp is placed across the colon above the anastomosis, and the integrity of the anastomosis is checked by irrigating the rectum with water under pressure. Leaks are repaired with silk sutures. (From Knight CD, Griffen FD: An improved technique for low anterior resection of the rectum using the EEA stapler. Surgery 88:710, 1980; with permission.)

with handsewn reconstruction, the recurrence and survival rates should remain the same. Lower lesions have higher local recurrence rates because of the more limited lateral resection, just as has been observed with abdomino-perineal resection for very low lesions. In patients with lesions high enough to be

candidates for hand-sewn anastomosis, the stapler enables the surgeon to provide a greater margin of resection below the tumor. Cure of the patient's cancer should continue to be the overriding objective, and preservation of the sphincter a secondary consideration.

Table 49-4. Incidence of Clinical Leaks with Stapled Colo-Rectal Anastomoses

Series, Year	n	Number leaks	% Leaks
Cutait and Cutait, 1986[12]	140	10	7.1
Fazio, 1984[13]	162	5	3.0
Fazio, 1985[14]	84	1	1.2
Feinberg et al, 1986[4]	79	6	7.6
Gordon and Dalrymple, 1986[8]	143	1	0.7
Kennedy et al, 1983[15]	174	8	4.6
Polglase, 1986[16]	120	13	10.8
Thiede et al, 1986[17]	301	16	5.3
Trollope et al, 1986[6]	205	3	1.5
Knight and Griffen, 1987	64	1	1.5
Totals	1472	64	4.3

Table 49-5. Incidence of Clinical Stenosis with Stapled Colo-rectal Anastomoses

Series, Year	n	Number Stenoses	% Stenosis
Cutait and Cutait, 1986[12]	140	3	2.1
Fazio, 1984[13]	162	1	0.6
Fazio, 1985[14]	84	0	0
Feinberg et al, 1986[4]	79	0	0
Gordon and Dalrymple, 1986[8]	143	2	1.4
Kennedy et al, 1983[12]	174	1	0.5
Polglase, 1986[16]	120	8	6.6
Thiede et al, 1986[17]	301	2	0.6
Trollope et al, 1986[6]	205	6	2.9
Knight and Griffen, 1987	64	2	3.1
	1472	25	1.6

REFERENCES

1. Ravitch MM, Steichen FM: A stapling instrument for end-to-end inverting anastomosis in the gastrointestinal tract. Ann Surg 189:791, 1979.
2. Knight CD, Griffen FD: An improved technique for low anterior resection of the rectum using the EEA stapler. Surgery 88:710, 1980.
3. Julian TB, Ravitch MM: Evaluation of the safety of end-to-end (EEA) stapling anastomoses across linear stapled closure. Surg Clin North Am 64:567, 1984.
4. Feinberg SM, Parker F, Cohen Z, et al: The double stapling technique for low anterior resection of rectal carcinoma. Dis Colon Rectum 29:885, 1986.
5. Griffen FD, Knight CD: Stapling technique for primary and secondary rectal anastomoses. Surg Clin North Am 64:579, 1984.
6. Trollope ML, Cohen RG, Lee RH, Cannon WB, Marzoni FA, Cressman RD: A 7 year experience with low anterior sigmoid resections using the EEA stapler. Am J Surg 152:11, 1986.
7. Knight CD, Griffen FD: Techniques of low rectal reconstruction. Curr Probl Surg 20:391, 1984.
8. Gordon PH, Dalrymple S: The use of staples for reconstruction after colonic and rectal surgery. In: Principles and Practice of Surgical Stapling. Ravitch MM, Steichen FM, eds: Chicago-London-Boca Raton: Year Book, 1987:402–431.
9. Polglase AL, Hughes ESR, McDermott FT, Pihl E, Burke FR: A comparison of end-to-end staple and suture colorectal anastomosis in the dog. Surg Gynecol Obstet 152:792, 1981.
10. Penninckx FM, Kerremans RP, Geboes KJ: The healing of single and double-row stapled circular anastomoses. Dis Colon Rectum 27:714, 1984.
11. Wong J, Cheung H, Lui R, Fan YW, Smith A, Siu KF: Esophagogastric anastomosis performed with a stapler. The occurrence of leakage and stricture. Surgery 101:408, 1987.
12. Cutait DE, Cutait R: Stapled anterior resection of the rectum. In: Principles and Practice of Surgical Stapling. Ravitch MM, Steichen FM, eds: Chicago-London-Boca Raton: Year Book, 1987:388–401.
13. Fazio VW: Advances in the surgery of rectal carcinoma utilizing the circular stapler. In: Neoplasms of the Colon, Rectum, and Anus. 1st Ed. Spratt JS, ed: Philadelphia: WB Saunders, 1984:268–288.
14. Fazio VW, Jagelman DG, Lavery IC, McGonagle BA: Evaluation of the Proximate-ILS circular stapler. Ann Surg 201:108, 1985.
15. Kennedy HL, Rothenberger DA, Goldberg SM, et al: Colocolostomy and coloproctostomy utilizing the circular intraluminal stapling devices. Dis Colon Rectum 26:145, 1983.
16. Polglase MS: Anterior resection for carcinoma of the rectum. In: Principles and Practice of Surgical Stapling. Ravitch MM, Steichen FM, eds: Chicago-London-Boca Raton: Year Book, 1987:373–387.
17. Thiede A, Jastarndt L, Schröder D, Schubert G, Hamelmann H: Prospective and controlled studies in colorectal surgery: a comparison of hand-sutured and stapled rectal anastomoses. In: Principles and Practice of Surgical Stapling. Ravitch MM, Steichen FM, eds: Chicago-London-Boca Raton: Year Book, 1987:432–462.

CHAPTER 50

COLO-ANAL PROCEDURE FOR RECTAL NEOPLASMS

Robert W. Beart, Jr.

The colo-anal anastomosis for rectal neoplasms is enjoying renewed popularity.[1] This operation offers an attractive alternative to a difficult low anterior anastomosis or an abdomino-perineal resection and end colostomy. Improved understanding of the surgical approach and physiology of defecation have resulted in a technically superior and functionally enhanced alternative to colostomy.[2] Although in our institution a large number of these procedures have been performed since the early 1950s,[3,4] since 1976 we have reported 29 and performed more than 70 colo-anal procedures with a modified technique that does not require a diverting stoma and has superior functional results.

INDICATIONS

Patients with neoplastic lesions of the rectum are generally best treated by surgical excision of the lesion. If the lesion is small, transanal excision may be possible. If a benign lesion is large, or if the patient would theoretically benefit from a perirectal lymphadenectomy, trans-abdominal excision is recommended. Removal of the tumor is rarely a problem. If a malignant lesion impinges on the anal canal, abdomino-perineal resection may be necessary to remove the tumor. However, if the anal canal is not involved, then removal of the anus, levators, and ischio-rectal fat has not been shown to enhance survival. Once the mass is removed trans-abdominally, technical limitations may prevent restoration of intestinal continuity; surgeons have frequently removed the anus because of technical inability to restore continuity.

The availability of the circular stapler has simpli-

fied rectal anastomosis,[5] but because it is not helpful in extraordinarily low and difficult situations, and because of concern that the use of this instrument may in some way contribute to an increased risk of local recurrence of the tumor,[6] we have increasingly turned to the use of the colo-anal anastomosis for low rectal neoplasms. In addition, this procedure has been useful in treating failed low anterior anastomoses, high rectal vaginal and rectal urethral fistulas, and radiation injuries to the rectum.

TECHNIQUE

With the patient in the combined lithotomy-Trendelenburg (Lloyd-Davies) position, mobilization of the sigmoid and rectum is performed in the standard abdominal manner. A wide lymphadenectomy is carried out. The sympathetic nerve fibers coursing over the sacral promontory are usually, although not always, sacrificed. Throughout the pelvic dissection, firm traction on the rectum helps to identify tissue planes. The lateral rectal attachments are bluntly or sharply divided close to the lateral pelvic wall. The hypogastric vessels are bared, but a lateral lymphadenectomy is not routinely performed. Anteriorly, the dissection is carried to the distal margin of the prostate in the male and well down onto the vagina in the female. Laterally, all stalks are divided that limit mobilization of the rectum when it is placed on tension. Posteriorly, the dissection is carried well past the coccyx to the point where the rectum passes through the levators. A soft muscular area of 2 to 3 cm can be felt between this point and the coccyx when the dissection is properly completed. Major blood vessels are ligated, but in about 80% of patients, few vessels are encountered in the proper planes of dissection. Inspection around the lateral aspects of the vagina or prostate is necessary to rule out troublesome venous oozing. After completion of the dissection, a laparotomy pack is placed firmly in the presacral space to help define the transanal extent of dissection.

If there is adequate length of colon, some choose to fashion a small pouch from the sigmoid or descending colon.[7,8] We have rarely found enough bowel to do this, but it makes sense to create a small reservoir based on our understanding of the physiology of the ileo-anal procedure.[9] The reservoir may be particularly important if muscular sigmoid is used as opposed to more capacious and less muscular descending colon. Prior to finishing the abdominal dissection, one should check the length of the colon. The point of mesenteric dissection and future anal anastomosis should reach well past the pubic symphysis. If it does, then anastomosis to the anus should be relatively easy. At the conclusion of the procedure one again checks for adequate length by making sure that the bowel in the pelvis conforms to the sacral hollow. If it does not and there is some "bow stringing," more mobilization of the left and transverse colon is necessary.

Occasionally, ligation of the left branch of the middle colic artery and ligation of the inferior mesenteric vein will be necessary to obtain adequate length. Blood supply to the colon is usually well maintained by the marginal artery of Drummond. At this point a J-pouch can be added if there is adequate bowel length. This is simply created by identifying the apex of the pouch and making a small colotomy. Through this colotomy, one or two linear dividing and anastomosing staple lines can be placed to create a pouch of 5 to 10 cm in length. The colotomy site is then anastomosed to the anal muscles.

Upon completion of the pelvic dissection and mobilization of the colon, attention is turned to the perineal procedure. A bivalve Smith-Buie retractor is introduced into the anus, exposing the dentate line. A betadine-soaked sponge is placed into the rectum to help eliminate viable tumor cells that might be present. Two Gelpi retractors are placed at right angles to each other with their teeth at the dentate line, thus effacing the anus (Fig. 50-1). The Smith-Buie retractor is then removed. The bulge produced by the trans-abdominally placed laparotomy pad should be easily palpable and clearly visible within several centimeters of the dentate line posteriorly. This pad is above the levator muscles and represents the upper limit of the future mucosal dissection.

The endo-rectal mucosal dissection is begun posteriorly (Fig. 50-2). We rarely use a submucosal injection of saline or epinephrine containing saline, but

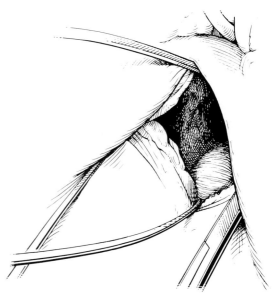

Fig. 50-1. Two Gelpi retractors are placed at right angles to each other with their teeth at the dentate line, thus effacing the anus.

other surgeons feel it enhances the ease of the dissection and decreases the blood loss during the dissection. The layer of loose connective tissue just beneath the mucosa is entered. By blunt and sharp dissection the mucosa is circumferentially dissected free to the level of the laparotomy pack. The length of the

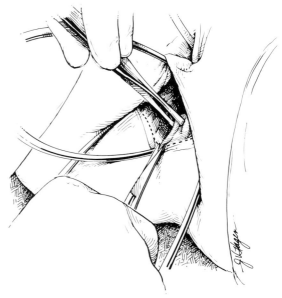

Fig. 50-2. The endo-rectal mucosal dissection is begun at the dentate line posteriorly by elevating the mucosa from the sphincter muscle.

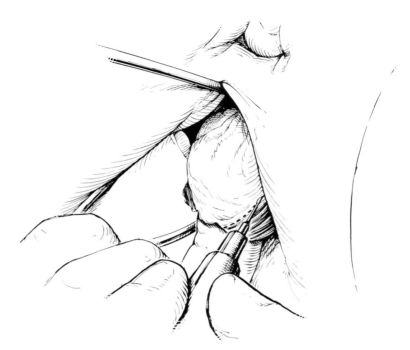

Fig. 50-3. After the mucosa is elevated circumferentially, an incision is made in the posterior rectal muscle and a finger is inserted into the presacral space, filled by the abdominally placed laparotomy pad, which is now removed. The rectum is then transected circumferentially from the back to the front.

dissection is essentially to the top of the surgical anal canal. The muscular wall of the rectum is transected into the laparotomy pad, thereby entering the presacral space. The laparotomy pad is removed from above. A finger is passed into the presacral space and used to guide the remaining dissection (Fig. 50-3). The muscular wall is divided laterally on both sides, leaving the rectum attached anteriorly. A finger is then placed between the rectum and either the prostate or vagina, and traction exposes the anterior rectal muscle, which is transected with the cautery. This last transection frees the rectum circumferentially. It can be pulled through the anus to the point where the transected mesentery is exposed beyond the anal margin.

The bowel is grasped above the point of mesenteric dissection with an Allis clamp and is then transected at that level (Fig. 50-4). Four absorbable sutures (2-0 chromic) are placed through the full thickness of the bowel wall, into the internal sphincter, and finally through the anoderm at the dentate line (Fig. 50-5). Placed in this way in each of the four quadrants, they firmly anchor the bowel at the level of the internal sphincter and prevent mucosal ectropion. The proximal bowel, between each one of these sutures, is then attached to the anoderm at the dentate line with interrupted absorbable sutures. A total of 16 sutures are usually necessary to complete the anastomosis. The use of a UR6 needle facilitates work in the anal canal. Exposure during the anastomosis can be best maintained by sewing the anterior half of the anasto-

mosis first. Goligher has described the use of the circular stapler to complete this anastomosis. Although clearly this is technically feasible, there seems to be little advantage over the hand-sewn technique.

Finally, the suture line is checked by the surgeon's finger. One can feel defects more easily than see them. The skin defects, left after the Gelpi retractors

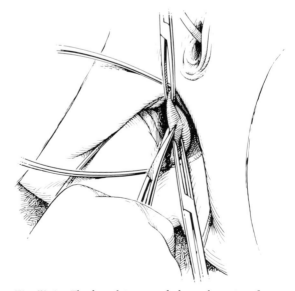

Fig. 50-4. The bowel is grasped above the point of mesenteric dissection and is transected at that level between Allis clamps.

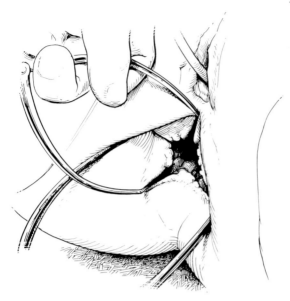

Fig. 50-5. The end of the neorectum is sutured to the internal sphincter and anoderm with absorbable sutures.

are removed, are left untouched. Attention is then turned again to the abdomen, where two suction drains are placed in the presacral space and brought out through the left lower quadrant of the abdomen. Tension on the bowel is relieved as noted above. If there is excessive tension, pelvic inflammation due to radiation or sepsis, or any question of bowel viability, a protective right transverse loop colostomy should be created prior to abdominal closure.

Postoperative management is much the same as with any patient with low anterior anastomosis. The drains are removed as stooling begins and drainage decreases. Patients may experience some incontinence initially as they begin to use the new rectum. Psyllium can be used to thicken the stool once the patient is eating well. Lomotil or codeine may be used to decrease stool frequency. Most patients will initially note increased stool frequency and urgency. Within several months, frequency and urgency should decrease and most patients experience 1 to 3 bowel movements per day with normal continence.

RESULTS

We have reported a small series of 29 patients. Our experience seems typical of the literature. There were 24 men and 5 women. The mean age at operation was 61 years. Indications for the operation included carcinoma of the rectum in 19 patients, radiation injury in 5 patients, villous adenoma in 3 patients, and complication of prior surgical procedures

in 2 patients. Three patients had a pre-anastomotic reservoir constructed. The mean length of hospitalization was 14 days.

There was no operative mortality. Transient urinary retention occurred in 10 patients. No patient required prolonged self-catheterization. One patient had an anastomotic dehiscence, yielding a leak rate of 3.4%. Four patients, for technical or functional reasons, were considered failures (14%). With increasing experience, this percentage clearly decreases. Among the cancer patients, one of 18 had a local recurrence, suggesting that a high degree of local control was achieved.

The mean stool frequency of all patients was 3 per 24 hours. This frequency appears to decrease with followup after the surgical procedure.

DISCUSSION

The proper role of colo-anal anastomosis remains to be defined. Experience with the procedure has been increasing but is generally scant, in large part because of the availability of the circular stapler making alternate approaches possible. Until recently, the colo-anal procedure accounted for less than 2% of sphincter-saving procedures at our institution.[1] We and others have documented that colo-anal anastomosis and, more recently, colon pouch-anal anastomosis, can be performed safely and efficaciously, and can restore enteric continence in selected patients with benign or malignant rectal disease.[1,8,10–13]

We have found the colo-anal anastomosis helpful for radiation injuries and large villous tumors of the rectum.[1,12,15] We have also found the colo-anal procedure helpful in the management of patients with a severe anastomotic stricture or with chronic anastomotic leaks requiring fecal diversion. In management of carcinoma, colo-anal anastomosis has traditionally been restricted to those patients in whom it was technically difficult to perform a safe anastomosis very low in the pelvis, but in whom acceptable margins of resection could be obtained by anterior mobilization.

Our experience supports the findings of others that colo-anal anastomosis can be performed safely.[12,16,17,18] There were no operative deaths in our series. Transient urinary retention occurred in 34% of our patients. Ninety percent of patients with urinary tract complications were in the group treated for rectal cancer. This suggests that extent of dissection, rather than type of anastomosis, may be the most significant factor in predicting the occurrence of urinary retention. Most patients regain normal bladder function.

Anastomotic stricture occurs in about 30% of our patients, but can usually be easily managed by outpatient and self-dilation. Many series note that 25 to 30% of patients require an enema to initiate defecation.[11,17] It is unclear in these series if this is related to the presence of outlet obstruction. The frequency of difficulty in initiating defecation appears greater if a reservoir is incorporated, and may reflect a manifestation of a motility disorder. We have not noted this problem in our patients who have had predominantly straight anastomoses without a pre-anastomotic pouch. Evaluation of this subset of patients with manometry and defecography should help define the problem.

Most important, survival following colo-anal anastomosis for cancer seems comparable to that in series using low anterior or abdomino-perineal approaches.[10,19,20] Theoretically, the risk of distant recurrence should not be influenced by the choice of procedure. The risk of local recurrence was 7% (1 in 19) in our series and has not been excessive in any series.

Functional results have been good and may be enhanced by the addition of a pre-anastomotic reservoir.[7,8] It remains unclear as to whether the reservoir compromises the initiation of defecation. Urgency and frequency of defecation are a problem early after a colo-anal anastomosis. Several authors have shown that decreased capacity and compliance of the pulled-through proximal colon correlates directly with increased stool frequency and decreased continence. Keighley and Matheson demonstrated a marked reduction in the neorectal capacity of their colo-anal patients compared to preoperative values.[13] Lazorthes et al. found that the capacity was greater when a reservoir was constructed than when the end of the colon was anastomosed directly to the sphincters.[8] They were able to demonstrate a significant correlation between the maximal tolerable volume of the neorectum and the stool frequency. Functional results in their series were good; 86% of the patients had fewer than three stools per day, at the end of one year. Unlike the ileal pouch, the colon reservoir need not incorporate limbs longer than 7 or 8 cm. The role of preservation of the distal rectal mucosa remains unclear. Martin has suggested that improved sensation results if this mucosa is preserved, but the physiology of this has not been defined.[21]

CONCLUSIONS

Colo-anal anastomosis is safe, efficacious, and preserves anal continence in a variety of difficult situations in which it is impractical or unwise to attempt anastomosis of the colon directly to the full thickness of the rectum. Moreover, the functional results after colo-anal anastomosis are good and compare favorably with those reported after low anterior anastomosis. In the management of rectal cancer, local recurrence rates appear to be as low as those reported for anterior resection. These encouraging clinical and functional results of colo-anal anastomosis should prompt careful but wider application of the technique in selected patients with complicated benign and malignant rectal disease.

REFERENCES

1. Drake DB, Pemberton JH, Beart RW, Dozois RR, Wolff BG: Coloanal anastomosis in the management of benign and malignant disease. Ann Surg 206:600–605, 1987.
2. Lane RH, Parks AG: Function of the anal sphincters following colo-anal anastomosis. Br J Surg 64:596–599, 1977.
3. Black BM: Combined abdominoendorectal resection. Arch Surg 63:406–416, 1952.
4. Waugh JM, Black MA, Gage RP: Three and five year survivals following combined abdominoperineal resection, abdominoperineal resection with sphincter preservation and anterior resection for carcinoma of the rectum and lower part of the sigmoid colon. Ann Surg 142:752–757, 1955.
5. Beart RW, Kelly KA: Randomized prospective evaluation of the EEA stapler for colorectal anastomoses. Am J Surg 141:143–147, 1981.
6. Rosen C, Beart RW: Local recurrence of rectal carcinoma after hand-sewn and stapled anastomoses. Dis Colon Rectum 28:305–309, 1985.
7. Parc R, Tiret E, Frileus P, Moszkowski E, Loygue J: Resection and colo-anal anastomosis with colonic reservoir for rectal carcinoma. Br J Surg 73:139–141, 1986.
8. Lazorthes F, Fages P, Chiotasso P, Lemozy J, Bloom E: Resection of the rectum with construction of a colonic reservoir and colo-anal anastomosis for carcinoma of the rectum. Br J Surg 73:136–138, 1986.
9. Taylor BM, Beart RW, Dozois RR: Straight ileoanal anastomosis vs. ileal pouch-anal anastomosis after colectomy and mucosal proctectomy. Arch Surg 118:696–701, 1983.
10. Enker WE, Stearns NW, Janov AJ: Perianal coloanal anastomosis following low anterior resection for rectal carcinoma. Dis Colon Rectum 28:576–581, 1985.
11. Nicholls RJ: Rectal cancer: anterior resection of perianal coloanal anastomosis. The results in 76 patients treated by Sir Alan Parks. Bull Cancer (Paris) 70:304–307, 1983.
12. Goligher JC, Duthie FJL, DeDombal FT: Abdomino-anal pull-through excision for tumors of the mid-third of the rectum. A comparison with low anterior resection. Br J Surg 52:323–325, 1965.
13. Keighley MRR, Matheson D: Functional results of rectal excision and endoanal anastomosis. Br J Surg 67:757–761, 1980.
14. Jeffrey PJ, Hawley PR, Parks AG: Colo-anal anastomosis in the treatment of diffuse cavernous haemangioma involving the rectum. Br J Surg 63:678–682, 1976.
15. Parks AG, Allen CL, Frank JD: A method of treating post irradiation rectovaginal fistulae. Br J Surg 65:417–421, 1978.
16. Goligher JC: Use of circular stapling gun with perianal insertion of anorectal purse-string suture for construc-

tion of low colorectal or colo-anal anastomoses. Br J Surg 66:501–504, 1979.

17. Kratzer GL, Mata J: Review of the pull-through operation for rectal cancer. Dis Colon Rectum 22:120–122, 1979.

18. Bacon HE: Cancer of the rectum: pull-through operation. Penn Med J 66:33–38, 1963.

19. Wilson SM, Beahrs OH: The curative treatment of carcinoma of the sigmoid, rectosigmoid and rectum. Ann Surg 183:556–565, 1976.

20. Goligher JC, Duthie HL, DeDombal FT: Abdominoanal and pullthrough excision for tumours of the mid-third of the rectum. Br J Surg 52:323–335, 1965.

21. Martin LW, Fischer JE: Preservation of anorectal continence following total colectomy. Ann Surg 196:700–704, 1982.

CHAPTER 51

CRITICAL EVALUATION OF STAPLED COLO-RECTAL ANASTOMOSIS

F. Sandei, R.V. Bardini, G. Leoni, G. Reginato, and A. Peracchia

The use of stapling instruments has extended the field of primary and difficult reconstructive procedures, especially in colo-rectal surgery, in which very low anastomoses have become possible with preservation of the anal sphincter. With increasing experience, surgeons have observed a reduction in operative time and tissue trauma, as well as shortened exposures of the open bowel to the peritoneal cavity, and hence a diminished opportunity for contamination. The various techniques have been standardized and can be incorporated in the curriculum of a surgical teaching and training program.

However, the handling of the instruments has to be carefully mastered to ensure their optimal use for the various operative techniques. Satisfaction with the instruments could be jeopardized by the occurrence of problems related to the faulty or inappropriate use of the instruments, such as pelvic abscess or suture-line dehiscence due to a poorly executed mechanical anastomosis.

MATERIALS AND METHODS

From January 1980 to December 1987, various colon resections followed by colo-rectal or ileo-rectal reconstruction were performed in 94 patients with the stapling instruments at the Surgical Clinical Institute I of the University of Padova. The patients were equally distributed between men and women (47 in each group) and had an average age of 62.4 years (range: 36 to 85 years). A total of 95 anastomoses were accomplished; 93 were between the colon and rectum, and 2 were between the ileum and the rectum. An additional anastomosis occurred in one patient in whom it was possible to do a second anterior resection after recurrence of carcinoma.

Of the 95 anastomoses, 57 were end-to-end (60%), 19 were end-to-side (20%), and 19 were side-to-end (20%). All patients underwent operation for carcinoma. The average distance of the neoplasm from the anal margin was 16.1 cm, with a range of 7 to 30 cm. For each of the anastomotic techniques, these values were as follows: for end-to-end anastomoses, the average was 15.7 cm with a range of 7 to 30 cm; for end-to-side anastomoses, the average was 10.1 cm with a range of 7 to 13 cm; and for the side-to-end anastomoses, the average was 19.1 cm with a range of 10 to 30 cm.

In 47 operations, we preferred the use of the EEA instrument with the 31-mm cartridge in 37 patients, and the 28-mm cartridge in the remaining 10 patients. In 7 patients we used the ILS-29, in 2 patients the compression AKA-II, and in 1 patient the SPTU. In the 19 end-to-side anastomoses, the rectum was closed with the TA-55. In the group of 19 patients with side-to-end anastomoses, the colon was closed 14 times with the TA-55, once with the TA-30, once with the YOT-40, and three times with interrupted manual sutures. The rectal purse-string suture for end-to-end anastomosis was accomplished with the ASP-50 special instrument in 45 operations, manually in 10 cases, and by a transanal manual technique in the remaining 2 patients. For the side-to-end anastomosis, the ASP-50 was used 17 times; a manual purse-string was accomplished twice.

The circular anastomosing instrument was placed through the rectum in 55 operations for the end-to-end anastomoses and 17 times for the end-to-side anastomoses. On two occasions the instrument was placed from above through a colotomy for the end-to-end anastomoses; in the 19 operations with side-to-end anastomoses, the instrument was placed through the open, redundant loop of colon.

In 24 cases (25.2%), it was the judgment of the operating surgeon that individual reinforcing sutures were necessary (8 end-to-end anastomoses = 14.0%, 6 end-to-side anastomoses = 31.5%, and 10 side-to-end anastomoses = 52.6%). All operative sites were drained with one drain on the left, posterior to the anastomosis, and the second one on the right, anterior to it. In 40 patients an ano-rectal tube was placed across the anastomosis.

The staging of the various carcinomas was done according to the classification of Dukes-Astler-Coller.

INTRA-OPERATIVE AND POSTOPERATIVE COMPLICATIONS

We observed four intra-operative technical incidents (4.2%) as follows: incomplete end-to-end anastomosis posteriorly with the EEA-28 on one occasion was treated by manual sutures in two layers without a proximal colostomy. On two occasions (1 end-to-side and 1 end-to-end anastomosis), the EEA-31 instrument was closed insufficiently, with a resulting defective staple formation and incomplete circular transection of the purse-stringed bowel. This problem was solved by performing a manual anastomosis with protective colostomy in the patient with the end-to-side anastomosis and by resecting the defective end-to-end anastomosis and creating a new end-to-end anastomosis with the EEA-31. Finally, in 1 patient with a planned end-to-side anastomosis using the EEA-28 instrument, a second lesion or an insufficient margin of resection was discovered proximal to the colon purse-string suture. An additional segment of colon was resected and the anastomosis was accomplished end-to-end with the EEA-28 instrument.

A diverting colostomy was necessary with end-to-end anastomosis because of minimal leakage of methylene blue in 4 patients, and in a proximal colon filled with feces in 1 patient who underwent operation under emergency conditions. In the end-to-side anastomoses, one protective colostomy was done for a methylene-blue-positive test; a second was done for proximal dilatation of the colon with feces.

Postoperatively, we observed the following complications: 2 anastomotic leaks and 9 fistulae (11.6%), and 12 strictures (12.6%); of 11 patients with cancer recurrence (11.6%), an abdomino-perineal resection was necessary in 10. In 1 patient it was possible to achieve yet a second anterior resection.

MORTALITY

Of the 94 patients, two died from complete separation of the anastomosis and 1 from pulmonary embolism (3.2%). This series of patients underwent operations by 7 surgeons performing anywhere from 3 to 34 operations each. However, examination of the results does not show a significant difference among these surgeons with regard to preference for a given instrument, number of protective colostomies, or incidence of complications.

DISCUSSION

Circular anastomosing instruments facilitate some of the more difficult steps in colo-rectal surgery, such as the very low anastomosis with preservation of the anal sphincter and improved early function at this low level of anastomosis.[1–6] The use of staples created the potential for different types of intra-operative and postoperative complications of which surgeons have to be aware.[1,3] Some of these complications relate more to inexperience or lack of attention by the surgeon, and are not necessarily inherent to the instruments or their use.

Comparing overall results obtained with manual and with mechanical sutures, the difference in the rate of complications is not statistically significant.[3] A major condition for success with both techniques is the painstaking local preoperative preparation of the colon and systemic, prophylactic antibiotic treatment of the patient. We believe that the irrigation of the rectum with Betadine, especially in low anastomoses, is particularly important before the introduction of the EEA instrument through the anus.

Other points of importance to be checked by the surgeon are: whether the assembly and functioning of the circular stapling instrument are satisfactory; whether placement of the instrument into the two bowel ends that have been satisfactorily mobilized is correct; whether joining of the bowel ends is without tension; and whether the bowel ends have comparable diameters. A safe distal line of resection is at a level 3 cm from the tumor.[24] Preservation of the pubo-rectalis muscle is essential to avoid postoperative problems with fecal incontinence. A carefully executed purse-string suture is of the utmost importance and can be achieved manually or with a special SP-50 clamp, depending on the individual anatomic findings and the preference and experience of the surgeon. More recently, the double-stapling technique of Knight, consisting of the intersection of a linear TA-55 staple line closing the rectum by a circular end-to-end colo-rectal anastomosis, has become popular and appears to add great safety to the critical step of placing a purse-string or closing suture on the distal rectal stump.

The transanal placement of the instrument, as well as its extraction after the anastomosis, has to be accomplished without any force or difficulty. Furthermore, the size of the instrument cartridge should be perfectly adapted to the lumen of the bowel to be anastomosed, which in general is the diameter of the proximal colon rather than the diameter of the rectal stump (usually somewhat larger and more muscular than the proximal colon end). After achieving the anastomosis, checking of the integrity of the two tissue doughnuts obtained, as well as testing the completeness of the anastomosis with the injection of methylene blue, have appeared important in our experience. If there is minimal leakage of methylene blue, then a protective colostomy should be done, or a new anastomosis performed if the leakage is important.

CONCLUSIONS

The use of stapling instruments in colo-rectal surgery has made for standard anastomoses with perfect geometry, albeit at the price of some inherent complications, depending on the learning curve of individual surgeons and the departments in which they work. However, the use of these instruments for low colo-rectal or even colo-anal anastomoses is beyond comparison with alternative methods for this purpose, such as "pull-through" procedures or, even more so, permanent colostomy after abdomino-perineal resection.

To avoid the intra-operative mishaps or errors in technique that may lead to postoperative complications, the surgeon has to control every step of instrument assembly and functioning, placement of purse-string sutures or their alternatives, and introduction, closure, and extraction of the instruments.

In general, anastomotic leaks may manifest themselves in the first 2 or 3 postoperative days; if this occurs, the clinical picture is usually critical and should usually lead to re-intervention and all the steps necessary to control this acute complication. In other instances, less severe, a leak will only be evident by a blind fistula, usually on x-ray control with contrast some 7 to 8 days after the operation. In such cases a non-operative treatment with adequate drainage may be all that is necessary.

Anastomotic strictures are late complications, occurring some 2 months after operation. In our experience, we have not found a correlation between anastomotic leaks, fistulae, and strictures. Most of the strictures are asymptomatic and are found usually by digital rectal examination or by endoscopy. They are almost invariably treated by one or several dilatations with great success. We have never had to re-operate for an anastomotic stricture.

The recurrence of cancer remains the most vexing problem. To a large extent the problem is one of choice between anterior resection and abdominoperineal resection. In our experience, cancer recurrence has always been localized, often to the anastomotic site, even if the tissue doughnuts had been free of tumor at the time of the original anastomosis. It is probable that the source of these recurrences has to be found in the presence of microscopic foci of tumor in the lymphatics of the colo-rectal walls or in the peri-rectal fat tissue. It is possible that with the advent of preoperative endo-rectal echography a more complete assessment of the extramural extension of a rectal tumor is possible, which in turn would lead to a more adequate operative procedure, reducing the risk of early postoperative cancer recurrence.

BIBLIOGRAPHY

1. Adloff M: Les "Gags" des anastomoses mécaniques. VII Con Soc Franc Chir.
2. Adloff M, Arnaud JP, Beehary S: Stapled vs sutured colorectal anastomosis. Arch Surg 115:1436–1438, 1980.
3. Beart RW, Kelly KA: Randomised prospective evaluation of the EEA stapler for colorectal anastomosis. Am J Surg 141:143–147, 1981.
4. Ballantyne GH, Burke JB, Rogers G, Lampert EG, Boccia J: Accelerated wound healing with stapled enteric suture lines. An experimental study comparing traditional sewing techniques and stapling device. Ann Surg 201:360–364, 1985.
5. Brennan SS, Pickford IR, Mary Evans Pollock AV: Stapler or sutures for colonic anastomoses—a controlled clinical trial. Br J Surg 69:722–724, 1982.
6. Cade D, Gallagher P, Schofield PF, Turner L: Complications of anterior resection of the rectum using the EEA stapling device. Br J Surg 68:339–340, 1981.
7. Cady J, Godfroy J, Sibaud O, Mercadier M: La désunion anastomotique en chirurgie colique et rectale. Etude comparative de suture manuelle et mècanique à propos d'une série de 149 résections. Ann Chir 34(5): 350–356, 1980.
8. Deliére Th, Moller E, Brun JG, Patel JC: Colectomies par résection-anastomose intégré pièce en place utilisant les sutures mécaniques linéaires. Presse Méd 17(3):675–677, 1984.
9. Détry R, Kestens PJ, Secchi M: Experience with the EEA stapler for colorectal anastomosis: early and late results. Dig Surg 1:2–5, 1984.
10. Fegiz G: Rectal cancer: restorative surgery with EEA stapling service. Int Surg 68:13–18, 1983.
11. Goligher JC: Recent trends in the practice of sphincter-saving excision for rectal cancer. Ann R Coll Surg Engl 61:169, 1979.
12. Goligher JC: Use of circular stapling gun with peranal insertion of anorectal purse-string suture for construction of very low colorectal or colo-anal anastomoses. Br J Surg 66:501, 1979.
13. Goligher JC, Lee PWR, Macfie J, Simpkins KC, Lintott

DJ: Experience with the Russian model 249 suture gun for the anastomosis of the rectum. Surg Gynecol Obstet 148:517, 1979.

14. Graffner H, Fredlund P, Olsson S-A, Oscarson J, Peterson B-G: Protective colostomy in low anterior resection of the rectum using the EEA stapling instrument—a randomized study. Dis Colon Rectum 26:87–90, 1983.

15. Halsted WS: End to end suture anastomosis of the large intestine by abutted closed ends and puncuring of double diaphragm with an instrument passed per rectum. Johns Hopkins Hosp Bull 32:98, 1921.

16. Morgestern L: The intestinal anastomosis with end-to-end stapling instrument progress and problems. Arch Surg 116:141, 1981.

17. Murphy JB: Cholecysto-intestinal, gastro-intestinal, entero-intestinal anastomosis and approximation without sutures. Med Rec 42:665, 1892.

18. Nicholls RL, Broido P, Condon RE, Gorbach SL, Nylus LM: Effect of preoperative neomycin-erythromycin intestinal preparation on the incidence of infectious complication following colon surgery. Ann Surg 178:453–462, 1973.

19. Pélissier E, Bachour A: Bilan de 172 anastomoses colorectales manuelles et mècaniques. Chirurgie 110:650–654, 1984.

20. Rovati V: Anterior resection of the rectum: stapled vs sutured anastomoses. Coloproct 5:305, 1986.

21. Sandei F, Lovascio D, Leoni G, Peracchia A: Le anastomosi colo-rettali. Studio funzionale. Riv It Coloproct 3:2, 1984.

22. Schaffer CJ, Giordano JM: Complications associated with EEA stapler in performance of low anterior resection. Am J Surg 47:426, 1981.

23. Scher KS, Scott-Conner C, Jones CW, Leach M: A comparison of stapled and sutured anastomases in colonic operations. Surg Gynecol Obstet 155:489–493, 1982.

24. Smith LE: Anastomosis with the EEA stapler after anterior colon resection. Dis Colon Rectum 24:236–242, 1981.

25. Steinhagen RM, Wealkley FL: Anastomosis to the rectum. Operative experience. Dis Col Rect 28:105–109, 1985.

26. Turbelin JM, Arnaud JP, Welter R, Adloff MA: Etude comparative des surfaces anastomotique obtenues par utilisation des sutures mécaniques en chirurgie digestive. J Chir (Paris) 117(10):541–546, 1980.

27. Waxman BP: Large bowel anastomoses. II. The circular staplers. Br J Surg 70:64–67, 1983.

Index

Page numbers in *italics* are figures; page numbers followed by "t" are tables.